MARITAL THERAPY

Strategies Based on Social Learning and Behavior Exchange Principles

Marital Therapy

Strategies Based on Social Learning and Behavior Exchange Principles

By

NEIL S. JACOBSON

Assistant Professor,
Department of Psychology,
The University of Iowa

and

GAYLA MARGOLIN

Assistant Professor,
Department of Psychology,
University of Southern California

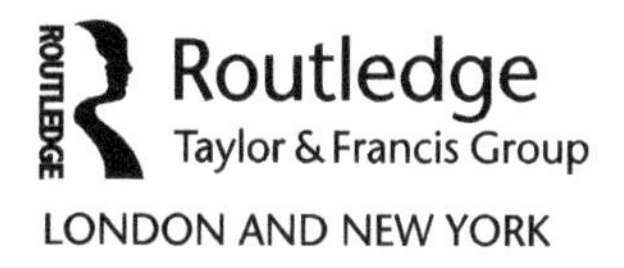

LONDON AND NEW YORK

First published 1979 by Brunner/Mazel, Inc.

Published 2014 by Routledge
2 Park Square, Milton Park, Abingdon, Oxfordshire OX14 4RN
711 Third Avenue, New York, NY 10017

Routledge is an imprint of the Taylor & Francis Group, an informa business

Library of Congress Cataloging in Publication Data

Jacobson, Neil S. 1949-
Marital therapy.
Bibliography: p.
Includes index.
1. Marital psychotherapy. 2. Socialization. 3. Behavior therapy.
I. Margolin, Gayla, 1949—joint author. II. Title.
RC488.5.J35 362.8'2 79-728

ISBN 978-0-87630-199-9 (hbk)
ISBN 978-1-138-00435-1 (pbk)

Foreword

It was only a decade and a half ago that social learning theory was rising phoenix-like from the ashes of Hullian learning theory. The renewed enthusiasm was in part a reflection of the writings of H. J. Eysenck and J. Wolpe. However, the particular impetus within social learning was provided primarily by B. F. Skinner in a series of volumes beginning with *Behavior of Organisms*. It took some time for his translations of reinforcement theory to make their appearance in the general realm of social engineering. Those were indeed exciting times. Each new visitor coming through the campus at the University of Oregon brought news of some startling new application of operant procedures to some long-standing clinical problem. At first, it seemed that there was not any problem that could not be solved. Many of us went out into the field to apply the existing social technology to problems of severely brain-damaged children, autistic children, psychotic adults, depressed adults, etc.

Some of our creative pioneers in social engineering, such as Richard Stuart, also applied the technology to problems of distressed married couples. However, even a casual reading to Stuart's early publications suggests that he added a great deal to the enterprise other than that which he described in his journal articles. For example, he introduced the idea of contracting and the ideas of social exchange; more than that, he brought to therapy his own inestimable clinical skills. These were not described in any of his reports.

At that time, our group at Oregon was working with families of severely aggressive children. We were teaching parents simple child management skills—or at least that is what we thought we were doing. Our follow-up data revealed the fact that some families no longer practiced family management skills after termination of therapy. Clinical follow-up with these people revealed that some of them were involved in severe marital conflict, often leading to separation and divorce. Caught up in the enthusiasm of that time, we decided it would be a simple matter to alleviate these problems. One had only to apply the notions inherent in social learning principles; the distressed couples would be relieved and our follow-up data would look as it should.

One of my most gifted graduate student therapists, Hyman Hops, was available at that time. He and I collaborated in applying what we thought were the existing techniques of contracting and social exchange theory to two different couples. It was also decided that an attempt would be made to measure changes in the couples. This necessitated altering an existing observation code system being used with families of aggressive children in order to fit this new problem. It was tailored to describe problem-solving interactions among distressed couples. The data were collected before and after treatment as one means of deciding what the impact of treatment had been. In that same context, we were concerned about the effect of generalizing from the videotape measures of problem-solving skills to the home. We freely plagiarized some ideas from Eric Houghton, who in turn received them from Og Lindsley. That involved collecting daily reports from a couple about specific behaviors occurring at home.

Our perceived success in working with these two couples seemed infectious. In any case, it contaminated our colleagues working with us on a Navy sponsored laboratory research program. That research group then spent the next two years collaborating in an effort to improve the extremely primitive criterion measures and introduced other new instruments such as the Marital Interaction Inventory. By that time, the group was comprised of Robert Weiss and his graduate students John Vincent, Tom Wills, and Gary Birchler. We set about the task of making explicit what the therapy process really was. The two years of effort led to some pilot reports describing both laboratory studies and the first set of ten cases treated by that group.

In my opinion, the most notable thing that came from the first effort was the fact that those early papers stimulated the attention of both Gayla Margolin and Neil Jacobson. I was astounded to find that a student in North Carolina, Neil Jacobson, had taken those papers and translated them into an elegant comparison design, which showed a successful outcome for the treated group. This was a daring venture, particularly in view of the fact that even within our own group I am not sure that we would have agreed on what the treatment procedures really were. Certainly, none of our descriptions would do the task justice. The fact that

Neil was able to do this speaks more to his clinical acumen than to the clarity of procedures described either by Stuart or the Oregon group. That he has since gone on to replicate the effect with some new therapists makes a preliminary believer out of this writer.

There is little doubt that at this time Jacobson and Margolin are the preeminent spokespeople for the social learning approach to marital problems. They have earned that position as a result of both their published scientific work and this current volume. I think that in many ways this volume signifies a new era in what has been called behavior modification. The modern look can also be found in the work of persons such as Alan Marlatt at Washington, Thomas Borkovec at Pennsylvania State, James Alexander at Utah, Robert Wahler at Tennessee, Gerald Davison at Stony Brook, and my colleague John Reid. These people characteristically emphasize multilevel assessment and a hard line on the necessity for replication, for comparison designs, and for follow-up data. That point of view is not new—it has been the trademark of Boulder model clinical psychologists for some time. In addition, however, one will find in their writings that the existing engineering technology is thought to be a necessary but not sufficient means for producing behavioral change in distressed couples. The techniques described here are the familiar ones of establishing contracts and contigencies and training in communcation and problem-solving skills. As the reader will see, these techniques are eminently teachable. The fact that they are described here and that they are teachable suggests that clinical technology has stepped forward a long way from the arcane mysteries which characterized psychotherapy efforts in the late 1950s and early 1960s.

The aspect of this work which sets it clearly in the forefront is the emphasis upon soft clinical skills as being a necessary, and again not sufficient, component for effective treatment. I think the authors would agree that the novice who simply employs the technology without a commensurate set of soft skills is probably not going to be sucessful in working with distressed couples. In taking this candid stance, they do, of course, expose themselves to attack by radical behaviorists. On the other hand, by verbalizing what it is that characterizes a sound clinical practice, they are bringing into the picture a set of variables which themselves need to be measured and understood if we are to get on with the business of building a better means for treating people.

It is both a pleasure and a privilege to write a foreword to a book of this caliber. I see it as the first in a beginning series of publications that will define yet another chapter in the development of clinical practice.

GERALD R. PATTERSON

Preface

Marital therapy has become an ever more popular treatment modality in the past ten years. In part this is probably due to the increasing requests for therapeutic assistance on the part of distressed couples. Although there is little evidence that more distressed marriages exist today than 20 years ago, couples do seem to be seeking more from their long-term relationships than they once did. The increasing ease of divorce, the Women's Movement, and other factors have conspired to produce more fastidious marital partners. As a result, there is an ever-increasing demand for the services of clinicians trained in handling the wide-ranging problems associated with many marriages.

This book presents a model for treating the problems of distressed couples. We have tried to integrate an extensive discussion of treatment techniques and strategies with a theoretical framework based on laboratory research in experimental and social psychology.

The model to which we adhere is a social learning model; we are behaviorists. We believe that behavior therapy and marital therapy have much in common, and that nonbehaviorists who read this book will find that much of what they do in their everyday practice in treating couples closely resembles the most common strategies which comprise behavioral marital therapy. In this area, the divisive debates between behavioral and psychodynamic therapists seem to diminish and become transformed into at least a tentative rapprochement. We have tried to systematically present treatment techniques which are familiar to most practitioners of marital therapy within a coherent theretical framework. In addition, the book elucidates a methodology for analyzing distressed relationships which will hopefully assist nonbehavioral as well as behavioral practitioners. Thus we hope that readers of diverse backgrounds and orientations will find the book helpful in their clinical work with couples.

A few words about how the book is organized:

Chapter 1 provides background material into the laboratory foundations of behavior therapy. This background material is a prelude to the presentation of a theoretical model of relationship distress.

Chapter 2 introduces the basic principles of therapy which follow from the theoretical framework in Chapter 1, and discusses the similarities and differences between behavioral and nonbehavioral approaches to marital therapy.

Chapters 3 through *9* consist of detailed explications of clinical strategies for treating couples, beginning with the initial interview and assessment phases of therapy, continuing through early treatment phases, and elaborating on various techniques such as communication training, problem-solving training, contingency contracting, behavior exchange procedures, cognitive restructuring, and paradoxical directives. Chapter 7 includes a manual for couples to be used in conjunction with therapy. Chapter 9 covers a number of specific problems and issues which commonly confront the marital therapist: treating deficits in sexual and affectionate interaction, integrating marital therapy with a partial focus on child problems, and treating partners where one spouse is clinically depressed. Also discussed in this chapter are problems of physical aggression, jealousy, and issues related to divorce and separation, along with the treatment of couples consisting of one highly affiliative and one very independent partner.

Chapter 10 reviews the outcome research that has been completed in recent years.

Chapter 11 presents two case studies, one very successful and one not so successful.

A comment about our use of the pronoun "he" is needed. Although it is not appropriate to use "he" when referring to a therapist, we have, for reasons of convenience, done so on occasion, while acknowledging the inequity of this usage.

We would like to pay special tribute to Andy Christensen, who reviewed and critiqued the original draft of each chapter for us. His feedback was invaluable, and contributed significantly to subsequent improvements. We would also like to express gratitude to Bob Weiss who, although not directly involved in the writing process, made the book possible with his pioneering work in the area. More importantly, Bob taught one of us (Gayla Margolin) how to do marital therapy, and his influence is pervasive throughout the book. Gerald Patterson also deserves special thanks for his important role in creating the field of behavioral marital therapy, and laying the theoretical foundations for the social learning approach as applied to family interaction. Jerry's encouragement and support helped us reach the conclusion that we could write this book. Several of our students used the problem-solving manual when it was in its raw form, and provided us with insightful suggestions: At the risk of omitting some individuals, we particularly remember the help we received from Audrey Berger, Dave Fordyce, Mercedes Dallas, Diane Tucker, Dorothy Anderson, and students from our marital and family therapy practica.

Judy Freedman and Steve Rottman also critiqued and provided useful feedback on certain chapters. Several people were enlisted in the task of typing various drafts of the manuscript: Pam Young, Holly Waldron, Eileen Wetrich, Ann Hulme, Barbara Noss, and Barbara Tzur-Jenks.

Most of all, we would like to acknowledge each other. Since we began this project together 15 months ago, collaborating despite a 2,000-mile distance between us, we have learned that the experience of writing a book with another person can be fulfilling, fun, and reasonably effortless. It is hard to imagine how either of us could have done it alone.

GAYLA MARGOLIN
NEIL S. JACOBSON

April, 1979

Contents

MARITAL THERAPY

Strategies Based on Social Learning and Behavior Exchange Principles

CHAPTER 1

Marriage and Marital Distress from a Social Learning Perspective

DAN AND SANDRA had known each other since junior high school, and had been married for seven years at the time they sought therapy. Their history as a couple traversed 13 years, and exhausted each of their heterosexual vitae. They grew up in the same neighborhood in a small, rural town.

Although Dan and Sandra were both highly intelligent and destined for successful professional careers, they were naive and deficient when it came to the skills of maintaining a long-term relationship. As they grew from adolescence to adulthood together, there were no mentors to tell them that conflict is inevitable when two people live together and sleep together, or that sexual lovemaking becomes boring after 2,000 repetitions of ten minutes of foreplay followed by the missionary position. This couple relied primarily on one another for their apprenticeship to the lifelong endeavors of love and intimacy. They each confirmed for the other the mistaken notion that love is a qualitative state, that when one is "in love," a relationship proceeds smoothly, quite independently of events as mundane as the daily exchange of pleasing and displeasing behavior, or effective communication. In essence, Dan and Sandra were deficient in a variety of skills, skills that are necessary for a relationship to remain satisfying over a long period of time. Since they did not understand the need for skills in a relationship, and since they assumed that a happy, vital marriage would automatically follow from the state of being "in love," they were unable to correct the gradual deterioration of their relationship.

The difficulties began almost as soon as Dan and Sandra began to live together. Although they had been close companions for six years prior to their marriage, and had been sleeping together regularly for two of those years, they had never lived together. Their fantasies about marriage being a perpetual honeymoon were quickly vitiated by financial difficulties in their first year. Financial obligations produced a new arena for their interaction, and led to their first significant exchanges of punishing behavior. For example, Dan insisted upon making unilateral decisions on important financial matters; Sandra did not comment on this practice, although she became angry as a result of it. Sandra occasionally purchased expensive items without first consulting Dan, a practice which angered him although he did not comment on it. The sudden occurrence of displeasing behavior was not discussed. Both Dan and Sandra were terrified by their respective discoveries of the other's imperfections: did it mean that they were no longer "in love"? Like many couples, they hoped that the conflicts would disappear if they were simply ignored; somehow, to acknowledge them and attempt to resolve them would be to inject them with more reality. As long as they were not acknowledged, the veneer of a perfect marriage, a ruse in which they both had an investment, was maintained. This is the precedent that was set in the early stages of their marriage. It became their habitual strategy for handling conflicts. In the ensuing years, significant conflicts arose in other areas. Each discovered displeasing personal habits engaged in by the partner. As displeasing behaviors proliferated, their overall satisfaction with the relationship plummeted.

Other factors conspired to exacerbate this gradual, unacknowledged mounting of aversive behavior. Previously rewarding interactions became stale and habitual: sex became boring, their continued practice of the same few shared activities (dining out, going to movies, gardening) ceased to create the enjoyment that it had in the past. Their conversation, confined to the same limited content areas, proved less rewarding. What seemed to be happening was that behaviors which had once provided great benefits and rewards produced gradually diminishing returns. Rather than expanding their repertoires to include new sources of satisfaction and new provisions for beneficial exchange, they relied on the same stale behaviors, hoping myopically that "love would conquer all." They did not realize that a relationship requires continuous attention and care, and must be rejuvenated and stimulated by varied and occasionally novel rewards. Since their conception of a successful marriage required that they adhere to a doctrine of mutual dependency, they also deprived themselves of the relief that many couples derived from independent activities and friends. For Dan and Sandra, love meant that everything they needed for a happy life is provided by the marriage partner. This ideology precluded their acknowledgment that the other's capacity for producing sufficient rewards was in any way limited.

By the time this couple acknowledged their difficulties and sought assistance from a marital therapist, their long-term neglect had led to a noticeable depletion of mutual rewards. On a day by day basis, they provided few reinforcers; they offered long lists of changes they would like to see in their partner's behavior, based on the years of accumulated but unacknowledged complaints. They lacked a variety of relationship skills, most notably an inability to talk to one another about these conflict areas. Their problem areas thus included communication, disagreements over finances, a lack of common interests, and dissatisfaction with sex. More specifically, Sandra yelled at Dan when she wanted him to comply with her requests; Dan avoided initiating intimate conversation about his feelings and concerns, seldom praised or complimented his wife, and tended to preempt Sandra's rudimentary attempt to negotiate change by refusals to discuss such matters. Sandra continued to spend money impulsively. Dan continued to insist on hegemony in financial matters. Sex was infrequent and plagued by a lack of spontaneity and diversity.

Finally, it should be noted that the couple did not present a specific list of grievances when they first entered the therapist's office for their initial interview. Instead, they expressed vague discontent in terms of a "loss of individuality," an "inability to feel," and an "emptiness" about the marriage.

Only after a thorough, persistent behavioral analysis were Dan and Sandra's concerns translated into the specific list described above. This social learning description of their evolving marital distress, along with the treatment strategies which follow from such an analysis, comprise the subject matter of this book. Our immediate focus in this chapter lies in the theoretical underpinnings of an analysis which produces the type of case description presented above. Although the body of this book is devoted to clinical strategies for treating couples, we believe that it is impossible to understand and effectively utilize a social learning perspective in marital therapy without a foundation in theory.

The chapter begins with a brief discussion of the basic principles of learning which are implicit in a social learning analysis. Then, we will describe a behavioral or social learning model of relationship distress. The parallels between the general model and our analysis of the above case will become evident in this presentation.

BASIC CONCEPTS AND PRINCIPLES OF LEARNING

Since behavior therapy has been associated with principles of learning derived from laboratory research in experimental psychology, it is appropriate to begin an introduction to a behavioral analysis of marital conflict by outlining some of these basic laboratory-based principles. A distinguishing characteristic of a learning perspective is the assumption that the most important determinants of behavior can be found in the external environment. By analyzing those environmental events which systematically covary with an individual's behavior, it is often possible to make specific and accurate predictions about the recurrence of subsequent behavior. Since prediction is thought to be one of the fundamental goals of a behavioral science, the ability to predict behavior solely through knowledge of the individual's environment provides reasonably strong support for the utility of a model which ascribes supreme importance to the organism's environment as a causal determinant of behavior. Behavior modification or, as it is often called, behavior therapy, has extended this analysis one giant step further by asserting that, through a behavioral analysis of the relationship between an individual's behavior and his/her environment, it is often possible not only to identify the factors that are accounting for the problems that compelled the individual to seek therapeutic assistance, but also to design treatment programs which will put an end to the client's suffering.

Environmental Determinants of Behavior

Consider an individual who is behaving in some environmental context. If our goal is to categorize the events which impinge upon and influence this individual's behavior, we are able to define a number of *types* of events which have the potential for such controlling influence. The environmental events which influence behavior are usually called *stimuli.*

One important distinction is between stimuli which occur temporally prior to the behavior in question and stimuli which follow the behavior. Controlling stimuli which occur prior to the behavior being analyzed are usually referred to as *antecedent stimuli* or simply *antecedents.* Some antecedents reliably elicit specific behavior, and are thus referred to as *eliciting stimuli.* Behavior which is elicited by particular antecedents typically has a reflexive quality to it and is often thought of as involuntary. People with phobias experience intense anxiety reactions when confronted with the phobic stimulus: a snake phobic will become anxious when presented with a snake; someone with a public speaking phobia will become terribly frightened when forced to enter into a public speaking arena; an agoraphobic individual may become overwhelmed with anxiety as soon as she/he ventures outside the home. Notice that the antecedent stimuli, in these instances, vary from very discrete, clearly identifiable aspects of the environment to entire situational settings.

It becomes immediately apparent that many of the important eliciting stimuli in the environments of human beings are not inherently compelling, but have developed their eliciting potential as a result of the person's experience or learning history. The process by which formerly neutral stimuli acquire eliciting potential as a result of experience is known as *classical* or *respondent conditioning.* This phenomenon was first identified by the Russian physiologist Ivan Pavlov in his well-known experiments with dogs. The most famous of Pavlov's experimental demonstrations involved training dogs to salivate in the presence of a formerly neutral stimulus, such as a light or a tone. By pairing a natural eliciting stimulus (meat) with a neutral stimulus over a series of trials, the latter gradually acquired eliciting properties. Eliciting stimuli which become compelling due to their association with natural eliciting stimuli are called *conditioned stimuli.* A person who has a serious automobile accident may develop an anxiety reaction to automobiles; in this case the automobile has become a conditioned stimulus for anxiety. In Freud's classic case of Little Hans, Hans developed a horse phobia after being at the scene of an accident involving a horse-drawn carriage; one explanation of this phobia, consistent with the model presented here, is that the horse became a conditioned stimulus for fear (Wolpe & Rachman, 1960).

Classical conditioning plays an extremely minor role in marital interaction, except in the production of certain sexual dysfunctions. As a result these phenomena will receive little emphasis.

Another type of antecedent stimulus which serves a different kind of controlling function is known as a discriminative stimulus (S^D). A discriminative stimulus is a cue which tells the person that a particular type of behavior, if performed, is likely to be followed by a positive consequence. Discriminative stimuli are signals which indicate the likely outcomes of particular behavior. They can be distinguished from eliciting stimuli in that they do not serve a direct controlling function, i.e., they do not elicit behavior, but rather that they provide the person with information that certain behaviors, if emitted, will yield positive outcomes. As in the case of eliciting stimuli, discriminative stimuli range from the very discrete to the exceedingly complex and subtle. A green traffic light tells us that the act of driving through an intersection is likely to yield a safe crossing. When a spouse arrives at home to a candlelight dinner and a seductive, affectionate partner, she/he can safely conclude that a sexual initiation will meet with positive results. Conversely, a red traffic light indicates the likelihood of a punishing consequence if the intersection is crossed, be it an automobile accident or a ticket from a vigilant police officer. Similarly, an amorous spouse who arrives home to a grumpy, irritable partner is unlikely to initiate sexual advances. These stimuli, which suggest that specific behaviors are unlikely to yield positive outcomes, are symbolized by S^{Δ}.

Thus far, we have confined our discussion to stimuli which occur prior to the behavior in question. But one of the major categories of controlling stimuli involve those which follow rather than precede behavior. The consequences of behavior often serve as the primary determinants of the rate at which behavior recurs in the future. A stimulus which increases the probability of behavior which it follows is a *reinforcer.* Reinforcement describes the process by which certain behaviors occur at a subsequently higher rate as a result of their being followed by a specific environmental stimulus. When a husband's complaints about his work situation increase in frequency once they are reliably followed by a wife's expression of solicitation and concern, it is said that the wife is reinforcing the husband's complaining.

Technically, in order to demonstrate that reinforcement has occurred, the behavior in question must be demonstrated to increase in frequency when followed by a particular stimulus, and decrease in frequency when the stimulus is withdrawn. In order to be certain that the wife's solicitation and concern reinforce the husband's complaining, it must be shown that the latter occurs at a relatively high rate when followed by the former, and seldom occurs when the wife ignores the complaining behavior. This exemplifies a subtlety to the definition of reinforcement. A reinforcer is defined empirically on the basis of its effect on behavior. No stimulus can be designated a reinforcer until it has been shown to effectively increase the rate of specific behavior. Thus, the terms reinforcement and reward are not synonymous. A stimulus can be rewarding in the sense that someone might report that he likes or is attracted to it; yet it may fail to function as a reinforcer. A spouse may report that she/he greatly enjoys backrubs. However, a marital therapist may be quite disappointed to discover that a backrub following the husband's washing the dishes has no effect whatsoever on the likelihood of his washing the dishes in the future. Although the backrub is rewarding to the husband, in relation to the target behavior of dishwashing it is not a reinforcer.

In contrast to a reinforcer, a *punishing stimulus* is an event which decreases the likelihood of a behavior which it follows. If an alcoholic husband stops drinking after his wife develops the tactic of throwing a shoe at him whenever he enters his home intoxicated, it is said that the wife effectively punished her husband's drinking behavior.

Reinforcers can be either positive or negative. Up until now, all of our examples have depicted positive reinforcement, the process by which *presentation* of a stimulus results in an increased rate of some particular response. We can now add to our set of definitions the process of *negative reinforcement,* in which the *termination* of some stimulus leads to an increase in the frequency of behavior which precedes this termination. If a husband can turn off his wife's verbal abuse by telling her that he loves her, we can say that his affectionate remarks are reinforced by the cessation of the wife's verbal abuse. Notice that negative reinforcement differs from positive reinforcement in that an aversive consequence serves as the controlling stimulus. Notice also that negative reinforcement differs from punishment: whereas the former describes a process in which behavior is *strengthened* by the termination of an aversive stimulus, the latter describes a process by which behavior is *weakened* by the presentation of an aversive stimulus.

Most of the important interpersonal behaviors which will interest us in our discussion of adult relationships have acquired their reinforcing or punishing properties through learning and experience. We will be primarily focusing on the reinforcing effects of one spouse's interpersonal behavior on the partner. Such control occurs by the systematic presentation (or termination) of rewarding and punishing stimuli. We are emphasizing that behavior is influenced not only by the presentation of stimuli, but also by the absence of stimuli. *Extinction* defines the process whereby reinforcing stimuli are withheld after certain responses. The husband may refuse to sleep with his wife when she initiates sex in a certain way. To the extent that sexual activity is reinforcing to her, the husband is effectively extinguishing her undesirable sexual advances.

Now that we have defined the primary categories of stimuli which exert a controlling influence on behavior, we can focus on the behavior which is a function of such controlling stimuli. The term *response* refers to identifiable units of behavior. Although organisms behave continuously, for experimental purposes this continuous stream of behavior is often arbitrarily and operationally punctuated into discrete response units. To correspond to our categories of controlling stimuli, responses can be categorized into those which are largely elicited by antecedent stimuli, and those which are determined by their consequences. The former are called *respondents,* the latter *operants.* In lay terms, respondents often correspond to involuntary behavior; operants often correspond to what we think of as voluntary behavior. Respondents are often detectable only by technical recording equipment or verbal reports on the part of the person; operants are usually visible or audible to an observer. A wife who walks in on her husband engaging in sexual activity with another woman may report dizziness, an accelerated heartbeat, and "jealous feelings." These are respondents. Her response to the situation may be to yell and scream, threaten to mutilate the other woman, or file for divorce. To the extent that such responses are reinforced by a cessation of this extramarital sexual behavior, these responses can be thought of as operants. The type of learning which occurs as a result of the relationship between behavior and its consequences is called *operant conditioning.*

As organisms interact continuously with their environment, their behaviors are constantly being affected by the presence or absence of rewarding and punishing stimuli. It is possible to describe the *contingencies* of reinforcement in well-controlled experimental settings, that is, the exact relationship between behavior and its consequences. By this we refer to the frequency of reinforcement, defined either in terms of its rate per unit time (interval schedule) or the ratio of response to reinforcement (ratio schedule). The important point is that most adult behaviors are not reinforced continuously, that is, every time the response occurs, but somewhat less frequently. A response need not be reinforced continuously for it to remain strong; in fact, intermittent reinforcement often renders a response even more resistant to extinction. This phenomenon is probably due to the relative difficulty in distinguishing between reinforcing and nonreinforcing environments during an intermittent reinforcement schedule. When a behavior is being reinforced continuously, a person will readily perceive an environmental change when reinforcement is withdrawn; since the onset of extinction is readily apprehended, the behavior will quickly cease. However, in an intermittent reinforcement situation, it is much more difficult to detect an environmental change resulting from the onset of extinction, and behavior will weaken much more gradually. The aperiodic nature of most adult reinforcement contingencies complicates the task of identifying relevant contingencies in marital relationships.

Now that we have described the process by which behavior is controlled by its consequences, let us reintroduce the discriminative stimulus to our behavioral analysis. An S^D tells us that reinforcement is likely, given the enactment of a certain response. By combining the information provided by the numerous S^D's and S^Δ's in the environment, discrimination learning becomes possible. Operant behavior then is not only a function of its consequences, but also subject to the stimulus control of these antecedent discriminative stimuli. The amorous spouse's initiation of sexual activity is more likely to occur when certain cues in the environment are present (e.g., seductive behavior emanating from the partner), but only because these cues allow the spouse to predict the likelihood of reinforcement for such initiation with some degree of certainty. Thus, the association between discriminative stimuli and certain reinforcers collectively serves a controlling function. Behavior that is responsive to such cues is said to be under stimulus control; yet it is the reinforcers reliably associated with such S^D's which maintain the latter's cueing function.

As we mentioned, behavior is continuous. It occurs in sequence rather than as a series of isolated, random, discrete responses. We speak of orderly behavior, consisting of a series of responses occurring together in reliable sequence, as *response chains.* In a response chain, each re-
in reliable sequence, as *response chains.* In a response chain, each re-
sponse serves as an S^D for the subsequent responses in the chain, and the entire chain is reinforced by the event which follows completion of the yet the process of acquiring such complicated sequences of responses is often gradual and tedious. It is often necessary for each aspect of the chain to be individually reinforced before the chain has become well-established. The process of reinforcing successive approximations to the ultimately desired response chain is an example of *shaping,* a process which accounts for a large proportion of the complex learning that occurs in humans. As we shall see, shaping plays a pivotal role in the success with which spouses are able to modify displeasing excesses or deficits in their partners' behavior. For example, when a wife is dissatisfied with her husband's participation in household tasks, she may demand sweeping changes in his behavior, in which case he is likely to respond negatively, since the demand for change will be perceived as overwhelming. However, if the demand for change is gradual and moderate, and successive approximations to the desired level of participation are reinforced, the process of change is smoother and more likely to be effective.

Person Variables

Our analysis would be incomplete if we were to confine our attention to the influence of the environment on behavior. Most behaviorists acknowledge that controlling influence on behavior can come from within the organism as well as from the external world. Constitutional factors provide constraints on learning, and render the acquisition of specific behaviors relatively easy or difficult. Cognitive variables also must be included in a comprehensive analysis of the determinants of complex human behavior. People talk to themselves, they appraise their environments, and they make attributions and interpretations of their world. These self-statements, appraisals, and attributions mediate and moderate the effects of environmental stimuli on behavior, and can serve either as eliciting or discriminative stimuli. Attributions on the part of one spouse regarding the "intent" of the partner's behavior can moderate the reinforcing effects of that behavior. The husband who hugs his wife will be effectively reinforcing her only if she attributes his behavior to such desirable motivating factors as "love." If she perceives his affection as serving a manipulative function, for example, "he is just trying to get me to iron his shirts," the behavior is less likely to be reinforcing. Emotional reactions can be elicited by specific self-statements, which often serve as interpretations of an environmental event. When Jackie arrived home at 1:00 a.m. from a play rehearsal, Michael was very upset because he interpreted her tardiness as evidence of her "involvement with another man." These thoughts triggered an emotional response, whereas alternative appraisals would have been less likely to result in an emotional reaction. For example, if her absence had been interpreted as evidence simply of her "having a good time with the girls" or "working overtime on the play," an emotional reaction would have been less likely. The inclusion of cognitions as possible mediators of behavior will have important implications for the analysis and treatment of distressed relationships.

A Behavioral-Exchange Model of Relationship Discord

Now that we have introduced some basic learning principles we will present a model of relationship discord based primarily on similar experimentally-derived laboratory principles. The model assumes that the behavior of individuals in a marital relationship can be made explicable by focusing on the social environment of each spouse. In particular, each spouse's behavior in an intimate relationship can be viewed as largely a function of the consequences provided for that behavior by the partner. The tendency to emit rewarding as opposed to punishing behavior in a marital relationship, one's subjective feelings of satisfaction with a relationship, and one's tendency to remain in a relationship are all viewed as functions of the environmental consequences as provided by the partner. Since each spouse is providing consequences for the other on a continuous basis, and since each partner exerts an important controlling influence on the other's behavior, the marital relationship is best thought of as a process of circular and reciprocal sequences of behavior and consequences, where each person's behavior is at once being affected by and influencing the other.

The model is consistent with the revisionist, mediational behaviorism of the 70's in its inclusion of cognitive constructs and its attempt to conceptualize the way in which spouses appraise the relationship in order to judge the adequacy of its outcomes. It is a model which attempts to incorporate not only the environment provided by the context of the relationship, but also influential variables occurring outside of the relationship, which affect both one's tendency to remain in the relationship and one's subjective feelings of satisfaction with the relationship. As we shall make explicit in the paragraphs below, the model not only utilizes principles derived from the experimental psychology laboratory, but also borrows from social psychological theories of dyadic interaction. Finally, the model is not only a cross-sectional one, attempting to describe the current interaction of a distressed couple in reinforcement terms, but also a developmental, longitudinal model, attempting to describe the antecedents of relationship distress as the latter develops over time.

Positive Reinforcement

Simply stated, a distressed relationship is one in which there is a scarcity of positive outcomes available for each person in the relationship (Stuart, 1969). Couples who exchange very low rates of rewarding interactional stimuli provide the simplest case of this phenomenon. However, when one considers that couples are capable of punishing as well as rewarding one another, the picture becomes more complicated. If the frequency of rewarding exchanges remains constant, relationship distress can still develop due to an increase in the rate of punishing interactional exchanges. There is experimental evidence that rewarding and punishing exchanges are relatively independent of one another in intimate relationships (Wills, Weiss, & Patterson, 1974). Thus it is quite conceivable that either of these manifestations of relationship distress can occur in isolation. The third possibility, of course, is that both low rates of rewarding exchanges and high rates of punishing exchanges exist concurrently in a distressed relationship. Experimental evidence, although scanty, is consistent with the proposition that distressed couples, relative to nondistressed couples, exchange relatively low rates of pleasing behavior, high rates of displeasing behavior, or both (Birchler, Weiss,

& Vincent, 1975; Gottman, Markman, & Notarius, 1977; Gottman, Notarius, Markman, Bank, Yoppi, & Rubin, 1976; Vincent, Weiss, & Birchler, 1975).

By rewards and punishments, we are including all stimuli generated by one partner which have either a pleasing or displeasing effect on the other. For any relationship the effective stimuli will be idiosyncratic, and impossible to specify on an a priori basis. Couples provide benefits of all kinds: sexual, affectionate, communicative, and instrumental.

Given that each couple has an idiosyncratic set of effective reinforcers, it may nonetheless be possible to describe certain topographical classes of reinforcers which are of general importance to most couples (Jacobson, 1978e). For example, there is some evidence that affectionate and communicative acts tend to be more salient than instrumental behavior (household, financial, child-rearing activities) for most couples (Jacobson, 1978e; Wills et al., 1974). There is also some evidence that companionship *per se* is not reinforcing for distressed couples, although shared activities do appear to exert a reinforcing influence on nondistressed couples (Jacobson, 1978e). We would predict that, in addition to topographical differences between the most powerful reinforcers in distressed and nondistressed relationships, the two groups can be distinguished by the valence of effective reinforcers. It is expected that happy couples tend to function according to a *positive control* system, whereas *aversive control* predominates as the behavior-maintaining mechanism in distressed couples. That is, behavioral frequencies and day-to-day satisfaction in happy couples are primarily a function of the frequency of partner-provided positive reinforcement, whereas for distressed couples satisfaction is controlled by negative reinforcement, the presence or absence of punishing behaviors.

Reciprocity

We are attempting to describe not only the behavior of an individual within a relationship, but also the characteristics of the relationship as a whole. One important contribution of the systems theory perspective is the assertion that the behavior of marital partners is interdependent (Haley, 1963; Minuchin, 1974; Steinglass, 1978). It is impossible to understand the behavior of one member of a marital dyad independently of the other. Similarly, the members of a marital relationship are constantly influencing and controlling one another, so that it is arbitrary and downright misleading to interrupt the flow of interaction and assign singular causal importance to one person's behavior. The processes of influence and control in a marital relationship are mutual, reciprocal, and circular. Couples behave lawfully, and it is possible to describe this lawfulness. *Reciprocity* defines an important dimension of this lawfulness, namely the tendency for couples to reward each other at approximately equal rates (Patterson & Reid, 1970). This correlation can be seen at a number of different levels. First, on a moment by moment basis, one might ask the question, is one spouse more likely to reward the partner, given that he has just received a reward from the partner, than at other times? That is, in an ongoing interaction sequence, is the probability of a reward more likely immediately following a reward from the partner? The answer to this question seems to be "yes" (Birchler, 1973; Gottman, Notarius, Markman et al., 1976; Gottman et al., 1977), although this phenomenon seems to be equally characteristic of distressed and nondistressed couples. The same question can be asked regarding punishing behavior: Is a punisher from one partner more likely immediately following a punisher directed to the partner than at other times? Again, the answer seems to be "yes," and here the degree of reciprocity is even stronger (Birchler, 1973; Gottman, Notarius, Markman et al., 1976; Gottman et al., 1977). Furthermore, there is some evidence that negative reciprocity is particularly characteristic of distressed couples.

One might also describe reciprocity in terms of the correlation of rewarding and punishing exchanges over an extended period of time. This description can be thought of as a question of "base rates": Are spouses more similar to one another than they are to other couples in their rate of exchange of rewarding and punishing stimuli? Again, the answer seems to be affirmative. On days when one spouse reinforces the other at a high rate, the rate is likely to be reciprocated by the partner. On days where one partner emits few rewarding stimuli, it is likely that few rewarding stimuli will emanate from the partner (Birchler, 1973; Wills et al., 1974). This correlation can be found in both distressed and nondistressed relationships. As far as punishing stimuli are concerned, reciprocity seems to hold only for distressed couples (Birchler, 1973).

Finally, over an extended period of time, rates of rewards exchanged by spouses are highly correlated (Birchler, Weiss, & Vincent, 1975; Robinson & Price, 1976). This means that, over time, the exchange of rewards is balanced in long-term relationships. A spouse who gives a lot, gets a lot; a spouse who gives a little, gets a little.

To summarize, reciprocity of positive exchanges is no more characteristic of nondistressed than distressed couples, but does seem to be a law which describes the interaction of all couples regardless of the degree of distress. This association is apparent in ongoing interaction, on a moment by moment basis; but it is also apparent if one follows a couple over a long period of time. This latter relationship has been described by Gottman, Notarius, Markman et al. (1976) as a "bank account" model of marital exchange, whereby couples "invest" in the relationship by giving rewards to one another, which over time balance each other and thereby maintain the current rate of rewarding exchange. This aspect of reciprocity says nothing about any given interchange between a couple, nor does it preclude nonreciprocal exchanges at any given point in time.

It is when we examine the degree of reciprocity in punishing exchanges that we find another basis for distinguishing between distressed and nondistressed couples. Distressed couples reciprocate punishment to a greater degree than do nondistressed couples. These findings prompted one of us to comment, in another context, that "some nondistressed marriages are characterized by one-sided coercive relationships that are nevertheless stable and in which spouses deny any dissatisfaction or distress" (Jacobson & Martin, 1976, p. 542). Following this line of reasoning, distress is more likely to become acute and acknowledged when the victim of coercion rebels and begins to reciprocate aversive control.

Gottman's "bank account" model also explains this discrepancy between distressed and nondistressed couples. When the ratio of rewards to punishments in a relationship is low, as is the case with distressed couples, one is more apt to "balance the checkbook" regularly, to keep score. One would then expect greater reciprocity in distressed couples. However, this particular notion would also predict greater reciprocity of positive behaviors in distressed than in nondistressed relationships; as we mentioned, this finding has not emerged from research investigations.

It does appear that, in general, distressed couples are relatively dependent on immediate, as opposed to delayed, rewards and punishments (Jacobson, 1978e). Since happily-married couples are accustomed to receiving a consistent, high rate of rewards from one another, nonreinforced behavior or inequitable exchanges can be tolerated in the short run, since their shared reinforcement history offers promise of long-term equality and continued rewards. Perhaps this freedom from control by a partner's immediate consequences is an operational definition of "trust" (Jacobson, 1978e). In contrast, unhappy couples experience rewards from one another only in sparse and erratic doses. Their satisfaction level might be described as labile and rapidly fluctuating according to the moment-by-moment changes in the rate of punishment provided by the partner.

The high reactivity and dependence on immediate consequences which we are positing for distressed couples suggest that each spouse's response to changes in the frequency of the partner's behavior should be rapid and extreme. In concordance with research findings, we would predict that increases in the rate of punishing behavior in one distressed partner should lead to large corresponding increases in the other's rate of punishing behavior, whereas less marked and perhaps negligible changes would be expected in happy couples following an escalation in one partner's delivery of punishment. However, we would not expect this elevated reactivity in distressed couples to apply to escalations in rewarding behavior; that is, increases in the frequency of positive behavior in one partner following the other's elevation should be no more striking in distressed than in nondistressed couples. This is because, despite their greater reactivity, distressed couples are also expected to be less sensitive to the partner's provision of positive behavior. By selectively focusing on and tracking negative behavior, distressed spouses often ignore and fail to process the partner's delivery of rewards. This selective tracking counteracts the reactivity to immediate behavior. Our suggestion is consistent with current research findings, but has yet to be tested directly.

Thus, a behavior exchange model of relationship distress emphasizes both the *rate* of reinforcing and punishing exchanges between partners and the juxtaposition or covariance between each partner's emission of such behavior. Marital distress can be described not only in terms of a reduced reward/punishment ratio, but also in terms of an increased reactivity to the partner's aversive behavior.

Social Exchange and Relationship Satisfaction

In this section we add to our theoretical model some of the contributions from social psychological exchange theories (Homans, 1961; Thibaut & Kelley, 1959). We have already seen that a marital relationship is an interdependent one. Couples constantly emit stimuli which have reinforcing or punishing effects on the partner. Each possible combination of behavioral exchanges yields an outcome for each partner. These outcomes collectively determine one's tendency to emit rewarding behavior in future encounters, one's level of satisfaction in the relationship, and one's general tendency to continue in the relationship. One factor which determines the outcome of a particular interaction is the receiver's appraisal of his/her potential outcomes in alternative relationships, or the outcomes accruing as a result of being alone. The more positive each spouse estimates his/her options outside of the relationship to be, the more positive the outcomes in the relationship need to be in order to justify continuance of the relationship.

It is here that our model becomes cognitive. We are asserting that the reinforcing effects of interactional sequences in a relationship depend upon the valence of the partner's behavior, and the receiver's *estimation* of his/her outcomes in alternative relationships. Spouses evaluate their current relationships by processing stimuli received from the partner, by monitoring their experience of the partner's behavior as it interacts with their own, and by comparing the end products with various alternatives. The outcomes associated with a satisfying relationship are not identical to the outcomes necessary for a continuance of the relationship. People who perceive themselves as having attractive options outside of the relationship will demand more positive outcomes for the continuance of that relationship than will individuals who view their alternatives to the relationship as limited and restricted. A relationship which is minimally rewarding may be nevertheless quite stable and persistent if the participants perceive their positions as providing them with no equally satisfactory alternatives. However, since these relationships are not particularly rewarding, costs will usually be kept to a minimum, and the relationship will likely stabilize at a point where little rewarding interaction occurs between the couple. This explains the apparent paradox involved in couples who seem, to an observer, to be involved in an unsatisfying relationship, yet the participants have no intention of terminating it. Similarly, young attractive couples who perceive themselves as having many viable options at their disposal are likely to have little tolerance for relationship problems. The comparative ease of separation and divorce contributes to the lowered threshold for tolerance of relationship difficulties present in young couples.

Thus, at any given point in time, each member of a marital dyad retains an overall degree of satisfaction with the current relationship. Each member also possesses classes of both rewarding and punishing behaviors, each carrying a certain probability of emission. Finally, on the basis of comparing the outcomes of the present relationship with one's estimation of the outcomes to be derived from alternative potential relationships, the partners will maintain some degree of commitment toward remaining in the relationship. The first two of these stances are assumed to be contingent upon reinforcement derived directly from the relationship; the latter depends primarily upon factors outside of the relationship.

It would be vastly oversimplified to suggest that each behavior in the repertoire of marital partners is maintained by specific reinforcing stimuli from the spouse on a point-for-point basis. Rather, it seems more realistic to posit a summation process such that classes of positive relationship behavior are maintained by a number of partner-initiated behaviors which are experientially summated by the receiver and integrated into an overall experience of the partner's behavior. That is, in a relationship each spouse responds on the basis of his/her experience of the partner, based on the partner's behavior. Elements of the partner's behavior are processed and integrated by the receiver over a given period of time, and large classes of reinforcing behavior are directed toward the partner to the extent that the receiver's overall experience of the relationship is reinforcing at given points in time. This is not to say that there are not specific, discrete response-reinforcement relationships controlling some relationship behaviors; certainly there are. For example, one partner's tendency to communicate his day's activities to the partner may be under the control of the partner's response to his initial overtures. Eye contact, interested questions, and verbal support may reinforce such conversation, whereas yawning, looking away, and verbal interruptions may punish such communicative endeavors. However, in addition to these discrete functional relationships there are overriding cumulative happenings which must be taken into account in a behavioral analysis of relationship satisfaction.

This learning model is most similar to paradigms in experimental psychology which emphasize the correlation between responses and reinforcement over time, rather than discrete functional relationships between a given response and a particular reinforcer (e.g., Baum, 1973; Herrnstein, 1970). These models depict the organism as responding to clusters of reinforcers which accumulate over time. Rate of responding is thought to be a complex function of the way reinforcers are spread out over the environment and over time. Maximum predictability is believed to be attained through an analysis of these correlations between responses and reinforcement.

Perhaps an example will illustrate our hypothesis about marital reinforcement. Let us assume that, for a given couple, the wife's affection is controlled not by the husband's immediate response to that affection but by her overriding experience of the relationship at a given point in time. The probability of her being affectionate varies according to the husband's provision of various reinforcing behaviors, say over the previous week. Many types of behavior on the husband's part are functionally equivalent, and the only requirement is that a collection of such behaviors occur at a sufficiently right rate, or at a sufficiently high ratio to punishing behavior, to prompt affectionate behavior on the wife's part. It may be that active communication is one way of meeting these minimum standards so that if the husband has been spending a large amount of time talking to the wife over the past week, the probability of her affection is increased. Initiation of social activities with other couples might be another important factor, so that if the husband has planned an enjoyable evening outside of the home, the wife's inclination to be affectionate may be increased. Punishing behavior emanating from the husband may dilute her experience and counteract the impact of his reinforcing behavior. For example, if in the middle of the previous week the husband insulted his wife in public the negative valence may be so great as to neutralize the impact of his animated conversation during the remainder of the week. All of these factors contribute to the likelihood of the wife's behaving in an affectionate manner. If we knew enough about the weightings, both positive and negative, given by the wife to various aspects of the husband's behavior, and if we knew the rates of these weighted behaviors, we should be able to predict the likelihood of the wife's behaving with affection toward her husband.

The model holds that there is a strong relationship between satisfaction in a relationship and the tendency to behave in a pleasing manner toward one's spouse. Those relationship behaviors which are under the control of large classes of functionally similar partner behaviors are probably barometers for relationship satisfaction. Other behaviors, which may be related to very discrete, specific, immediate environmental consequences, are probably weaker predictors of satisfaction. The important point is that couples act on their marital environment to summarize and integrate the information provided by the partner, and that this cognitive processing affects the participant's subsequent responding, as well as his current evaluation of the quality of the marriage. These evaluations and response tendencies are not static, and in fact are constantly being modified by new information and new experiences.

The Development of Marital Distress

Thus far our presentation of the behavioral exchange model has described the reciprocal relationship between responses exchanged by marital partners, and the patterns thought to be indicative of distress. But current interaction patterns are the culmination of months or years of continuous interacting, and it is important to identify the antecedents of marital distress in addition to analyzing its current manifestations. One can think of a long-term relationship as a developmental process. This process begins during an initial relationship formation stage. With increasing intimacy, or degree of association, couples must adapt to new circumstances and new relationship requirements. The couple that persists in a satisfying relationship is able to adjust to these changing circumstances and change behavior when such change is necessitated. The need for change and adaptation can stem from either demands within the relationship or developments external to the dyad. Couples decide to live together, marry, bear children, move to new locations, and change jobs; they are also subjected to changing social and political climates. Finally, all couples must cope with their differences, and the conflict which is an inevitable concomitant to a long-term intimate relationship. During these periods of transition and changing circumstances, couples face their sternest tests, and their collective reaction to these stresses can be thought of as crucial to the subsequent degree of relationship distress.

Assuming some initial attraction between two people, the first phase of a relationship is characterized by a mutually high rate of rewarding exchanges. Many factors contribute to this initially dense exchange of reinforcement. First, because of each person's attraction to the other, which is often based on minimal information or knowledge of the other's behavior, they draw selectively from their repertoires those behaviors which are deemed likely to be received as pleasing. Their concern with minimizing costs is subservient to the goal of producing and maintaining positive feelings in the other. Participants monitor their own behavior, and attend to the task of pleasing the partner, while simultaneously suspending the usually important requirement that the exchange of pleasing behavior is balanced and reciprocated by the partner. The result is often a preponderance of maximally rewarding interactions, producing the effects which are typically described as the euphoria during the honeymoon stage of a relationship. Second, the restricted range of interactional opportunities present in the early stages of a relationship ensures a high rate of pleasing exchanges for an additional reason. Couples spend most of their time engaging in pleasurable activities together, without having to make any of the costly sacrifices that will later be necessary. There are no financial decisions to make, no household or child-rearing responsibilities to negotiate and minimal concern with the constraints on one's freedom of action which are often associated with the commitment to a relationship. Third, during the early stages of a relationship the partner's reinforcing power is often at its maximum. The novelty of the sexual, communicative, and recreational stimulation ensures that each partner's capacity to reinforce is at its peak. Fourth, each partner's cognitions play a part in maximizing the reinforcing experience of a relationship's early stages. Both members form expectations about areas of the relationship not directly experienced as yet; they predict the likelihood of continued satisfaction in the future. The high output of initial positive exchanges leads to expectations of further rewards in the untapped arenas of mutual experience. In this way, the other person is "idealized." Cognitions regarding the other person enhance the latter's reinforcing value, because whatever gratification is currently being derived is augmented by the anticipation of further rewards in an expanded domain of interactional opportunities. The partner's capacity to provide gratification is inappropriately generalized. Seldom are the future *costs* of further relationship involvement adequately anticipated.

These early stages notwithstanding, for every couple the honeymoon eventually ends. As couples widen the arena of interaction, it becomes increasingly difficult to produce only those elements from one's repertoire that are rewarding. Inevitably, the "other side" of each fallible human being becomes visible to the partner, and the rate of rewarding exchanges thins, and is augmented by displeasing behavior. Differences between spouses, which were either ignored or not discovered during the honeymoon phase, assume greater importance and become sources of displeasure. The distressing realization that the other is not always going to be pleasing or rewarding leads to more realistic appraisal of the person's present or future capacity to provide benefits. This can lead to a readjustment of expectations, and the renewal of a highly satisfying, although different, relationship. However, it can also sow the seeds of dissatisfaction and distress.

Against this backdrop of inevitable disappointment and conflict, the struggle to maintain a satisfying relationship begins in earnest. The collision between expectation and reality is the first barrier to the couple's quest for intimacy. From this point on, the potential antecedents of marital distress are numerous. In the paragraphs below, we will outline some of the more common ones.

Behavior Change Deficits

Given the inevitability of conflict in a long-term relationship, couples are distinguished not by its presence or absence but by their mode of response to it. When partner A first discovers that some aspect of partner B's behavior upsets him, A must find a way of responding to this discovery. Some couples initiate an early precedent for speaking openly and directly about conflict, and solve relationship conflicts decisively. They learn that an inherent cost in a successful marriage is the periodic necessity for sacrifice and compromise. In order for a relationship to be viable and mutually satisfying over a long period of time, partners must accommodate to one another, and at times do things that, in an ideal world, they would prefer not to do. Thus, it is often necessary for partners to modify their behavior *simply* because the current state of affairs is upsetting to the spouse. Some couples learn this lesson well. For those who do, problem-solving and behavior change skills serve a prophylactic function, preventing the accumulation of unsolved problems and lingering resentments.

However, some couples are not so lucky. For these couples (like Dan and Sandra), conflict is seen as a catastrophe rather than an inevitability. To acknowledge and openly deal with conflict is viewed as tantamount to admitting to a "bad" relationship, or it is viewed as evidence that they are no longer "in love." Conflict is ignored, remaining covert. Unfortunately the effects of unattended conflict are irrepressible, and satisfaction will be cumulatively impaired. Once conflict is finally acknowledged, the areas of discord are so numerous and multifaceted as to appear insurmountable. Johann and Marianne, the couple in Bergman's "Scenes from a Marriage," typify this maladaptive response to conflict. Like all couples, they faced the inevitable costs of marriage: the constancy of married life, impositions on each person's behavioral options, and the like. However, each had an overriding investment in maintaining harmony, and an injunction against openly acknowledging conflict pervaded their married life. When the areas of conflict were finally admitted to, it was too late to save the marriage.

Other couples develop a superficial ability to "communicate" about problems, but they spend their problem-solving time with an unproductive focusing on insight and understanding. Feelings are expressed, but needed changes are not agreed upon or implemented, solutions are not forthcoming. All of us are familiar with couples who openly and honestly communicate about their relationship, yet separate to the surprise of many. Often a scrutiny of their history reveals a lack of accommodation and change in response to conflict, despite their open communication.

The most blatant example of faulty behavior change strategies involves couples who develop coercive methods to modify the other person's behavior. Either actively, by physical or verbal abuse, or passively, through withdrawal and the withholding of rewards, such spouses attempt to gain compliance and behavior change through applying punishment and negative reinforcement. More will be said of this phenomenon in the next chapter. For now, suffice it to say that these strategies are often tempting because of their short-term efficacy. Punishing stimuli can be quite compelling, and often lead to dramatic, immediate changes in behavior. As our discussion of reciprocity indicated, however, punishment tends to beget punishment for some couples; once coercion is used as a behavior change tactic, it tends to be reciprocated in an ominous, self-perpetuating cycle.

In summary, one important antecedent of relationship distress is a deficit in couples' ability to generate behavior change or relationship change. Deficits in behavior change skills can be lethal, since the need for change is present, at one time or another, in even the most compatible of relationships.

Reinforcement Erosion

We have already mentioned that the novelty of a new partner's stimulus value tends to maximize each person's reinforcing capabilities in the early stages of a relationship. Over time, it is not uncommon for the partner's reinforcing potential to diminish, simply due to habituation. In order to counter such satiation effects, many couples expand their repertoires of reinforcing behaviors. The more varied the reinforcing behaviors, the less dependent the relationship is on a given class of reinforcers. Happy couples can be quite creative in expanding their repertoires to cope with the reduced potency of old behaviors. As sexual encounters become more common and thereby lose some of their excitement, couples expand their sexual repertoires to include new, novel ways of making love. Couples also develop new common interests and avocations, both to maximize their engagement in shared pleasurable activities and to provide themselves with new topics of conversation.

Unfortunately, many couples (like Dan and Sandra) do not alter their repertoires sufficiently to cope with the erosion problem. Thus, they continue to interact in the routinized, restricted ways that proved to be rewarding in the past, but that now have lost much of their magic. The relationship becomes dull and boring, and the development of such a state perplexes and frightens the participants. This is one of the most common sources of marital discord, and also one of the most gradual. Seldom do couples seek therapy strictly in response to this process, since acute stress and crisis are relatively absent. But the continued ability to provide rewards can act as a buffer against other acute stressors, and the absence of such reinforcing power is often implicated in a marital crisis with other more clear-cut precipitants. Therapists are often insensitive to the indirect role of this subtle erosion process, and the importance of including strategies in therapy designed to increase each partner's reinforcing capabilities.

This raises an important theoretical issue which carries with it implications for both the assessment and treatment of marital discord. For any couple exchanging a low rate of rewards, it is appropriate to ask whether the problem is one of actually withholding rewarding stimuli, or one of providing the same stimuli that were once reinforcing but have now lost their potency. The question is basically one involving the assessment of each spouse's current *reinforcement value* for the other. A marriage in which the spouses perform ineffectually but are at least attempting to provide benefits is a very different problem from one in which reinforcement potential is high but the rewards are being withheld.

Stimulus Control Deficiencies

As relationships develop over time, couples develop "rules" to govern their behavior over the diverse, expanding range of interactional modalities (Jackson, 1965; Weiss, 1978). These rules are often unacknowledged and implicit, yet they exert powerful control over the behavior of both participants. They can be thought of as "norms" which reduce the uncertainty and enhance the predictability of members' behavior. Without these rules, relationship behavior would be unorganized, chaotic, and unpredictable. Decisions would be made anew in every situation, and couples would be in a perpetual state of negotiation and decision-making.

Some relationships can be characterized as possessing lacunae in their normative structure. Perhaps rules have been established to cover an insufficient number of variegated interactional possibilities. For example, if norms are not established to define each person's duties and responsibilities regarding household management, each time something has to be done the couple must arrive at a decision about who is going to do it. The possibilities for conflict are multiplied under such arrangements. Every relationship needs a division of responsibilities and tasks which ensures that each spouse will be preeminent in some domains, with the corresponding rewards and costs inherent in such primacy.

It is also possible for the rule structure to be adequate at one point in a relationship, but later insufficient as a result of a couple's entry into a new phase. If the normative structure adapts to the new phase, and if new rules are added or old ones sufficiently modified, the couple will experience a minimum of discord during the transition phase. In contrast, couples who rigidly adhere to obsolete sets of rules will experience a great deal of stress and conflict during such transitional periods, and the conflict may not abate until they respond adequately to the new situational demands. For example, in the traditional marriage, the birth of a child usually led to greatly increased demands on the wife, while the changes demanded of the husband were generally minimal. First, the wife expanded her domain of power and responsibility to include nurturance of the child, whereas the husband's duties remained relatively constant. Second, the wife was less available to reward the husband with either affection or communication. Conflict was likely in this situation unless the husband expanded his role in the home to remove some of the burden from the wife. Furthermore, the rules regarding when and how the wife was to provide direct benefits to the husband had to be altered in such a way that the husband was able to accept less, at least temporarily, and the wife could tolerate giving less without feeling guilty and inadequate as a wife. The changes in the normative structure of the marriage can be thought of as new rules; without them the relationship is in trouble.

Skill Deficits

A number of diverse skills are necessary to provide continued satisfaction in a relationship. Problem-solving and behavior change skills are one example that have already been mentioned. But other types of communication skills are also important in a relationship. Spouses need to be able to express their feelings, both positive and negative. They need to provide support and understanding to one another (Weiss, 1978). In the sexual realm, they need skills to maintain a viable sex life, particularly after the initial novelty has ended. Various instrumental skills are also necessary, including child-rearing, household and financial management, and the like. Notice that some of these skills are unimportant during a relationship's early stages, but assume increasing importance as time goes on. Any of these skill deficits can serve as antecedents for distress, either because they were absent from the beginning, or because they were unavailable at a subsequent phase of a relationship when they first became necessary.

Changes in the External Environment

For some couples the antecedents of distress stem from changes which occur outside of the relationship, which have little directly to do with anything that has transpired within the dyad itself. If environmental changes are such that alternatives to the relationship become attractive to the partner, stress may result in the relationship. This phenomenon relates to the standards against which each partner judges the suitability of a current relationship. We have already mentioned that spouses compare their current level of satisfaction with their assessment of the benefits to be derived either from alternative relationships or from the state of being alone. This comparison helps determine the likelihood of remaining in the current relationship.

One of the most heralded examples of an external factor impinging on the stability of a marriage is the appearance of a third party who offers one of the spouses the potential for a sexual relationship. A new person offers possibilities for rewards which are quite difficult for a spouse to duplicate. All of the benefits outlined earlier during our discussion of a relationship's early stages compete rather formidably with the rewards derived from one's marriage. To the extent that the new relationship is very attractive to the spouse, the rewards derived from the marriage must increase for the latter relationship to remain viable.

Career opportunities which compete with a marriage are not uncommon. It is not so much that career advancement is incompatible with devotion to a marital partner. Rather, as a career provides increasing rewards, some spouses will face conflicts over how to distribute their time, and may spend more and more of their time away from home engaging in career pursuits. At times spouses are faced with incompatible choices between their career and their relationship, as in the situation where one's career requires a relocation in a place which is unacceptable to the partner.

Another common environmental change which has affected many marital relationships in the last decade is the changing social and political climate, which has altered women's perceptions of their options. Women enmeshed in traditional marriages have begun to view less restrictive relationships, or even the alternative of being alone, as more desirable than a continuance of a marriage in which their opportunities for satisfaction are constrained by the adoption of traditional norms and roles. Many couples have faced a crisis whereby the relationship had to become more satisfying to the woman in order to neutralize the attractiveness of these alternatives. Usually, this has meant moving to a more egalitarian relationship.

In general, any attractive environmental alternative to the marriage figures into a spouse's evaluation of the latter. In any analysis of a marital dyad, it is important to include relevant exogenous factors which may be affecting either spouse's expectations or standards regarding the relationship.

Affiliative Versus Independent Preferences

Although we have been emphasizing environmental antecedents of relationship distress, it is also possible that individual differences between partners can lead to substantial difficulties. In particular we have been impressed by a particular incompatibility in partners' reinforcement preferences which often seems to be a powerful deterrent to marital satisfaction. This difference lies in the extent to which each spouse derives rewards from interpersonal closeness and intimacy, as opposed to independence and interpersonal distance. Some people display characteristic preferences, which transcend any particular relationship, for a relatively high rate of interpersonal contact. Moreover, these people often prefer "intimate contact" such as affection, conversation about feelings, and the like, to simple companionship and shared activities. Finally, these people find the scarcity of these events aversive. There are also people who characteristically prefer relatively low rates of interpersonal contact, a low ratio of intimate contact to simple companionship, and often prefer to be alone. Excessively high rates of interpersonal contact are experienced as aversive to these people. When these two types are matched in a marital relationship, the capacity for conflict is great.

Eidelson (1976) has presented data which suggest that at early stages of relationship development, couples with these different preferences are unlikely to be in conflict. The high rate of reinforcement takes precedence over either partner's excessive requirements in this area. However, as the degree of association intensifies, partners' discrepancies begin to emerge as a source of conflict. Most typically, the affiliative partner increases the demands for intimate contact in consonance with the onset of reticence on the part of the more distant partner. With this process, a vicious cycle of approach-avoidance ensues, which gradually renders the relationship less satisfying to both members.

One might legitimately question the wisdom of mutual choice in such a couple's initial decision to become a couple. However, it is quite common for people to be attracted initially to those who possess attributes and skills which they themselves lack, particularly when the costs of these differences are not apparent. These sources of attraction become sources of conflict only when the requirements of marriage force each spouse to reconcile his/her behavior with that of the partner. Differences between people on the dimensions of affiliation/independence have been singled out here not because they represent the only individual difference which produces marital conflict, but rather because the existence of pairs mismatched on this dimension is common, and can often generate acute distress which, once initiated, seems to be self-perpetuating.

SUMMARY

The behavior exchange model of marital distress is based largely on principles of learning derived from laboratory research in experimental psychology. These principles categorize the various environmental stimuli which can influence behavior, and also delineate the various ways that behavior can be a function of such stimuli. More recent learning models have included cognitive or mediational events in their formulations. For the past 20 years, learning principles have been applied to clinical problems with impressive success.

Marital distress is viewed largely as a function of the *rate* of reinforcement (and/or punishment) directed by marital partners toward one another, and the *relationship* between each person's delivery of reinforcement and punishment. Distressed couples not only deliver relatively low rates of reinforcement toward one another (and/or relatively high rates of punishment), but they also tend to reciprocate the presentation of displeasing or punishing stimuli. Cognitive events are believed to play an important role in this process. Couples base their emission of pleasing and displeasing behavior on a summation of salient displeasing and pleasing stimuli delivered by the partner. Their overall experience of the relationship at any given point in time, based on the partner's behavior, determines not only their rate of positive and negative stimuli, but also their degree of satisfaction with the marriage. Each spouse's appraisal of alternatives to the present relationship also enters into the equation, primarily by determining the minimum level of satisfaction required for maintenance of the present relationship.

Marital distress can result from any one of a number of antecedents, the most important of which are the following: deficits in problem-solving and behavior change skills, reinforcement erosion, stimulus control deficiencies, skill deficits, exogenous factors which increase the attractiveness of alternatives to the marriage, and discrepant preferences in regard to the degree of intimacy desired.

CHAPTER 2

General Considerations

BEHAVIORAL MARITAL THERAPY has already come to be associated with a technology which includes 1) training couples in communication skills, 2) contingency contracting, and 3) the application of reinforcement principles to increase positive relationship behavior (Jacobson & Martin, 1976; Stuart, 1969; Weiss, Hops, & Patterson, 1973). A perusal of our table of contents suggests an encouragement of this tendency to define marital therapy as the application of these techniques to the problems of distressed couples. We devote an entire chapter to each of these three technological strategies. And it is true that our model, depicted in the previous chapter, suggests that certain general strategies will be applicable to a wide variety of distressed couples. For example, the notion that many distressed couples are ineffective at either solving relationship problems or modifying the behavior of the partner carries with it the implication that, given the existence of effective techniques designed to teach couples skills in either problem-solving or behavior management, these techniques will prove useful for a substantial number of such couples.

However, in many ways it is inconsistent with the spirit and the tradition of behavior therapy to define it as the application of specified techniques (cf. Goldfried & Davison, 1976; Yates, 1970). Although at one time many people thought of behavior therapy as a set of techniques such as systematic desensitization and assertive training, techniques apparently derived from some form of learning theory (Wolpe & Lazarus, 1966), over the last decade the definition has been progressively altered in two ways. First, the principles from which behavioral techniques are derived have gradually expanded from various learning theories to experimental psychology in general, and more recently from experimental psychology to any area of psychology. There is now some consensus that any experimentally-based principle, whether it be from experimental psychology, cognitive psychology, or social psychology, which can be applied to clinical problems, results in a clinical intervention which can be considered behavior therapy. Here, the definition has been modified from the application of a set of techniques to the application of a set of principles. The transformation redefines behavior therapy as *applied general psychology*.

The treatment of relationship problems reflects this change in emphasis from techniques to principles. While learning-based procedures have predominated in the literature on helping couples change, social psychological principles have also played a major role in the development of intervention strategies. As Chapter 1 emphasized, *social exchange theory*, e.g., Thibaut and Kelley (1959), has been a seminal influence on behavioral formulations of marital distress. Theories of cognitive consistency and causal attribution also figure prominently in the derivation of treatment strategies. The bottom line for the theoretical antecedents used to construct a treatment program for marital distress is that, to some degree, the validity of the theories has been established by controlled investigation.

Second, in recent years, primarily due to the influence of operant psychology, behavior therapy has come to be defined as a method of inquiry, an approach to analyzing clinical problems and designing intervention strategies which transcends the specific techniques that are applied.

This method of investigation is described in detail by various authors (e.g., Sidman, 1960) and involves a *functional analysis* of the client's presenting problem behaviors. During the initial assessment phase, a careful analysis of the relationship between the problem behaviors and the environment is conducted, and this analysis leads to a set of hypotheses about the antecedent stimuli and consequences which are controlling the behavior in question. These hypotheses then lead to an intervention strategy designed to alter the behavior in desirable ways. Assessment of the behavior continues throughout the treatment phase for the purpose of carefully evaluating the effects of the intervention. This assessment ideally consists of continuous measurement of the identified target behavior; in addition, steps are taken in the experimental design to establish the functional relations between the treatment applied and the altered behavior. In the event that treatment is unsuccessful, the continuous assessment procedure allows for early detection of this failure, and a revised analysis leads to a reformulated intervention (Hersen & Barlow, 1976).

For the practicing clinician, defining behavior therapy by the experimental procedures used to analyze individual cases is both prudent and practical. Prudent because every client has a unique learning history, and the presumptuous application of techniques to a given case based on a similarity between the topography of a client's problem and other client problems known to have been successfully treated by that technique might overlook idiosyncracies of a particular case which would render such a decision inappropriate. The complexity of behavior-environment interactions precludes cookbook applications of techniques without such a careful analysis.

The procedures for analyzing behavior-environment relationships with couples are described in detail in Chapter 4. However, for purposes of the present discussion, we will consider a few cases which illustrate the complexity of such behavior-environment interactions, and justify the need for careful, continuous analyses of such interactions.

Bob and Sarah systematically avoided discussing their relationship problems. They described their few attempts at conflict resolution as "all out war." Apparently as a result of these unsuccessful interactions, the husband put up with a great many dissatisfactions rather than risk the overt conflict that the direct confrontation of such dissatisfactions would entail. The first impulse of a technique-oriented behavior therapist would be to provide this couple with intensive training in problem-solving skills. However, a careful pretreatment assessment revealed that this couple was very effective at problem-solving. In the therapist's office, when the couple was told to solve a particular relationship problem, for example, the husband coming home late for dinner, they reached agreement efficiently and amicably. The solution was implemented immediately, without coaching from the therapist, and by the next week, which was really the first week of actual therapy, the relationship was already much improved. This couple possessed sufficient problem-solving skills and was simply not using them. Their anticipation of arguments was based on past discussions which had occurred only after months of avoidance and accumulated resentment. Rather than reflecting an inability to discuss problems together, their fights reflected their unwillingness to use their skills after allowing the problems to proliferate for long periods of time. Instead of requiring training in communication skills, this couple needed environmental programming such that their already existent skills would be brought under the stimulus control of their normal daily routines. By introducing certain rituals into their daily lives, such as a regular time set aside for problem-solving, the environmental prompts were installed, and problem-solving began to occur regularly. Now problems were dealt with immediately and efficiently during this regularly scheduled time. It would have been costly, time-consuming, and not to the point to embark on an intensive training program in problem-solving with this couple. A careful analysis of behavior-environment relationships avoided such a clinical error.

A second example involves Al and Laura, who presented with the husband's complaint of "secondary impotence." For the past year, on about half of the couple's attempts at intercourse, the husband had been unable to attain an erection. The couple had read the work of Masters and Johnson, and were both psychologically-minded and intelligent. They insisted that their marriage was functioning well in all other respects, and particularly patted themselves on the back for their willingness to communicate openly about problems when they did present themselves. Somewhat surprisingly, data which they collected at home during the initial assessment phase revealed that unsuccessful intercourse generally followed discussions "about the relationship." When asked to "discuss their relationship" in the therapist's office, they exhibited a highly intellectualized, psychodynamically oriented style of discussion, featuring much speculation regarding the childhood origins of their "hang-ups." They never actually "problem-solved" at all, and change agreements were never reached. The apparent relationship between intimate conversation and unsuccessful sex was tested through an intervention strategy aimed at altering their problem-solving interaction according to the guidelines enumerated in Chapter 7. Specifically, the wife was coached to refrain from "mind-reading" and not use motivational inferences in discussing Al's behavior. They were both taught to listen to each other more completely and to demonstrate, through paraphrasing and reflecting each other's remarks, that they had been listening to one another. Once they were able to problem-solve effectively, the husband's erectile difficulties vanished, and did not recur through a one-year follow-up.

In both of these examples, a less than adequate assessment would have lead to the inappropriate application of techniques. For these couples, behavior therapy meant a fine-grain idiographic study of the stimuli which controlled their marital responding, and a treatment program tailored to the results of this analysis. Many mistakes will be avoided if the marital therapist remembers that behavior therapy implies a method of analysis, and that judgment about the appropriate intervention should be withheld, pending the revelations provided by such an analysis.

Thus, in approaching relationship discord, the behavioral clinician has many ways to define his role. He can view himself as one who uses certain techniques, such as communication training, contingency contracting, or sex therapy, to improve relationships. Alternatively, he can view himself as one who applies experimentally-based principles from general psychology to marital problems. Finally, and ideally, he will view himself as one who engages in an experimental analysis of a couple entering therapy, and base his treatment decisions on this analysis. Although he may end up using certain standardized techniques on a majority of occasions, the proper balance of their application, and decisions about when to deviate from such techniques, can be determined only through the experimental analysis.

So far, we have focused on three definitions of behavior therapy which have some general applicability to a wide range of clinical problems. Now we wish to complicate matters further by adding an additional definition of behavior therapy. This will be a somewhat arbitrary attempt on our part to operationalize a behavioral approach to working with couples by identifying a number of themes which cut across the various intervention strategies consistent with a behavioral framework. Hopefully, these themes will provide some conceptual unity and clarity to the rather heterogeneous set of possible options that the behavioral clinician has before him when working with couples.

POSITIVE TRACKING

At every point in time, from the initial contact with a couple to the termination of treatment, the strengths of the relationship are emphasized, and treatment is characterized as a way of building on these strengths. The specific strategies for accomplishing this end will be elaborated in subsequent chapters, but here a few general points will be made. Couples often enter therapy with a biased perspective on their relationship. Because significant problems have existed for some duration by the time the couple finds their way to a therapist's office, and because these problems in most cases have become exacerbated over time, couples tend to progressively focus on the negative aspects of their relationship. By the time that they enter therapy, they are truly out of touch with the good things, and as a result, verbalize more hopelessness than their situation warrants. The perspective offered by the therapist that there are indeed strengths in the relationship, and that these strengths are to be broadened in therapy, can often be therapeutic in itself, because such a perspective cuts into couples' hopelessness and provides for anxiety reduction (cf. Frank, 1961). As couples begin to replace their negative scanning with positive tracking, their perspective on the relationship changes, and they are better able to focus on collaborating with one another in improving the relationship.

In the initial interview, positive tracking is encouraged by focusing many of the questions on positive aspects of the relationship. Assessment should also emphasize a monitoring of the positive. For example, Stuart and Stuart's (1973) precounseling inventory asks each spouse to list ten things the partner currently does which are pleasing. In addition, baseline data collected by couples in the home should include monitoring of "pleasing" spouse behaviors. In presenting a couple with the results of a pretreatment assessment, relationship strengths should be given equal time. Throughout therapy, relevant positive interchanges between spouses, both within sessions and between sessions, should be emphasized. For example, the therapist must relentlessly point out the distinction between a spouse's "intentions" and his/her "actions." Confusion of these two labels often leads spouses to infer malevolent motivation from their partners' undesirable behavior; this makes the attribution more pejorative. It is not nearly as bad in a spouse's eyes when the partner "screws up" as it is when he is seen as intentionally behaving negatively. The consistent attribution of good intentions, despite inappropriate behavior, aids in the task of positive tracking.

POSITIVE CONTROL

Behavioral couples therapy assumes that many couples who fail to deal effectively with conflict use aversive control strategies in their ineffectual attempts to alter the behavior of one another. In a problem-solving discussion, such tactics would be exemplified by punishing verbal and nonverbal responses. One spouse may "demand" immediate compliance from the partner, as in the example provided by the wife who opened a problem-solving session by telling her husband that "I'm not going to tolerate your laziness anymore; you better do something about it." Threats are an additional aversive control strategy common in distressed couple communication. A husband who continuously felt rejected by his wife in the bedroom issued the following threatening ultimation: "I'm going to find someone who appreciates me unless you shape up." An abundance of critical remarks is also quite common among distressed couples; such remarks constitute aversive control strategies by virtue of their *frequency* of *occurrence* as opposed to their *intensity*, as in the case of threats and demands. Nonverbal behaviors can also function as aversive stimuli in a problem-solving situation; the strategic avoidance of eye contact, the utilization of eye-rolling and expressions of disgust, the tendency to glare at one's partner, all represent some of the less subtle forms of "coercion" so common in the problem-solving repertoires of distressed couples.

Aversive control strategies can be spotted in the daily routines of distressed couples. A classic hypothetical example of "coercion in everyday life" involves the wife who is cooking in the kitchen, and notices that the garbage is overflowing. Since removal of the garbage is the husband's responsibility, she marches into the living room to request that the garbage be removed immediately. The husband, meanwhile, is relaxing in the living room reading the newspaper. The wife begins by neutrally requesting that the husband "please take out the garbage." The husband responds: "I'll take it out later; I'm in the middle of something now." Since the wife feels that immediate action is necessary, she presses the issue; furthermore, since the benign request went unheeded, she escalates the degree of aversiveness, by changing her words and injecting an irritable tone: "George, the garbage needs to be taken out now!"

H: In a few minutes.
W: I need the space, George. Do it now! (*Demand*)
H: If it has to be done now, do it yourself.
W: It's not my job, goddamnit! Do it now!
H: No!!! Get off my back!

At this point the wife pulls out her ultimate weapon from her bag of tricks, the threat. For many more severely distressed couples, the ultimate threat is physical violence, which is the most dangerous consequence of a coercive interactional chain. But for this middle class couple, the ultimate threat is more tempered, although as we shall see, it serves the same function as a physical threat: "Either you take out the fucking garbage, or you're on your own as far as dinner is concerned." At this point, George rises from his easy chair and swiftly removes the garbage. In doing so, he has reinforced his wife's use of this aversive control strategy; in fact, he has reinforced the entire chain of gradually escalating aversive stimuli. The wife is more likely to use such strategies in future attempts to gain compliance from her husband. The husband, in turn, has been *negatively reinforced* for compliance, since his wife turned off the demands and threats subsequent to his compliant behavior. Although both partners are reinforced, the reinforcement came at great cost. Not only are they angry at one another, but a destructive behavior change strategy has been strengthened.

All of the above examples share the use of compelling aversive stimuli to try to bring about change in the relationship. Often, the stimuli are so compelling that short-term changes are successfully brought about as a result of their use. Thus, couples are reinforced for the use of such strategies. The costs of these strategies are long-term and insidious. Aversive control strategies tend to multiply over time, and they tend to be reciprocated by the other partner. We saw in the "garbage" example that neither spouse was "happy" despite the apparent effectiveness of the wife's intervention and the husband's compliance. As aversive control becomes the predominant mode of behavior change strategy in a marriage, satisfaction plummets.

Behavior therapy with couples is predicated on the desirability of teaching couples to use positive control strategies in their attempts to bring about change in the relationship. By positive control, we mean using positive reinforcement rather than negative reinforcement or punishment. Positive control strategies, if used correctly, are just as efficient as aversive control strategies in the short run (cf. Skinner, 1953), and promote marital satisfaction in the long run. Unfortunately, our culture seldom practices positive control in its attempts to control its citizens. On the macro level, our legal system is based on an aversive control model, with punishment (fines and imprisonment) used contingent upon violations, and avoidance of punishment the only consequence of obeying the law. On the micro level, child-rearing practices rely primarily on aversive control procedures. Children are punished by their parents for behaving inappropriately, and seldom systematically reinforced for behaving appropriately. When positive reinforcement is used, it is often inadvertently made contingent on inappropriate behavior, as when a parent provides attention to a child following a temper tantrum.

In light of our society's propensity for punishment and negative reinforcement, it is not in the least surprising that couples frequently adopt such strategies when change is desired in their relationship. The chapters in this book will illustrate a consistent focus on helping couples change these strategies. At the beginning stage of therapy, where couples are provided with general instructions for pinpointing changes that they would like to see occurring, the focus is on increasing desirable behavior rather than decreasing undesirable behavior, and couples are encouraged to reinforce their partners' approximations toward desired change. The focus on increasing positives rather than decreasing negatives is based on the emphasis on positive control. Negative behavior can be directly decreased only by introducing extinction or aversive control procedures. Therefore, a focus on such behavior would necessitate programming additional aversive control procedures into repertoires already replete with such tactics.

The focus on positive control continues during problem-solving and communication training with the focus on increasing both verbal and nonverbal behavior which is supportive of the partner's problem-solving efforts. Similarly, in the use of contingency contracting (see Chapter 8), the emphasis is on specifying positive consequences for compliance with a change agreement. If negative consequences are used at all, they play a subsidiary role in the maintenance of behavior change.

In addition to the use of positive reinforcement, positive control strategies place heavy emphasis on the principle of *shaping*. Shaping refers to the application of reinforcement to successive approximations of the behavior that is ultimately desired. For example, when Helen requested that John increase his rate of "talking about his feelings" in the relationship, she began with a request which only approximated the amount of feeling expression that she desired. Her initial request was easier for John to honor than a more stringent directive, and she was encouraged to reinforce him for this change, although it was less than what she had previously wanted. Once the intermediate level of feeling expression was occurring with sufficient frequency, she increased the required amount of feeling expression, and withheld reinforcement until this new rate was achieved. Distressed couples often demand sweeping changes instantly, and the partner's difficulty with the extent of change demanded is not taken into account. Couples must learn in therapy to settle for less than what they want initially, in order that they be more likely to receive what they want in the long run. Moderating one's demands to fit the current capabilities of the partner is an important step in the improvement of a relationship.

RECIPROCITY

Despite recent controversy regarding the concept of reciprocity in regard to long-term adult relationships, it is generally agreed by behavioral theorists that, over a long period of time, members of a cohabitating dyad reward and punish each other at equal rates. The implications of the reciprocity notion for treatment are vast, and convincing couples to believe in the principle, or at least to temporarily suspend their disbelief, is critical. Chapter 5 will include a detailed discussion of this problem. For now, let it suffice to say that couples' willingness to collaborate with one another, and with the therapist, depends, to a large extent, on each spouse's acceptance of his/her sharing of the causal role in the generation and maintenance of marital problems. Quite often spouses enter therapy with two major misconceptions, based on their ignorance of the degree of reciprocity present in their own relationship. First, each spouse views himself as a passive victim of the partner's undesirable behavior, and is relatively insensitive to his/her own input into the relationship problem. Second, since both spouses hold this view, each greatly underestimates his/her own power or control over the behavior of the partner, and, therefore, feels powerless to effect change. It is as if each partner has a theory about what is wrong with the relationship and each theory designates the other person as prime mover.

Acceptance of a reciprocal, interactional cause-effect model, where both partners continuously control the behavior of one another, and maintain undesirable behavior, immediately alters the entire context within which the relationship problems are viewed, and serves as a springboard for change. Not only does such acceptance lead to a greater sensitivity of one's own impact on the problems, but it suddenly makes behavior change seem possible. The insight that a spouse has power and control over the behavior of the partner, and can influence the other's behavior through altering one's own, can be tremendously liberating for a distressed couple; feelings of hopelessness about the other person's current behavior can be quickly abated if spouses can be convinced that they are part of what is maintaining the odious behavior. In addition, spouses now have a reason to change other than altruism; if they accept the reciprocal relationship between their behavior and the behavior of their partner, they can often be persuaded to initiate changes because those changes will lead to desirable changes on the part of the partner and thereby increase their *own* relationship satisfaction. They are asked to change not for their partner, but actually for themselves as well as for the relationship. Since couples seldom enter therapy with a spirit of giving and altruism, they tend to be much more responsive to an appeal based on self-interest.

The entire therapy process assumes the principle of reciprocity. The initial clinical procedures, which involve each partner's experimentation with unilateral increases in "positive behavior," is an example. Problem-solving, communication training, and contingency contracting also follow from this notion. As we shall observe in subsequent chapters, there is no concept which is more salient to the behavioral treatment of couples than the principle of reciprocity.

FOCUS ON THE LEARNING OF RELATIONSHIP SKILLS

Unlike most forms of marital therapy, a behavioral approach attempts to teach couples a set of skills. These skills are designed not only to aid the couple in the resolution of their current marital problems, but perhaps more importantly, to help the couples subsequent to the termination of therapy, when new problems arise. In general, one might think of behavioral couples therapy as the opposite of crisis intervention. Whereas crisis intervention usually involves a therapist who temporarily steps into the life of a couple, suggesting ways to resolve problems, the behavioral couples therapist will in most cases systematically avoid such suggestions. The behavior therapist focuses on the process by which couples change in addition to the content of changes; he shows a couple not what to do, but how to do it. In this sense it is at its best a preventative approach, since couples who are successfully treated leave therapy with the means to solve their own problems in the future.

The skill focus means that in some ways the role of the therapist resembles that of a teacher. It is important to the long-term success of therapy that couples *learn* to the degree necessary for them to function independently of the therapist. Herein lies one of the most subtle, yet important distinctions between successful and unsuccessful treatment, a point which we will be returning to on many occasions. There is some risk in working with couples that what appears to be improvement is in reality little more than situation-specific responses to discriminative stimuli provided by the therapist. That is, couples behave desirably during therapy sessions, problem-solving and communicating effectively, complying with homework assignments, and reporting a happier relationship. Yet, this hypothetical couple may not have abstracted the principles behind the skills sufficiently to use them without therapist prompts. These couples might be thought of as having *learned* new skills, but as not having successfully *generalized* these skills outside of the situational context of the therapy sessions. They are unlikely to maintain their progress once therapy has terminated.

Behavioral investigators have documented time and time again failures of generalization from the laboratory-clinical setting to the real world. It has become increasingly clear that generalization can never be assumed, but must be systematically programmed into the clinical interventions. In treating couples, this means that the therapist must somehow impart to couples the means to solve their own marital problems. If he simply assumes control over a couple's interaction and solves their problems for them, for example, by dictating behavioral contracts, the couple will be rescued from their current crisis but left ill prepared to tackle future crises on their own. Throughout this book, we will be discussing strategies for skill training designed to foster both generalization of gains into the real world and long-term maintenance of gains subsequent to the termination of therapy.

THE DIFFERENCES BETWEEN BEHAVIORAL MARITAL THERAPY AND OTHER APPROACHES

The procedural similarities among various approaches to marital therapy are numerous. Despite rather fundamental differences in theoretical and conceptual formulations of marital distress, experts representing these various theoretical perspectives have achieved considerable homogeneity in their recommendations for how therapy should be conducted. This homogeneity is apparent when comparing the treatment strategies recommended by behaviorists to recent textbooks written by authors representing psychoanalytic (Ables & Brandsma, 1977; Sager, 1976), systems theory (Haley, 1976), and Rogerian (Guerney, 1977) perspectives. From our vantage point, all of these perspectives have tended to become increasingly behavioral in their advocacy of intervention strategies. We will briefly outline some of the isomorphic elements of these various approaches as a backdrop for our discussion of the fundamental differences between behavior therapy and other perspectives.

Gurman (1978) has eloquently depicted the divergence between theory and practice in the most influential psychoanalytic treatises on alleviating marital distress. Despite a theoretical model which attributes marital problems to unresolved unconscious conflicts present in one or both spouses, the psychoanalytic model has become increasingly pragmatic and eclectic in the designing of treatment strategies. Thus, Ables and Brandsma (1977), despite their ego analytic theoretical model, break with the psychoanalytic tradition in their emphasis on facilitating changes in the current behavioral repertoires of distressed spouses. Couples are urged to formulate their complaints in specific, behavioral terms, and state these complaints directly. They are trained to negotiate their differences and communicate more effectively in their endeavor to achieve behavior change. The targets of communication training are in many ways identical to the content of such a program as outlined in this book. Exploration of the past is minimized, and the role of the unconscious, despite its alleged causal importance in generating relationship distress, is seldom apparent in the treatment regimen.

Haley (1976), one of the pioneers in the development of family therapy from a systems theory perspective, has evolved to a position which is in many ways indistinguishable from that of a classic behavioral orientation. His emphasis on treating the presenting problem departs substantially from the pure systems view, espoused at one time by Haley himself, that "symptoms" should be redefined by the therapist in terms of their interpersonal context. While Haley's position continues to reflect the view that individual problem behaviors are merely manifestations of interpersonal pathology existing in the marital or family relationship, the focus in therapy is on modifying the presenting problem. Consistent with the now familiar refrain of behavior therapists, the success of therapy is to be determined on the basis of success in meeting treatment goals mutually negotiated by therapist and family, goals which reflect the family's presenting complaints. Rigorous assessment of therapy outcome, viewed by many as the sine qua non of behavior therapy, has also become a point of emphasis in this revisionist systems perspective.

Guerney (1977) has popularized an approach to marital therapy which focuses on teaching couples communication skills. This approach evolved from an experiential or Rogerian theoretical perspective in which couples are taught both receptive and expressive communication skills, with the ultimate goal of improving each spouse's capacity for empathic listening and aiding them in the direct expression of feelings. In part, the similarities between Guerney's treatment strategy and ours reflect our indebtedness to his model for recognizing the importance of such skills in effective relationship functioning. Thus, we have incorporated communication skills such as "reflecting" into the repertoire of skills which couples are taught. Some of our behavioral colleagues have also been clearly influenced by Guerney's work (e.g., O'Leary & Turkewitz, 1978). It is Guerney's *strategy* for teaching communication training skills which is most similar to a traditional behavior therapy program. The provision of feedback, the modeling of appropriate skills by the therapist, and the opportunity to rehearse these new skills (behavior rehearsal) have been the predominant strategies for skill training within a behavioral framework. Guerney has incorporated this strategy into his work with couples.

Notwithstanding the numerous similarities between behavioral marital therapy and alternative approaches, it is important to delineate the still fundamental points of divergence. With the exception of Guerney's work, most of the procedural similarities reflect movement on the part of alternative perspectives toward an essentially behavioral one. This increasingly ubiquitous behavioral focus threatens to obfuscate some rather basic tenets which, we believe, are still unique to behavioral marital therapy. These will be outlined in the paragraphs below.

Systematic Assessment

Behavioral marital therapy differs from each of the prominent alternative perspectives in its emphasis on systematic, multidimensional assessment, and the explicit relationship between assessment and treatment. As we will outline in Chapter 4, behavioral marital therapy utilizes systematic procedures to assess various dimensions of relationship functioning. Through various self-report inventories, a couple's subjective complaints are uncovered and operationalized in terms of each person's specific, behavioral excesses and deficits. Communication and problem-solving skills are assessed through direct observation, by applying standardized behavioral rating scales to the quantification of specific communicative responses based on the spouses' direct interaction with one another. Through data collected by couples in the home, an evaluation of the frequency of spouses' emission of pleasing and displeasing behaviors is included, along with an analysis of the relationship between various behaviors and each partner's subjective feelings of satisfaction with the relationship. On the basis of these and other assessment techniques, a treatment plan is formulated, one which is tailored to the idiosyncratic needs of the individual couple.

This assessment strategy can be contrasted with that of other approaches. Consistent with the psychoanalytic tradition which dictates that diagnosis can be made only after a number of treatment sessions, i.e., that diagnosis evolves from treatment, marital therapists of a psychoanalytic persuasion include no formalized assessment procedure (Ables & Brandsma, 1977). Rather, intervention begins immediately, and relies primarily on the material generated during the initial therapy sessions. Systems theory advocates, while putting greater emphasis on diagnosis as a precursor to and a determinant of treatment strategy, rely primarily on the clinical interview as their method of acquiring assessment information, despite the lack of empirically established support for the reliability and validity of information gathered solely from this format. Although systems theory advocates recognize the importance of information provided by direct interaction between family members, marital and family communication is evaluated in a subjective, unsystematic manner, devoid of objective coding systems and observations on the part of trained, but otherwise uninvolved observers (Haley, 1976; Minuchin,

1974). In addition, both Haley and Minuchin recommend interventions on the part of the therapist as a diagnostic device. By entering the family system and observing the family's response to the therapist's intervention, the family's characteristic way of dealing with stress can be observed. This tactic resembles the psychoanalytic adherence to diagnosis evolving from treatment intervention, and at this stage of our knowledge it is unclear whether or not the resultant behavior bears a systematic relationship to marital or family distress.

Finally Guerney's (1977) communication training approach assumes *a priori* that most relationship problems result from specific types of faulty communication. Therefore, all couples receive the same type of treatment, and the need for systematic assessment is obviated. The primary weakness of this nonassessment approach lies in the tenuousness of Guerney's basic premise. At present there is little reason to believe that relationship problems can be viewed as primarily reflecting a deficit in the specific communication skills upon which Guerney's program focuses.

Couple's Capacity for Commitment and Change

Behavior marital therapy has been criticized by some (e.g., Gurman & Knudson, 1978) for its assumption that distressed couples are sufficiently rational to cooperate in the collaborative endeavor of improving their relationship. According to advocates of both psychoanalytic and systems theories, irrational forces both unacknowledged by spouses and beyond their conscious awareness rebel against the therapist's attempts to direct couples in behavior change. Psychoanalytic theorists emphasize a process termed "collusion," whereby spouses unconsciously contract to protect one another from anxiety-inducing situations. This contract supposedly renders most distressed couples resistant to the therapist's efforts to induce change; in order to change, couples must confront the anxiety inherent in each person's unresolved internal conflicts. This view is related to the analytic notion that marital discord is the result of two neurotic (or worse) individuals who have joined together for neurotic reasons; psychosexual fixation or unresolved conflicts with the family of origin, rather than the dynamics of the current relationship, are emphasized as the central etiological factor in marital discord (Martin, 1976; Meissner, 1978). Couples' resistance to change is equally central to the systems theoretical perspective. The marital dyad is viewed as a stable system which functions in such a way that any attempt to destabilize it by attempting to induce change is met with resistance.

The implications of the concept of resistance vary from one theoretical perspective to another. The most radical position is adopted by Haley (1976), who assumes that any attempt to directly influence a couple in the direction of behavior change is likely to fail, since couples are not capable of acting in a controlled, rational manner in regard to important relationship issues. Therefore, couples are most responsive to subtle, covert directives which generate change without the couple's being aware of it. This is the primary justification for paradoxical directives (the use of paradox in marital therapy will be discussed more extensively in Chapter 5). The psychoanalytic position seems to be an intermediate one, as reflected by Ables and Brandsma (1977). Their view holds that sometimes couples are being controlled by their rational egos, while at other times unconscious, irrational forces predominate. When the former is true, couples are capable of conforming to a treatment program based on direct efforts to induce behavior change. However, when such techniques prove ineffective, the most likely culprits are the primitive, unconscious forces festering within each individual, which collectively collude to prevent change. To Ables and Brandsma, conjoint marital therapy is unlikely to prove fruitful in such instances.

There is a subtle but prevalent circularity in the notion of resistance, as propagated by both psychoanalytic and systems theory adherents. For example, Ables and Brandsma (1977) invoke the concept only after their treatment strategies have proven unsuccessful. This *post hoc* inference is then used to explain the behavior from which the inference was drawn in the first place. Thus, both logically and scientifically, the psychoanalytic position assumes a circularity and disconfirmability which is, to us, unacceptable: resistance is invoked to explain the same behavior from which its existence was inferred. What makes families resist change? Resistance! How do we know that resistance is operating? Because a family has not responded to the therapist's change efforts! The explanatory power of such a circular notion is questionable. Resistance to change seems to function for marital and family therapists as a way of rationalizing unsuccessful treatment. The presumption that couples will resist change has the potentiality of a self-fulfilling prophesy. If therapists expect couples to resist their change efforts, their in-session behavior will be significantly affected, and they are likely to generate resistance.

While behavioral marital therapists acknowledge that change is often difficult to generate, and that couples often express ambivalence about change both in their verbal and nonverbal behavior, they do not presume that these difficulties stem from an opposition to the goals of positive relationship change. *Rather, as a working assumption, BMT accepts couples' expressed desire for change at face value, and interprets the obstacles presented in the therapy situation as reflecting the costly nature of the process of change itself.* Behavior change in a relationship is quite often a difficult as well as a risky endeavor. After months or years of being punished for positive behavior, couples enter therapy with the set that they will withhold rewards from one another until they are convinced that they will be adequately compensated for their rewarding behavior. Given the inherent difficulties of altering well-established behavior patterns and the additional inhibitions generated by their recent interactional history, it is not particularly surprising that couples are reluctant to work toward behavior change. The therapist's task is to place couples in touch with the long-term benefits of their change efforts, and make these long-term contingencies more salient to the couple. When successful, the short-term costs of change can be sufficiently mitigated so that therapy can proceed. When, on the other hand, couples fail to comply with their homework assignments, or when couples refuse to collaborate in a problem-solving situation, it usually means that the short-term consequences remain dominant. The therapist has failed in subordinating these interests to the goals of an improved relationship.

It is true that some couples, even after weighing the long-term benefits of struggling for change with the short-term costs of the change process, will decide that the costs exceed the potential benefits. This decision may have been made prior to seeking therapy, or it may be reached as a consequence of the first few therapy sessions. Here resistance to change may be real, but it is based not on the preeminence of unconscious irrational forces but from a conscious rational appraisal of costs and benefits. Few people would sustain a costly effort to sacrifice in the service of a relationship which, even at its best, does not exceed the level of satisfaction provided by alternatives to the relationship.

Finally, it should be added that behaviorists adamantly deny that marital discord necessarily, or even typically, reflects pathological or neurotic marital partners. Since factors produced within the relationship are generally viewed as the causal factors in marital discord, we assume that healthy individuals, as well as disturbed individuals, can enter into conflicted relationships. We are all potentially at risk for marital problems.

The Salience of Behavior as Behavior

Psychotherapy, as we mentioned in a previous chapter, has a tradition which denigrates the importance of overt behavior. This tradition has influenced the field of marital therapy, despite the practical focus on behavior changes adopted by various theoretical perspectives.

Marital therapy was initially practiced by therapists espousing a psychoanalytic orientation, and early papers on marital therapy focused extensively on the paradigmatic dilemma: since fundamental changes can come about only through insight into the unconscious, childhood roots of current maladaptive behavior, a short-term, behaviorally oriented treatment could not hope to generate permanent, sweeping changes in the personalities of marital partners; yet the demand for immediate changes in behavior constantly confronted the practitioner of marital therapy (cf. Olson, 1970). The compromise which was achieved acknowledged the inherent limitations of a practical approach, yet concluded that this crisis intervention orientation was necessary. This legacy continues in the writings of most contemporary psychoanalytic theorists, who acknowledge behavior change as a necessary goal, but argue for a long-term insight-oriented approach if the ultimate goal is to bring about fundamental, persistent changes in both members (Nadelson, 1978).

Systems theorists similarly minimize the importance of overt behavior in their view that maladaptive behaviors are best understood as metaphors, reflecting a more generalized pathology in the marital relationship (Bowen, 1976; Haley, 1963, 1976; Minuchin, 1974; Satir, 1967; Sluzki, 1978). Overt behavior is viewed as serving a communicative function, and is important only because, if accurately deciphered, it can lead to an understanding of the underlying relationship pathology.

BMT views the maladaptive behavior of distressed couples as its central concern. The behavior needs to be changed not because it is the only practical way of affecting more central aspects of relationship functioning, but simply because it is distressing to both members and directly generates subjective dissatisfaction with the relationship. Its focus on modifying overt behavior is based not on expediency, but on the premise that distressing behavior defines the distressed relationship.

Systematic Strategies for Changing Behavior

While most theoretical perspectives focus to a large extent on altering distressing relationship behavior, they vary considerably in procedures for bringing about such changes. Systems-oriented therapists rely on subtle, indirect suggestions and directives which are seldom explicitly defined for the couple as efforts designed to induce change. Their effectiveness is felt to be largely a function of their disguised nature since the couple will resist any directives which are explicitly defined as efforts to induce behavior change. The psychoanalytic approach, as represented by Ables and Brandsma (1977), attempts to induce behavior changes more directly through communication training and negotiation, yet sessions remain relatively unstructured. The primary vehicles for communication training are feedback provided by the therapist, and the prompting of alternative interaction patterns.

Behavior marital therapy is highly structured and explicitly didactic. It attempts to systematically teach couples relationship skills according to a prearranged format, with couples being appraised in advance of the procedures and rationales for each aspect of the treatment program. The strategies for the modification of interaction are based on a model attaching central importance to *behavior rehearsal,* the guided practice of explicitly defined behaviors. In this respect, behavior marital therapy resembles Guerney's (1977) training model.

In addition to being systematic and highly structured, behavior marital therapy endeavors to comprehensively cover the target problems defined at the conclusion of the assessment phase. Explicit efforts are made to transfer skills learned in therapy to the natural environment, and the program is structured to gradually render the couple autonomous and capable of functioning independently of the therapist. The attention to generalization is worth noting again, since other approaches, by comparison, seem to leave questions of maintenance to chance. Systems theorists assume that once the marital system is restructured, change will be sweeping and self-perpetuating. Thus, the primary focus is on generating initial changes with minimal attention to surveying all conflict areas, or taking steps to ensure generalization and maintenance. This belief in the self-perpetuating nature of change strikes us as a leap of faith lacking in empirical support. Couples can change temporarily in response to numerous factors; the comprehensiveness of their changes, and their subsequent persistence can be assessed only through careful follow-ups. Until proven unnecessary, it seems most prudent to adopt the comprehensive strategy, including the explicit programming of generalization, which characterizes behavior marital therapy.

Emphasis on Learning Principles and Environmental Contingencies

Behavior marital therapy can be differentiated from alternative approaches by its attempt to include behavior modification in the repertoire of skills taught to couples. The content of much of the training in a behavioral program includes many of the principles shown in other applied treatment settings to be effective ways to bring about behavior change. Thus, behavior marital therapy is not only oriented toward behavior change, but is also oriented toward training in behavior change skills. Couples learn to perform their own functional analyses of both their own and their partner's behavior. Similarly, they learn procedures such as shaping and the selective use of positive reinforcement, designed to help them function as change agents in their own marriage. Finally, they learn some of the skills in pinpointing, monitoring, and evaluating behavior change programs which characterize the field of applied behavior analysis. The goal of this training is to increase couples' expertise and autonomy, and to endow them with the capacity to treat themselves in the future.

SUMMARY

This chapter sets the stage for the remainder of the book by attempting to define the role of a behavior therapist working with couples. Four ways of defining this role are presented. First, the therapist can view himself as one who applies certain techniques, such as communication training and contingency contracting, to relationship discord. Second, the therapist can be thought of as using principles derived from general psychology in devising treatment programs for distressed couples. Third, the behavior therapist can define himself by his method, and thereby consider his task one of providing a functional analysis of relationship complaints. Fourth, the therapist can be somewhat arbitrary, and operationalize his role by defining behavior therapy as a set of themes which, regardless of the specific techniques used, are consistently applied to the treatment of relationship difficulties.

All four of these definitions have strengths and weaknesses. In part because this book emphasizes techniques, it is important to be aware of the dangers in applying such techniques in a cookbook manner, without practicing *behavior therapy methodology* and being aware of the broad experimental base from which techniques can be derived. The themes and principles enumerated above provide conceptual unity to upcoming chapters, and help in maintaining the link between clinical intervention strategies and their theoretical foundation.

Despite many practical similarities between behavior therapy and other approaches, the behavioral exchange model does lead to some fundamental distinctions. Behavior marital therapy uniquely emphasizes systematic, multi-dimensional assessment as a phase which precedes and is relatively distinct from the therapy phase itself. Behavior marital therapy assumes that couples are usually motivated to improve their relationship, although they may be ambivalent about the behavior changes defined as necessary in order to achieve that goal. Additionally, behavior marital therapy attaches primary importance to overt behavior as the defining characteristic of marital distress. Finally, in its relatively systematic, structured approach to treatment, and its emphasis on training couples in behavior change skills, behavior therapy retains a distinctive educational, skill-training format.

CHAPTER 3

Initial Interview

ONE OF THE MOST COMMON STEREOTYPES attributed to behavior therapists is that they are less concerned with relationship building than are other schools of psychotherapy. And it is certainly true that in the early years of behavior therapy, prominent writers in the field fostered this stereotype both by emphasizing the technological aspects of behavioral techniques and by conducting outcome studies which suggested that automated programs were as effective as real people in modifying phobic avoidance behavior (e.g., Lang, Melamed, & Hart, 1970). However, few advocates of behavior therapy deny the importance of relationship variables; in fact, these issues have been addressed more explicitly in recent years (e.g., Kanfer & Goldstein, 1975; Wilson & Evans, 1978). It is interesting, in light of these criticisms of behavior therapists, that in a widely cited comparative outcome study (Sloane, Staples, Cristel, Yorkston, & Whipple, 1975), behavior therapists were rated as significantly more empathic than psychodynamically oriented therapists by independent judges. In our discussion on the initial interview in behavioral marital therapy, we will argue that *the most desirable goal of an initial interview is not to gather assessment information but rather to set the stage for therapeutic change by building positive expectancies and trust in the couple, and by actually providing them with some benefits.* In keeping with recent emphases on the importance of relationship factors, the initial interview that we advocate is one where such factors are not only emphasized, but in fact determine the structure and content of the interview.

INITIAL INTERVIEW AS A METHOD OF BEHAVIORAL ASSESSMENT

Traditionally, in the behavioral literature the initial interview has been conceptualized as a way of specifying target behaviors, along with their antecedents and consequences (Mischel, 1968; Kanfer & Grimm, 1977; Lazarus, 1971; Rimm & Masters, 1974). In essence the initial interview is viewed as a vehicle for gathering relevant information that will lead to the formation of a treatment plan.

However, assessment and information-gathering may not be the optimal goals for an initial interview. First, the interview is not a particularly efficient way of conducting a functional analysis of a distressed relationship. In the absence of data comparing the interview with other methods of collecting marital assessment data (self-report inventories, behavioral observations, spouse-recorded behavior in the home), we will simply point out here that there are a variety of alternative methods of collecting such assessment information, all of which are described in the next chapter. Many of these methods have been shown to provide reliable, valid, useful information, whereas there is no evidence that the interview provides such information. Self-report questionnaires, such as Weiss' "Areas of Change Questionnaire" provide prompts for couples, as a result of which they need only to recognize their difficulties and identify them from a comprehensive list of relationship complaints.

Since couples are usually unskilled at defining problems in specific, discrete terms, it is generally difficult and time-consuming to generate such a list in an open-ended interview setting. In addition, some problem areas, such as sexual functioning, are embarrassing to many couples, and they often find it easier to respond to a questionnaire requesting sexual information than to provide such information in an initial, conjoint interview. Finally, in assessing communication, asking couples to discuss their communication is less desirable than simply observing them. Although such observation occurs in an initial interview, the sample will be more indicative of their *in vivo* behavior if they are talking to each other about conflict-related items, with the therapist out of the room. Ideally, communication and problem-solving skills should be assessed using the types of standardized tasks elaborated in Chapter 4.

Thus, an initial interview is expendable as a means of obtaining assessment information. In addition, from a clinical standpoint, *an initial interview which focuses on the identification of target problems is potentially antitherapeutic.* Couples entering therapy usually have spent the preceding several months, if not years, focusing on the areas of conflict. This is most obvious in cases where couples exhibit a high rate of verbally abusive interchanges, focusing on their dissatisfaction. But it is just as true of couples who avoid discussing conflict-related topics, since these couples devote a great deal of cognitive time to ruminating over their dissatisfactions with one another. The emotional accoutrements of this "negative tracking" often include both intense anger at the partner, and feelings of despair and hopelessness. In most cases the dissatisfactions are exaggerated, the strengths ignored, and pessimism about the relationship accentuated. To begin therapist contact with a thorough delineation of the problem areas might serve to magnify these feelings of despair and hopelessness, and the couple is likely to leave the office feeling worse than when they entered. These feelings can be mitigated to some extent by other therapist remarks designed to induce positive expectancies; however, there is no need to focus on these problem areas in the first place, since the formal assessment procedures will accomplish that end at less risk to the initial formation of a relationship.

We are not advocating a total avoidance of assessment during interview time, but suggesting that this not be the primary focus of an initial interview. During later interviews, clarification of identified problem areas should, when necessary, be undertaken. Moreover, there are certain kinds of assessment information which are more efficiently derived from an interview; some of this information can be obtained during the initial interview. The important point is that any such inquiries should be consistent with the fundamental goals of the first contact: extinguishing feelings of hopelessness, generating positive expectancies, and inducing some positive interaction between the couple.

INITIAL INTERVIEW AS THE INITIAL THERAPY SESSION

It follows from what has been said that the initial interview with a couple is the first treatment session, even though some assessment material will be obtained in the process. The impact that the therapist has can create a set that will generate rapid progress, or it can create a hole out of which it may take weeks or months to dig. Worse yet, if the experience is sufficiently negative for the couple, they will not return. The therapist who can provide couples with some immediate benefit in an initial contact is at a tremendous advantage in two main respects: first, that initial experience will make an impression on the couple which may help sustain them through difficult times during the beginning treatment sessions; second, couples for whom the first contact has been positive are more likely to comply with the therapist's instructions regarding the collecting of assessment data. Creating such a set for compliance at the beginning renders continued compliance more likely.

When the couple leaves the office after the initial interview, they should view their relationship in a more positive way than when they walked in. They also should have engaged in some positive interaction with one another during the session, hopefully including laughter. Some of the confusion and uncertainty regarding therapy should be mollified. Finally, assuming that the couple has entered treatment hoping to improve rather than terminate the relationship, they should be at least relatively optimistic that such improvement will be forthcoming. The ways to accomplish these goals will comprise the content of the remainder of this chapter.

One more preliminary issue needs to be addressed at this juncture. Should a therapist enter into such an initial contact "blind" or would it be better to have couples complete some self-report questionnaires prior to this contact? This is a particularly important issue in an initial interview which is unlikely to uncover the problem areas in any real depth. There are both pros and cons to a couple's completing self-report forms prior to the initial contact. In favor of their completion are the obvious advantages accruing to the therapist who knows a bit about the couple prior to meeting with them. He can then structure the interview idiosyncratically, taking into account the characteristics of the particular couple, about which he is already somewhat familiar. The availability of such information prior to the initial contact further reduces the need to collect assessment information during the initial interview. The basic disadvantage of this strategy is that it necessitates a high degree of effort on the part of couples even before they have met the therapist. Completing self-report forms is often experienced as demanding and unpleasant. Thus, the first treatment-related experience is a negative one. Considering both sides of the issue, we think that the disadvantages outweigh the advantages. Within the first two weeks after the initial interview, when forms have been completed, data have been collected in the home, and communication has been evaluated, the therapist will have the necessary information to form a treatment plan. In general, it is not necessary to have obtained this information by the end of the first contact.

AN OUTLINE OF THE INITIAL INTERVIEW

In our initial interview format, the *content* is to obtain a developmental history of the relationship. In pursuing this goal, the therapist begins by structuring both the session and the entire assessment period for the couple, by summarizing what will transpire during the interview, and integrating the interview with the remainder of the evaluation period. Then a series of relatively open-ended questions are directed toward both spouses, the purpose of which, from the standpoint of content, is to obtain a developmental history of the relationship. The clinical by-products of such an inquiry, if conducted skillfully, are that couples develop a sense of confidence and trust the therapist; they feel more positively about their relationship than they have in a long time; they interact positively and even enjoy each other a bit; and some of their initial trepidation and confusion regarding the treatment process is alleviated. Of course, it is also necessary for the therapist to ask some questions designed to uncover the couple's purpose in seeking professional help. The therapist should terminate the session by offering some introductory remarks about the treatment approach, and then give the first homework assignment which is usually the completion of self-report questionnaires, and/or the collecting of baseline data in the home. Each of these aspects of the session will be discussed below.

Initial Explanation of the Interview and Assessment Process

Whatever the state of the relationship at the time the couple enters therapy, it is a safe bet that they are somewhat confused and apprehensive about the prospect of involving themselves in treatment, and have little idea what to expect. By beginning the session with an outline of what is to occur during the next hour, much initial anxiety is relieved. By augmenting this introduction with an overview of the entire evaluation phase, couples are further reassured, and are made privy to the impressive, thorough evaluation which will be undertaken *prior* to the formation of a treatment plan. Positive expectancies begin immediately, before the clients have been asked to reveal anything about themselves. The following provides an example of such an introduction:

Before we get started tonight, I want to tell you a little bit about what we'll be doing. My goal is to get to know you a little and I'll be asking you some questions about the past and the present to get an idea of what your relationship has been like over the years. Then I'll tell you a bit about me and what I do so that you can get to know me.

I want to make it clear that you have not committed yourselves to therapy by coming here tonight. There will be a thorough evaluation period before any of us have to decide whether or not we would like to work together. Tonight's interview is part one of that evaluation. After tonight I will give you some forms to fill out which will give me a great deal of information about the difficulties that you're having. After you have finished those and returned them to me, I will see you again. During that second visit I will evaluate your communication by having you talk to each other about some of the problems you've reported.

Then, at the conclusion of that second visit, I will give you another assignment which will require you to collect some information at home, so that I can get a better picture of what goes on between the two of you on a day-to-day basis.

So, I'm going to be getting four different kinds of information. Tonight I'll be asking you some general questions about the history of your relationship. The forms I give you tonight will tell me what each of you thinks your problems are. Then I'll get a sense of what your communication is like. Finally, the second assignment will tell me what happens on a day-to-day basis. Then I will put all of this information together and, at a third meeting, present you with my perceptions of what your difficulties are. I will also, at that time, outline a plan for helping you improve your relationship, if that is what you want to do. Then, and only then, will I ask you to commit yourselves to therapy. Hopefully, by that time you will know enough about me and how I work to decide whether you can make that commitment.

I confess that this is a rather long evaluation period. I wish I could be of some help to you right away, but I need this time in order to put all of the information together. Do you have any questions before I begin to ask you some questions?

How this introduction is presented to the couple is at least as crucial as the fact of its presentation. The therapist wants, first of all, to present this material in a manner consistent with the competence suggested by the content of the speech. He should appear relaxed, confident, and talk to the couple in a conversational, rather than a didactic tone. Warmth and affability should also be conveyed through eye contact, frequent smiles, and body language. The therapist should lean forward as he talks, and alternate the direction of his remarks so that both partners are contacted.

If the style conveys warmth and confidence, the clients will almost invariably respond positively and become more relaxed. It is very reassuring to be told that they have not as yet committed themselves to a treatment regime, since many people are ambivalent about treatment when they first make contact.

In answering couples' initial questions, the therapist should restrict himself to clarifying the points he has already made. Any attempt by either partner to complain or criticize the other should be gently, but firmly, cut off immediately. The clients must learn from the outset that any fantasies that they might have had about griping to a marriage counselor about their partner's atrocities will not be fulfilled. Similarly, questions regarding type of therapy, length of time, and the like should be deferred until later in the session. By deferring questions which would lead to a deviation from the therapist's stated structure, he is setting an important precedent: *the couple learns early that the therapist, not the couple, structures the treatment sessions.* He is in control. This has important implications for subsequent events in therapy, as we shall see in later chapters.

Brief Discussion of Current Difficulties

Before taking a developmental history, the interviewer should anchor himself in the present by inquiring about the immediate precipitants to the couple's decision to seek therapy.*

Why Are They Here?

Without detailed questioning regarding current difficulties, it is still possible to focus on a couple's initial reason for coming to a therapist at this time. The therapist might simply ask, if he does not already know, who initiated the contact, and why the initiation occurred at this particular time. Are they here to improve their relationship, to reach an amicable separation, or to receive help in deciding whether to remain together or to separate? Although most couples will respond to such a question with the first of the above mentioned alternatives, a therapist cannot assume that a couple has come with that intention. When both spouses are given an opportunity to respond to this type of query, reservations that either partner might have about seeking marital therapy are likely to surface. The therapist should not attempt to challenge those reservations; on the contrary, they should be taken very seriously, since

* We used to ask about the immediate precipitants following rather than preceding the developmental history. Audrey Berger is to be credited for initially suggesting the change in format. Since enumerating current difficulties is almost inevitably unpleasant for couples, terminating the interview on such a note may undo whatever benefits have been derived from the refocusing on more pleasant times which occurs during the developmental history. With the brief delineation of present circumstances occurring prior to the developmental history, the latter is likely to have a more potent impact on the couple.

they can provide clues to significant obstacles in the path of treatment success.

The course of treatment can be very different depending on how couples respond to this question regarding their reasons for coming to a couples' therapist. This book is most relevant for couples who are seeking the first alternative, that is couples who want to leave therapy with a more satisfying relationship. Some discussion of the couple who is undecided will be provided in Chapter 5; couples seeking therapy for the purpose of a smoother separation require a very different kind of treatment approach, and we will briefly touch on the topic of separation counseling in Chapter 9.

First Signs of Significant Problems after Marriage

It is useful to develop at least a cursory understanding of how these difficulties developed over time. This information often follows from a question such as the following: "I would like to ask each of you to recall when it was that you first began to think of the relationship as having significant difficulties. When was it, what made you feel that way, and what did you do about it?" In addition to providing important information regarding the antecedents of current difficulties, through each partner's response to this question the therapist begins to get a sense of the couple's initial attempts at behavior modification. Upon experiencing dissatisfaction with certain aspects of the partner's behavior, did the person remain silent, hoping that the problems would dissipate with time? Did the couple's early behavior change efforts consist of aversive control strategies? Were initial change efforts successful or unsuccessful? In the development of marital conflicts, it is most common for couples to avoid change efforts until the difficulties have become greatly exacerbated. By the time problems are actually confronted, their resolution is complicated enough to tax even those with sophisticated behavior change skills. Less commonly, couples confront their difficulties early in their development; unfortunately, in these instances the confrontations usually consist of sloppy behavior change operations, often emphasizing coercion and aversive control. Although recollection of such events is often unreliable and subject to various distortions, it is at times possible to determine the degree to which problem-solving deficits were associated with the development and exacerbation of marital conflict. Later, when the therapist presents the couple with his formulation of their difficulties, a rationale based on behavior change deficits is a great deal more credible to a couple if concrete examples of faulty problem-solving operations can be alluded to, and are shown to have existed even in the early stages.

Collecting a Developmental History

As soon as the couple has responded satisfactorily to the above question, it is time to shift to the developmental focus. Gathering a historical perspective on the relationship in the initial interview has both assessment and therapeutic implications. From the standpoint of information-gathering, a relationship history is more difficult to elicit in a questionnaire; yet it is extremely important for a thorough understanding of the relationship. Among other things, the history usually has milestones which probably have some prognostic significance, as we will explain below. From the therapeutic standpoint, taking a historical perspective is consistent with the goals of the initial interview, that is, to provide couples with some perspective on their relationship by refocusing their attention on past and present strengths; also, couples often interact positively and with humor while recounting historical issues.

How Did You Meet?

This is an optimal way to start an inquiry into the development of a relationship. In recounting their initial encounter, couples immediately alter their focus from current problems to much happier times. Often the initial meeting has never been discussed retrospectively. In asking detailed questions regarding time, place and circumstances of the initial meeting, the therapist aids the couple in reliving those first moments, which often seem quite amusing in retrospect. Couples frequently differ in their perceptions of what occurred during the initial encounter; but since the beginning of a relationship is usually an exciting, exhilarating experience, attempts to reconcile their disparate recollections during the interview are experienced as enjoyable by both partners, and lead to a positive interchange between them. The therapist can foster such an interchange by laughing along with the couple as they attempt to recall the nuances of their flirtations, and by emphasizing the romantic aspects of the experience. If this interchange is successful, couples feel better about the relationship already, and are more relaxed for the remainder of the interview; more seeds for positive expectancies have been planted.

What Was It That Initially Attracted You to Your Partner?

With this type of question, usually following smoothly from the first, couples open therapy by describing their partners in positive terms, an activity in which they may not have engaged for months or years. It is often difficult to elicit an enumeration of these positive qualities from distressed couples, so poised are they to criticize and blame one another for current difficulties. The therapist must pull relentlessly for this information, and interrupt any attempts on their part to transform the recollection into a put down. For example, one partner may state, "I thought that he was kind and gentle, but . . ."; the interruption by the therapist should occur immediately after the "but." "So, you thought that he seemed kind and gentle. Was there anything else about him that you liked?" In most cases, with the therapist's help, couples are able to list those initial behaviors which led them to become interested in their present partner. This exercise further counters couples' tendencies to bicker about and focus on their current difficulties. Like recounting the events of their first meeting, it is usually a positive experience.

Although there is as yet no data to support this contention, our guess is that the answers to this question have prognostic significance. Couples who enumerate a list of "positive" reasons for pursuing their partner, such as finding them sexually attractive, intelligent, or interesting, are often a better "risk" than couples who insist that they initially pursued their partners because they were depressed, lonely, rebounding from a prior traumatic relationship, and so on. If the relationship began with a certain degree of romantic investment, that experience often facilitates a commitment to renew or approximate those early experiences. Even though it is a rare couple who can regain the romantic feelings of an early relationship stage, having experienced such a stage often enhances their collaborative spirit.

Discussion of Courtship Period

Information regarding the early stages of courtship presents the therapist with a more detailed picture of the early interaction patterns and reinforcers. Often couples will talk spontaneously about this period after recounting their initial encounter along with their reasons for being attracted to the partner. Questions should be aimed specifically at elucidating such material if the information is not spontaneously forthcoming. We reemphasize that, in most cases, the couple who found one another extremely reinforcing during this period is more easily treated than the couple who remained together despite a mixed courtship period, or a courtship period in which the positive exchanges were minimal. For illustrative purposes, we will contrast the courtship phase of John and Helen with that of Ed and Polly, both examples taken from our case records. John and Helen met at a party, were extremely attracted to one another, and began to see each other regularly. They "couldn't get enough of each other" during the six months prior to their engagement; sexual relations were begun within the first month, and they spent their time sharing a number of pleasant activities and interacting as a couple with other people. Despite the ensuance of marital conflicts as soon as this couple began cohabitating, the relationship was so reinforcing during its early stages that they were eager for help in improving their current relationship. In contrast, Ed hoped, when he first met Polly, that her outgoing and extroverted behavior would help him overcome his tendency to be withdrawn and introverted. Both of them had puritanical upbringings, and as a result were naive and lacking in social experience. Their courtship lacked any real passion, and physical contact was completely avoided until the wedding night. This couple had no frame of reference for a happy marriage, since even at its best their interaction consisted primarily of being polite and inoffensive to one another. Therapy was considerably more difficult with this couple, and the early indicators provided by their initial developmental history prepared the therapist for the special treatment considerations necessitated by their less than reinforcing courtship.

Lest we oversimplify matters, there are certainly exceptions to the predictive power of courtship behavior. For example, some couples behave with passion and enthusiasm derived from quite unrealistic expectations regarding the other. These couples are reacting to fantasies about the partner rather than the partner's actual ability to provide positive and fulfilling experiences. As the reality of the partner's actions progressively replace the expectations and fantasies, the relationships become dissatisfying. Here the initial courtship bliss is based less on shared positive experiences than on the anticipation of such experiences, which were not to be realized. *In the collection of courtship information, the therapist must attempt to discriminate the extent to which the initial positive feelings were based on the other's provision of reinforcement, rather than benefits anticipated but not received.*

Circumstances Surrounding Decision to Marry (or Live Together)

As the interview continues, and some of its therapeutic goals have been reached, the focus shifts in the direction of information-gathering. The decision to alter the definition of the relationship (e.g., by getting married) is always a developmental landmark and its antecedents often provide valuable clues regarding the couple's current difficulties. Of particular relevance is the following question: *To what extent were factors other than direct relationship benefits responsible for the decision to increase the level of commitment?* Did the couple marry because the woman was pregnant (an increasingly less common reason nowadays)? Was parental pressure exerted? What kinds of misgivings or reservations did each partner entertain in regard to the idea of cohabitation? In general, the therapist's task becomes more difficult to the extent that the decision to marry resulted from factors other than those associated with positive behavior exchange. Moreover, in exploring each partner's reservations about marriage as they recall them, the rudiments of current conflicts can be uncovered.

Foreshadowing of Current Problems

A question which should be injected at about this stage of the interview is the following: "As you look back on that period (before the marriage), was there anything in your relationship that resembled or hinted at the difficulties you're experiencing now?" Often, couples have never scrutinized their early history as this question directs them to do; factors can be uncovered which help in reconstructing the evolution of relationship discord. These early precursors of conflict are part of the functional analysis, and can have implications for the formation of the treatment plan.

Miscellaneous Points of Information

In the course of a relationship history, the therapist should acquire specific bits of information that have potential etiological and prognostic significance. At times these questions must be addressed directly. Initial sexual adjustment is one such area. When did sexual encounters begin? If the couple committed themselves to one another without knowing each other sexually, sexual adjustment should be carefully scrutinized as a potential source of early dissatisfaction. If sexual difficulties are presented as a problem area, it is important to determine at what point in the relationship sex became unsatisfactory. If sex was mutually enjoyable for both partners at first, it might be that their inability to expand their technique resulted in boredom and resultant avoidance later. Or conflicts in other areas, such as communication, may have led to a deterioration of the couple's sex life. It is often difficult to tease out the cause-effect relationship of sexual problems and other relationship problems; a developmental overview of the sexual relationship can often yield some insight into this area. As we have already mentioned, much of the sexual assessment should be conducted via questionnaires since it is often quite embarrassing for couples to discuss such matters with a therapist whom they have just met. Discussion of the couple's sex life during the interview should be restricted to more general and historical information.

Prior experiences of either or both partners in therapy should also be discussed. Two ends are served by discussing such experiences early: First, since current expectations might be based on such experiences, the therapist can clarify similarities and differences between what they will be experiencing in marriage therapy and what they experienced in the past; second, the mentioning of prior experiences in therapy puts the therapist in touch with any previous psychiatric history on the part of either partner. Relevant details regarding any past history of behavior problems on the part of either should of course be pursued.

Finally, if the information is not forthcoming spontaneously, we will ask explicitly about current and past involvements in extra-relationship affairs. The most common source of deception in presenting a relationship history involves the avoidance of disclosing information bearing on this question: "Illicit contracts" (Weiss, 1978) result when these issues are not uncovered, and therapy will not progress, to the bemusement of the therapist. With some couples, an interview with each spouse individually is the only way that such information can be uncovered. The pros and cons of interviewing spouses individually for this purpose are discussed in Chapter 5.

Therapist's Introduction

At the conclusion of the initial interview the therapist should provide couples with a brief introduction to therapy, while reemphasizing that a decision as to whether or not therapy is indicated will be made only after all of the assessment data have been collected and analyzed. Enough should be said to allow couples to leave the first session with a general understanding of the framework within which they will be working. We usually explain the treatment is time-limited (8 to 12 1½-hour sessions) and oriented toward solving present problems rather than focusing on the past. We also inform couples that they will be given homework assignments between sessions, and that much of the success of therapy will be predicated on their consistent adherence to these assignments. Then we present some statistics regarding our success with couples, stating that 75-80% of the couples treated with this approach derive benefit. Finally, we explain our use of records and videotape equipment, reassuring them in regard to confidentiality.

This introductory speech serves two primary functions. First, it orients couples to therapy, allaying some of their anxiety and confusion; after asking questions for an hour, couples need some information which will allow them to anticipate coming events. We believe that such information, although admittedly scanty, increases the likelihood of their complying with subsequent phases of the assessment. Second, our presentation of crude outcome statistics facilitates positive expectancies on the part of the couple.

CONCLUDING REMARKS

There are many ways to conduct an initial interview. The format suggested here is certainly not the only acceptable one, nor is it, in our view, always the optimal one. But it is a format which we believe serves the dual functions of an initial interview well: It provides the therapist with needed information regarding the history of the relationship, including the antecedents of current problems; and it serves the therapeutic functions of an initial contact, by alleviating some of the anxiety accompanying the introduction of therapy, inducing positive expectancies, and providing the couple with some immediate benefit through the redirecting of their "negative scanning" to the assumption of a broader, more positive perspective on their relationship.

The most difficult aspect to discuss is one of the most important, namely, the style in which the interview is conducted. The therapist must inspire liking, trust, and confidence in the couple. To do this, the therapist must appear relaxed and self-assured, and present material that comes across as natural rather than didactic. Interest and concern can be conveyed by a variety of verbal and nonverbal responses, many of which have been extensively discussed in numerous discourses on psychotherapy. *We would like to emphasize two therapist dimensions which we think are particularly important in the inducement of positive expectancies: enthusiasm and confidence.* If the therapist appears excited by the prospect of working with this couple, and if he expresses excitement about the behavioral approach, couples are likely to respond positively.

In addition to these difficult to specify therapist variables, control of the interview is vitally important. A therapist who is able to maintain control of a couple's "in therapy" behavior is much more likely to influence their "extra-therapy" behavior. Highly structured interviews portend highly structured treatment sessions; couples learn quickly that the therapist is going to decide what happens in therapy during the next few months. Their potential for rebellion and resistance is likely to wane as a result, and the therapist's instructions will be followed more often. Control means that couples not be allowed to digress from the topic implied by the therapist's question, and that spouses are reinforced for sticking to the topic. Couples should not be allowed to interrupt one another; rather it is the therapist who grants permission for one partner to comment on a remark just made by the other. *And above all, the therapist must be able to enforce his own rules.* Stating that couples not interrupt one another, for example, and then allowing interruptions to occur can seriously jeopardize couples' confidence in a therapist. It implies that the therapist is not to be taken seriously, that he does not mean what he says. Moreover, instructions are made to seem capricious when they are not consistently upheld.

Variables such as enthusiasm, confidence, and control are nebulous and difficult to operationalize, in part because they depend at least as much on the manner in which an interview is conducted as they do on the verbal content of the therapist's inquiries and responses. Strategies for displaying these qualities will be elaborated in Chapter 5. For now, we will restrict ourselves to a few comments. Couples usually respond positively to an interviewer who appears very engaged in the interviewing endeavor. A dry, formal presentation often conveys the impression that the interviewer is unenthusiastic about the task and uninterested in the couple. Interviewers who are excessively preoccupied with their function as providers and consumers of information, and not sufficiently attentive to the couple are unlikely to form a positive relationship during this initial contact. The information functions of the interview must be integrated with a natural, informal conversational style. This is often quite difficult for beginning therapists who become preoccupied with the content of their questions and walk into the interviewing setting with copious notes on the questions they need to ask and the comments they need to make. They become stimulus-bound and miss important nuances of the couple's interpersonal behavior. Not only are they likely to neglect important clinical observations, but they may come across as insensitive. The interviewer must adopt a supportive in addition to an information-seeking stance. Generous use of reflections must be interspersed with questions and comments, although at the same time, while exhibiting support, the interviewer must avoid forming alliances with one partner at the expense of the other.

We may be justifiably criticized for placing so much importance on the initial interview. Certainly, therapy can fail miserably despite an auspicious initial interview; and it is possible to rebound from an inauspicious beginning. But we believe that a primacy effect is operating in couples' therapy. We also believe that maintaining the commitment and collaborative behavior of couples is a struggle, at least initially; the therapist must be seductive, he must sell the couple on therapy. Only after they are sold will the technology be maximally effective.

SUMMARY

In this chapter, we described our format for conducting an initial interview with a couple. Rather than relying on the interview as a primary source of assessment information regarding the couple's current problems, we view the first contact as more of a therapy session, with the collection of information playing only an auxiliary role. The goals of the interview are to orient couples to the assessment process, relieve anxiety and hopelessness, and create positive expectancies. In terms of content, the focus is on collecting a developmental history of the relationship. The focus on historical material redirects the attention of distressed spouses to periods where the relationship was more positive, providing them with a broader perspective and undercutting their tendency to selectively attend to the current problems. The developmental history is also important for diagnostic and prognostic purposes, and it involves information which is not easily obtainable from other sources.

CHAPTER 4

Assessment of Relationship Dysfunction

THE PURPOSE OF ASSESSMENT, from a behavioral point of view, is to provide the information that is necessary to: (1) describe problems in the relationship; (2) identify variables that control the problem behaviors; (3) select appropriate therapeutic interventions; and (4) recognize when the intervention has been effective. A thorough assessment is essential to the development of effective and efficient treatment programs and cannot be dismissed as pertinent only to the researcher. Without adequate assessment procedures, clinicians are left with the two options of either treating all couples in a uniform manner, or making treatment decisions solely on the basis of clinical impressions. Embarking on a clinical intervention without the benefit of assessment information is comparable to searching for an unfamiliar destination without using directions or a road map. Without the benefit of assessment data, the road to successful clinical results will be circuitous and treatment objectives will be obscured. While a thorough assessment necessitates postponing the initial therapeutic intervention, the time and effort invested in that assessment will be rewarded in effective treatment planning.

Unlike more traditional assessment procedures which attempt to identify unifying personality constructs, behavioral assessment procedures attempt to describe specific behaviors that need to be changed as well as to identify variables controlling those behaviors. A thorough description of problem behaviors can be obtained through a SORC analysis, which examines the following components: (1) *Stimulus* variables, which elicit or set the stage for the target behavior; (2) *Organismic* variables, which act as mediating factors (cognitive and psychological) to a person's overt behaviors; (3) *Response* variables, which are the specific samples of the maladaptive responses, and (4) *Consequent* variables, which are changes in the environment that follow the response variables and affect their frequency (e.g. Goldfried & Sprafkin, 1974; Kanfer & Saslow, 1969; Mischel, 1968). Together, these components offer a complete description of the problem situation if the following conditions are met: (1) the behavioral responses being evaluated sample certain behavioral tendencies, and (2) the behaviors are being evaluated in relevant situations. It is thus critical in designing a behavioral assessment to strive both for adequate representation of the appropriate stimulus situations, and for a close resemblance between behavioral samples and actual problem behaviors.

The functional analysis, mentioned in Chapter 2, is used to guide the intervention and evaluate treatment effectiveness. This analysis includes: (1) systematic observation of the problem behaviors; (2) systematic observation of environmental antecedents and consequences to those behaviors; (3) therapeutic manipulation of a condition that is functionally related to the problem behaviors; and (4) further observation to record change in the behaviors in response to the manipulation (Peterson, 1968). In essence the functional analysis supplies the therapist with information about what variables control the problem situation and what is the effect of manipulating a particular variable. The decision for selecting an appropriate therapeutic manipulation rests greatly upon what one discovers about factors that control the problem behavior. An intervention to reduce the frequency of a couple's arguments, for example, would vary substantially depending upon whether the arguments follow from spouses' spending too little time together or come from poor communication skills. In the first instance, treatment would focus on helping the couple define the level of intimacy necessary to avoid arguments. In the second, the focus would be on the acquisition of specific communication skills.

In general, marital relationships are particularly challenging to assess since they represent an infinite variety of behavioral and attitudinal data involving the two marital partners during their shared time as well as their independent time. With all of this potential information, one must first decide on which components of the relationship to evaluate. Traditional assessments of marriages narrowed the choices down to the dimensions of stability and happiness (e.g., Hicks & Platt, 1970). Stability can be measured at its lowest point when divorce becomes a public index of instability, but at less obvious extremes, it is more difficult to quantify. Since objective criteria for measuring happiness are also lacking, it too is difficult to quantify. To complicate the situation further, happiness and stability do not covary, i.e., a stable relationship is not necessarily a happy one.

However, social learning theory, with its roots in reinforcement and exchange principles, has provided an approach to objectifying marital assessment. The objective of marital assessment based on social learning theory is to explore the interface between the specific relationship behaviors that spouses perform and the subjective cognitions that spouses hold about relationship satisfaction (Weiss & Margolin, 1977). Such an assessment produces answers to the following questions: (1) What are the beliefs that each spouse holds about the relationship? (2) What is the nature of the day-to-day interaction of the couple? (3) What factors contribute to the central relationship problems? and (4) How do spouses attempt to bring about change in their relationship? Later on in this chapter we will describe the procedures that are available to answer each of these questions. First, let us consider several assessment objectives that provide a framework for this approach.

ASSESSMENT OBJECTIVES

Assessment Should Examine Discrete, Observable Behaviors

In behavioral assessment, the behaviors that are assessed are a subset of the actual behaviors that will be the target of the intervention. Thus, predictions from the test behavior to the criterion behavior require few assumptions (Goldfried, 1977). What this means, however, is that the behavior being tested, like the problem behavior, must be carefully operationalized. To assess a marital relationship, the therapist must help the couple clarify and objectify vague global concepts with which they are familiar into discrete observable behaviors. Global concepts, such as appreciation and consideration, are not altogether discarded but acquire behavioral referents which comprise that general concept. For example, a wife's complaint that her husband does not appreciate her is assessed only after specifying the behaviors that he emits (or could emit) that communicate appreciation to her, perhaps physical gestures of affection, saying he loves her, or asking about her day. Rather than relying on retrospective verbal reports that he had been more or less appreciative, these specific behaviors can be observed on an ongoing basis. Treatment would be a direct outgrowth of the assessment since it would focus on those specific behaviors that contribute to the wife's feeling appreciated but that occur at too low a frequency.

Assessment Should be Broad Based

The clinician must evaluate multiple aspects of marital functioning beyond those areas specifically defined by the couple as problematic. The objective of such a broad based assessment is to examine a wide range of couple interactions so that the therapist obtains a detailed analysis of both the strengths and weaknesses of a particular couple. To conduct this assessment we recommend that the marital therapist generate his/her own list of assessment questions that apply to most couples. The idiosyncratic concerns of couples not covered by this general assessment strategy would then necessitate additional assessment procedures.

There are several reasons why we favor an all-encompassing approach to assessment. The primary reason is that spouses typically are not the most qualified judges of their own marital functioning. They tend to identify problems from a narrow perspective that focuses selectively on the major sources of irritation (e.g., "It's all because he works too hard," "If only she would stop nagging me"). Often they are not proficient at attending to and identifying behaviors that would enhance the relationship, even though this information is equally important to developing an intervention strategy. In addition, it is not uncommon to find that the immediate complaints that spouses bring to therapy change over time. While broad based assessment would not prevent this from occurring, it could provide the therapist with a greater understanding of the overall scope of a couple's problems. With that knowledge the therapist can make decisions regarding the sequencing of intervention strategies rather than blindly attacking the problem that appears to be of greatest immediacy.

Finally, a broad based assessment has the advantage of getting couples to look at their relationship in new ways since they are asked to respond to questions and situations that they have not anticipated. This type of intensive assessment can lay the groundwork for introducing couples into the philosophy of a behavioral treatment.

Assessment Should Include Cognitive Variables

The therapist must be aware that the clients' cognitions play a critical role in the problems that they experience. Spouses enter therapy with numerous assumptions about what has caused their relationship problems, with evaluations of themselves and their mates as marital partners and with attitudes about the quality of the relationship. These cognitions play an important role in determining why a couple is seeking marital counseling and how the couple might respond to behavior change activities. For a couple to feel that the therapy experience has been worthwhile, it is important for each partner to change individual cognitions as well as behaviors.

In the assessment of cognitive processes, cognitions can be viewed either as behaviors per se or as part of a behavioral response chain (Meichenbaum, 1976). When we view cognitions as behaviors, we then assess whether spouses hold realistic assumptions and expectations regarding the relationship situations. When we view cognitions as part of a behavioral response chain, we are more interested in how cognitions function to control behavioral responses. For this latter purpose it becomes necessary to understand how a spouse's self-dialogue mediates his/her behavioral changes. Meichenbaum's (1976) description of his cognitive-functional model is perhaps the most succinct statement on the subject of cognitive assessment. He defined the purpose of cognitive assessment as discovering "which cognitions (or the failure to produce which key cognitions), under what circumstances, are contributing to or interfering with adequate performance" (p. 162). This question suggests that at times it might be of greater expediency to modify cognitions prior to or simultaneous to changing the behavior, rather than waiting for cognitive change to follow behavioral change.

Assessment Should be Ongoing

Assessment that is ongoing throughout the course of therapy, rather than solely for the purposes of pre- and posttherapy evaluation, is essential for treatment planning. Some patterns of couple interaction, which spouses may refer to as high or low "cycles," unfold only over the course of several weeks or longer. Periodic isolated observation of these cyclical behavior patterns can be misleading and, therefore, counterproductive to the formulation of an effective strategy of change. Continuous data are needed to understand the development of these behavioral patterns and to plan ways for the couple to control the downward phases of their cycles.

Ongoing assessment that is examined on a daily or weekly basis throughout the course of treatment also provides continuous feedback to both the couple and therapist as to the efficacy of the prescribed procedures. Together the couple and the therapist can actively monitor the effect that each intervention produces on relationship functioning. Interventions that prove to be ineffective can be modified or discontinued before several weeks have elapsed and the entire treatment is considered a failure. Furthermore, the couple's active involvement with ongoing data collection teaches them to recognize the correspondence between their own behaviors and their overall progress. This association forms the basis for their continued efforts towards behavior change.

It may already be evident that ongoing assessment can become indistinguishable from the actual intervention procedures. While this might detract from one intent of the assessment, i.e. providing a nonreactive measurement of change, it is highly consistent with the goal of teaching couples to monitor their own relationships and to implement change strategies as needed.

ASSESSMENT OPTIONS

Prior to examining the specific instruments that assess marital functioning, let us first present a framework for differentiating these instruments. There are five dimensions that define each assessment instrument: (1) *Observational Targets* (e.g., relationship perceptions, discrete behaviors or skills, interaction sequences), (2) *Observer Sources* (e.g., self, spouse, significant others, trained others), (3) *Observational Methods* (e.g., interviews, questionnaires, behavioral rating forms, checklists, tracking instruments, observational coding systems), (4) *Timing* (e.g., continuous, daily, one-time measurements), and (5) *Setting* (e.g., home, therapy session, social environment). At least one form of each of these five dimensions must be utilized for every assessment instrument. Carrying this concept to the limit, the most complete range of all possible assessment instruments would result in an extremely complicated five dimensional matrix involving several options for each dimension. We call this matrix to mind only to define the range of assessment possibilities and to provide perspective on those instruments that are currently available.

Table 1 displays which options of the five assessment dimensions have been applied to each of the four questions that are fundamental to marital assessment. This table presents an overview of the types of information used to answer each question and the manner in which the information is collected. To some degree the nature of the assessment question defines the types of options that will be employed to answer it (i.e., spouses' beliefs can only be derived by the spouses themselves). However, the table also serves as a reminder that marital assessment has thus far employed only a fraction of the realm of potential assessment choices. As we turn to our description of specific assessment instruments, the reader is forewarned that the number of available instruments is misleading. Although the total number is high, the instruments represent a limited range of assessment options.

TABLE 1

Assessment Options as Applied to Questions of Marital Functioning

Assessment questions	Assessment dimensions				
	Observational targets	Observer sources	Observational methods	Timing	Settings
1. What are the beliefs that each spouse holds about the relationship?	marital satisfaction and stability, areas of desired change and areas of marital strength, perceptions of self and spouse	self	questionnaires, interview	one-time measurements at pre- and/or postintervention	home, counseling session
2. What is the nature of the day-to-day interaction of the couple?	instrumental, affectionate and companionship behaviors	spouse, trained observer	behavioral checklists, multibehavior coding systems	daily measurements throughout therapy and/or at pre- and postintervention	home, social environment
3. What factors contribute to the central relationship problems?	target behaviors, antecedents and consequences of those target behaviors	self, spouse	behavioral diaries, behavioral checklists, tracking instruments	continuous or successive measurements during therapy and/or at pre- and postintervention	home, social environment, counseling session
4. How do spouses attempt to bring about relationship change?	negotiation skills	self, spouse, trained observer	behavioral tracking, sequential coding systems	one-time measurement at pre- and postintervention	counseling session

With this framework for assessment in mind, it is now possible to explore what marital instruments have been developed and how these instruments relate to our four assessment questions.

What Are the Beliefs that Each Spouse Holds About the Relationship?

As this question suggests, one function of marital assessment is to collect information from spouses, as separate individuals, in the role of evaluating themselves, each other, and the relationship between them. We will first examine the questionnaires used to answer this question and then explore how interviews are used to supplement the questionnaire findings.

The Locke-Wallace Marital Adjustment Scale (MAS) (Locke & Wallace, 1959) represents one of the most widely used inventories of global marital satisfaction. The short 15-item MAS contains items to rate: (1) the level of overall satisfaction, (2) the amount of disagreement between spouses in eight subareas of marriage (e.g., finances and recreation), (3) the extent of spouses' mutual activity and mutual decision-making, and (4) the nature of each spouse's personal retrospections about the decision to marry. MAS scores range from 2 (high marital distress) to 161 (high marital adjustment) with 100 as the accepted cut-off score between distressed and nondistressed couples. Reliability and validity studies on the MAS have shown this instrument to be internally consistent and to be an accurate discriminator between distressed and nondistressed couples. These psychometric properties have resulted in the MAS being a popular choice in the marriage literature as a device for screening marital distress vs. adjustment. However, a factor to be considered when using this instrument is the evidence indicating a correlation between the MAS and social desirability measures. Spouses who report high marital satisfaction on the MAS also tend to endorse social desirability factors (Edmonds, Withers, & Dibatista, 1972; Murstein & Beck, 1972). It is as yet undetermined how much of a liability this poses for using the MAS as a measurement of marital adjustment .

In recent years two new scales have been developed which are similar in format and content to the MAS. Kimmel and van der Veen (1974) revised the MAS to include a greater number of items and to eliminate the sex bias in MAS scoring. Spanier (1976) developed the *Dyadic Adjustment Scale* (DAS), to provide an instrument for assessing unmarried cohabitating couples as well as married couples. This scale contains 32 items which form four factors—dyadic satisfaction, dyadic cohesion, dyadic consensus, and affectional expression. Each item included in the final version of the DAS has been shown to discriminate between happily married and divorced samples. Spanier is to be commended for his attention to the methodological properties of the DAS. He presents substantial evidence supporting the reliability and validity of this new scale.

Weiss, Patterson and their colleagues designed two self-report inventories that answer our basic assessment question but are more applicable to a behavioral approach than the above mentioned questionnaires. The *Areas of Change Questionnaire* (A-C) (see Patterson, 1976; Weiss & Margolin, 1977) assesses marital satisfaction in terms of the amount of change a couple desires to bring about in their relationship. Weiss and Birchler (1975, p. 1) describe the A-C as a vehicle "to provide a more precise sampling of relationship satisfaction, defined in terms of change and accurate perception of whether a change in behavioral rate would be welcomed by the other." The A-C is comprised of two parts which contain identical listings of 34 items reflecting specific issues for a couple. Part 1 instructs the respondent to indicate whether she/he wants the partner to increase, decrease, or not change the rate of each behavior (e.g., "I want my partner to pay attention to my sexual needs"). Part 2 asks the respondent to indicate whether an increase, decrease, or no change would be pleasing to the partner (e.g., "It would please my partner if I paid more attention to his/her sexual needs"). Desired change is indicated in both sections along a 7-point Likert scale ranging from Much Less (−3), to No Change (0), to Much More (+3). The first two items from this inventory illustrate its format:

I want my partner to:

								Major Item
1. . . participate in decisions about spending money	−3 much less	−2 less	−1 somewhat less	0	+1 somewhat more	+2 more	+3 much more	☐
2. . . spend time keeping the house clean	+3 much more	+2 more	+1 somewhat more	0	−1 somewhat less	−2 less	−3 much less	☐

In addition to marking their responses along this scale, respondents also indicate, with a checkmark, those items that are of major importance for the relationship.

Scoring of the A-C provides several types of information. Simply surveying Part 1 of each spouse's questionnaire provides the total amount of change sought by each partner. However, the instrument is scored to compare data from Part 1 of one spouse's questionnaire and from Part 2 of the partner's questionnaire, thereby providing the amount of agreement and disagreement between spouses on which behaviors should be changed and the desired direction of that change. Agreements are scored when one partner seeks change and the other accurately judges the direction of that change. Disagreements are scored when: (a) one partner desires change but the other is either unaware of this or is incorrect in judging the direction of change, or (b) one partner assumes the other desires change but, in fact, no change is requested. A couple's Total Change Score is derived from the sum of agreements and disagreements; these scores can range from 0 (no desired change) to 68 (change desired for each spouse in every area). In a normative study on the A-C, Birchler and Webb (1977) reported total change scores of 28.0 and 6.9 respectively for distressed and nondistressed couples. There are also data to suggest that the A-C measures the same psychological construct as the MAS, i.e., the correlation between the two measures is quite strong ($r = -.70$) (Weiss, Hops, & Patterson, 1973). However, the A-C provides data of much greater utility than the MAS since it can be used to identify specific problem areas and to assess the level of difficulty associated with changing those areas.

The second instrument was designed by Weiss to measure the stability of the marital relationship. The *Marital Status Inventory* (MSI) (Weiss & Cerreto, 1975) was developed as an inventory of the progressive steps that spouses take in the dissolution of their relationship. The 14 specific MSI items range in intensity and comprise a Guttman scaling, such that engaging in step five along the sequence would necessitate having completed the first four steps. The series of steps involved in terminating a relationship include: (a) vague thoughts about divorce (e.g., "I have considered divorce or separation a few times . . ."), (b) specific thoughts (e.g., "I have considered who would get the kids . . ."), (c) overt behaviors (e.g., "I have discussed the issue seriously and at length with my spouse"), and (d) behaviors initiating divorce procedures (e.g., "I have contacted a lawyer"). Since this instrument is relatively new there are only preliminary statistics to indicate its validity. However, it is the only instrument that we are aware of that specifically examines a couple's likelihood of divorce. Questions about divorce are often asked in the interview situation but the MSI is a superior method for eliciting specific data of this nature. This instrument will be extremely valuable to marriage therapists if further investigation reveals that progression to a particular stage on the scale precludes successful couples therapy. Currently, it is a useful means of determining a couple's predisposition toward divorce before engaging in the therapeutic process.

Stuart and Stuart (1972) developed the *Marital Pre-Counseling Inventory* (MPI), an exceptionally comprehensive questionnaire to assess the strengths and requests of marital partners. In the accompanying counselor's guide to the inventory, Stuart describes three purposes of the MPI: (1) it provides clients with socialization into therapy by directing their observations to positive elements of their own and their spouses' behaviors; (2) it provides highly organized, comprehensive data relevant to therapeutic goals; and (3) it provides the counselor and clients with a periodic evaluation of therapeutic progress. The inventory contains 13 separate sections to meet these goals. Given the comprehensive nature of the MPI, we cannot go into detail about each of the scales. However, several scales are particularly useful in analyzing the strengths and weaknesses of the relationship in behavioral terms. Two sections, Positive Aspects of Spouse's Behavior and Acceleration Targets from Spouse, help the respondent focus in on those aspects of the partner's behavior which are already rewarding and which would be rewarding if they occurred more frequently. In the two sections that follow, labelled Acceleration Targets for Spouse and Self-Assessment, the respondent specifies ways that he/she is reinforcing to the partner and assesses his/her strengths. A comparison between these two sections and the previous two sections assesses whether each person is aware of what the partner views as his/her relationship strengths.

Further details about the 13 separate scales can be found in the manual that accompanies this inventory. In this manual, Stuart also provides some sparse data on the validity of the MPI. Having given the MPI to 400 couples at pre- and posttreatment, he found: (1) substantial reductions in the discrepancy scores for the Decision-Making Scale (i.e., spouses reported greater congruence between how they perceived decisions to be made and how they wanted decisions to be made); and (2) large increases in the General Satisfaction section (i.e., from mean pretreatment satisfaction ratings of 38% for women and 30% for men to mean posttreatment ratings of 81% for both sexes). Unfortunately, these two scales are two of the most subjective indices in this inventory. Thus the utility of this inventory as an outcome measure is not completely clear. However, the MPI is noteworthy in the amount of information it provides preparatory to beginning the counseling process. The following repeating themes of the inventory are particularly helpful in this regard: (1) the focus on positive relationship aspects; (2) the focus on a wide base of relationship resources; (3) the emphasis on self-change (e.g., "Please suggest ways in which a change in your own behavior might improve . . ."); (4) the attention paid to situational specificity by asking the respondent to respond to the same question across multiple situations, and to situational control through the Family Locator; and (5) the attempts to weight, through rank orderings, the personal importance of each problem area. In summary, while the MPI contains many positive features, further information is still needed regarding its suitability as an outcome measure and its capability to orient spouses to the behavioral approach.

Before turning to the interview as an additional means of answering the first assessment question, let us examine the utility of questionnaire data. For the therapist, questionnaires present a low-cost and low-effort method of gathering information. They also offer a vehicle for collecting information that can be uncomfortable and unproductive for the therapist to pursue during an interview (e.g., "Do thoughts of divorce occur to you more frequently than once per week?"). From the clients' vantagepoint, questionnaires are relatively effortless, at least in comparison to other assessment procedures. Furthermore, they often elicit the types of information that spouses are eager to communicate to the therapist. Inventories that can be scored have the advantage of being used as outcome measures to assess the amount of attitudinal change over the course of therapy. These instruments should also be considered as a means of collecting follow-up data.

However, let us not lose sight of the fact that the measurements we have just described are limited in their applicability to the behavioral approach. These instruments are the least informative of our measures in terms of what spouses actually do with one another and are the most susceptible to demand characteristics and social desirability factors. Yet the subjective data provided by the instruments are imperative to successful work with couples. These data help the therapist plan and conduct interventions that are meaningful to the couple. They also establish the basis for therapeutic rapport by providing a great deal of information useful for understanding each spouse's position. It is then up to the therapist to demonstrate that understanding to the clients and thereby procure the couple's attention and trust.

The Behavioral Interview

As we mentioned in the introduction to this section, the interview can be used to supplement and follow up on data gathered from the above mentioned inventories. While we have already discussed the intake interview in Chapter 3, that is not the only occasion during which we use the interview as a data collection vehicle. It is our experience that it is necessary to devote, at the minimum, part of the second scheduled session to gathering details about the couple's interaction. The rest of that session is then spent collecting an actual sample of their problem-solving and preparing the couple for further data collection at home, both of which are described later in this chapter. The session time that is used for assessment purposes is an opportunity for spouses to report verbally on their activities, thoughts, and feelings. The actual contents of these verbalizations tend to overlap into our second and third assessment questions regarding the couple's day-to-day interactions and the factors that contribute to their problems. However, since we view the information obtained through the interview as subjective impressions, we have chosen to discuss it with the other tools for assessing spouses' relationship beliefs.

What type of information does the interview provide that cannot be obtained through questionnaires? Linehan (1977) listed several advantages to the behavioral interview. Most importantly, the interview provides observational data. This is a particular strength of a couple interview in which the therapist obtains a first-hand view of how the partners interact with one another and how they present themselves as a couple to a third party. Furthermore, the therapist also derives information about the behavior of the individual partners, that is, the different manner in which they respond to the therapist versus the other spouse, the topics that elicit emotional reactions and the types of emotional responses displayed by each partner.

Secondly, due to the flexibility of the interview situation, the interviewer can follow leads and pursue information in greater detail. Oftentimes spouses do not answer open ended questions on inventories with enough detail to be useful. This can be due to their misunderstanding of the instructions, their distaste for putting personal reactions on paper, or their self-consciousness about their lack of literacy skills. Thus, even with the best instructions for well-pinpointed statements about desired relationship change, spouses may respond with an imprecise phrase such as "communication problems." Within the context of the interview, it is possible to shape spouses to describe their desired changes through specific statements instead of vague complaints if the therapist defines and illustrates the difference between the two types of statements. It is also possible to assist spouses in describing the behaviors they wish to accelerate rather than focusing only on decelerate behaviors. Requests that both are specific and deal with behaviors to accelerate present a more optimistic picture and are less punitive for the recipient.

Once behavioral targets have been defined, the interview can be used to gather detailed information about the environmental conditions that surround those behaviors. Even the most behavioral of the available questionnaires focuses only on identifying goals and ignores the additional information necessary to formulate a complete behavioral analysis. To fully understand each problem, it is necessary to ask each partner to provide a detailed analysis of all related factors. The therapist can prompt such an analysis by telling the clients to "imagine that you are directing a movie of these events. Describe how the scene would be set, what would lead up to the situation, who would be present, what each participant would be doing, and how the scene might end." Thus, the couple who gets into frequent arguments at dinner time would be asked for details to describe when each partner gets home, how they greet each other, what other family members are doing, what types of household commotions are occurring, etc., plus their personal cognitions regarding the demands each spouse experiences, the expectations that each spouse holds for this period of the day, and the factors that seem to affect the spouses' respective moods. Eliciting this type of detailed information from both spouses can be a tedious process. In addition, there may be questions about the accuracy of spouses' reporting. When describing a conflict-laden situation, there is a high likelihood that the spouses will view the situation quite differently. Having the other spouse present provides only a partial deterrent to inaccuracies of reporting. It is helpful to view these discrepancies as due to poor or selective observations, rather than intentional distortions. The therapist should verbally acknowledge the disagreements that occur, restate each spouse's perceptions, and not attempt to "get to the truth of the matter." Resolving discrepant impressions is impossible and the efforts expended in such an exercise are clinically counterproductive since they foster competition and blaming.

During the interview the therapist may also wish to pursue information that portrays the spouses' lives together in a more global context. In planning the treatment, it is very useful to know what typical weekdays and weekend days look like for a particular couple, e.g., how much time they can expect to have with one another, how they spend both their shared and alone time. These questions are necessary to examine what external stimuli might control the relationship problems. A couple's communication problems, for example, may not be the result of a skills defect but may be due to the fact that during the work week they see each other for only one waking hour per day. Questions about the nature of a couple's time together can also help determine the degree of flexibility in the spouses' lives, e.g., are they trapped in the house because they have no money for babysitters or because they have nowhere to go?

Similar to the therapist's role in the intake session, there are several ways she/he can make this information-gathering session therapeutic even though the specific behavioral interventions have not yet begun. Once again, maintaining a positive focus is critical. The therapist should include questions such as "What are some activities that the two of you enjoy doing?" or "Why do you like to be married to one another?" Through these questions, the therapist learns what is currently reinforcing and what could be used as reinforcements in future behavior change. Secondly, the therapist elicits from each spouse a public statement of praise for the partner. It is important, however, for the therapist to feel quite assured that the spouses will indeed be able to answer these questions. To ask such a question and incur silence is extremely punishing and should be avoided. The therapist should be very aware of the types of spouse behavior she/he reinforces. Spouses' statements that are suggestive of a positive or constructive cognitive set or that are serious explorations of the problems should be reinforced. Statements that are critical of the partner, that bait the partner, or that reenact past hurts should be quickly terminated. This will involve actively interrupting the criticizing speaker and refocusing that person on a more constructive exploration of the situation. To lessen the burden of constantly monitoring some spouses from using this time as a "bitch session," the therapist should share his/her goals for this session and make it clear from the outset that the session will focus on the present not the past. Although some of the session will be focused on problem situations, that does not necessitate criticism or blaming.

The therapist's own behavior provides a model as to how problems can be discussed constructively. Through accurate paraphrasing of each spouse's position, she/he can demonstrate how both partners have contributed to the problems and how they both suffer as a result of these problems. In a recent example with a couple who had been referred because the husband hit the wife during one of their frequent arguments, the therapist restated the event in the following way so that the blame for this incident was shared by both spouses: "So Edith, it sounds as though you were upset with what Hank was doing and expressed this by yelling obscenities and calling him names. And when that continued for a bit, it so infuriated you, Hank, that in a moment of what you called 'blind rage,' you hit Edith." In this summary statement the therapist focused on the chain of events and restated each person's participation in the escalation of aggression.

The therapist can further induce a nonblaming atmosphere by suggesting an alternative way of viewing the problem. The following statement was made to a couple after the husband had been labelled "uncaring" but this label did not correspond to the therapist's observations during the therapy sessions: "I've heard you say, Sally, that at times you feel as though Joe doesn't care. And yet, Joe, you've demonstrated several times how concerned you are about Sally. Perhaps we're faced with the situation of your not knowing how to show the caring that you actually feel, and therefore, are not getting credit for it." By defining Joe's problem as a skills deficit rather than as a lack of concern, we continue to view the absence of that behavior as a problem, but recognize Joe's good intentions, thereby giving him credit and elevating him in Sally's estimation. Such explanations have the advantage of reassuring the spouses that the problems defined are modifiable.

One additional procedure that the therapist can use to promote constructive use of this assessment period is to stress the fact that spouses can and, in fact, often will have differences of opinion. It is important for the therapist to demonstrate that she/he has not become unnerved by the spouses' disagreements or problems. Furthermore, by giving permission for these problems to occur, there is no need to attempt to resolve each one as it arises.

In summary, the interview can be a useful way for the therapist to receive information but the therapist must teach the spouses how to impart that information. It is our experience that throughout the course of treatment, some portion of each session is used for further assessment of a previously untouched aspect of the relationship or of the success of the previous intervention strategy. Thus, even with its shortcomings the interview is an assessment tool which we use extensively. The more initial effort that is devoted to teaching couples how to utilize the interview situation, the easier, more enjoyable and more constructive it becomes for everyone involved.

What Is The Nature of the Day-To-Day Interaction of the Couple?

The purpose of examining this question as part of your overall assessment package is to learn what pleasures the spouses engage in and what efforts they expend to maintain their relationship. This question functions to expand the assessment package to areas beyond what the spouses regard as their problems. While spouses are apt to describe their problems in terms of the large philosophical or emotional differences between them, couple problems are oftentimes due to insufficient efforts devoted to the maintenance of smooth relationship functioning. Before attacking the large and difficult issues that face each couple, the therapist needs to assess whether, by rearranging daily interaction patterns, the couple can relieve some of the marital tensions. Unfortunately, however, this assessment question has been largely ignored except for the random bits of information that therapists gather through interview questions. For the most part, spouses are the only ones who can provide a wide range of details about their daily lives together. To increase the utility of their reports, spouses need a standardized procedure whereby they can keep daily records rather than being asked at varying intervals for retrospective recollections. Although there have also been several attempts at having outside observers code couples' activities, these are quite restricted in scope, compared to observations by the spouses themselves. The limitations of observations by persons other than the partners are discussed below.

What types of relationship behaviors do we observe? How do we categorize the multitude of events that occur within a marriage? The marriage literature of the 60's (Hicks & Platt, 1970; Tharp, 1963) identified two separate domains of marital interactions: (1) instrumental behaviors, defined as those necessary for the relationship to survive as a socioeconomic unit (e.g,. taking care of the baby; doing the grocery shopping; bringing home a paycheck); and (2) expressive behaviors, defined as those which convey concern, caring, appreciation, and approval (e.g., verbal and/or physical expressions of affection, interest in the other's activities, etc.). Another category of relationship interaction is that of companionship behaviors or shared recreational time. Historically this category has gained importance as it has become increasingly common for relationships to be formed on a basis of shared interests and shared pleasures, rather than traditional role perceptions.

Weiss, Patterson and their colleagues (Patterson, 1976, Patterson, Weiss, & Hops, 1976; Weiss, Hops, & Patterson, 1973) were the first to examine relationship adjustment in terms of the rate at which rewarding and punishing behaviors were exchanged between spouses. Based on their extensive knowledge of relationship activities, this group of researchers designed an eight-page listing of specific pleasing and displeasing relationship behaviors. This lengthy instrument, called the *Spouse Observation Checklist* (SOC), spanned the instrumental-expressive-companionship dimensions by including the following categories of behaviors: Meals and Shopping, Childcare, Finances, Personal Appearance, Transportation, Housekeeping, Family Recreation, and Affection. Each category contained a listing of specific behaviors. For example, "Spouse helped in planning the budget" and "Spouse wrote a check without recording it" are examples of a pleasing and displeasing item included under Finances. All categories of behaviors, except for the area of Affection, were rated once per day as to frequency of occurrence and degree of "pleasingness," i.e., from —3 (strongly displeasing) to +3 (strongly pleasing). Affectional behaviors, which are more difficult to recall since they occur at high frequencies and for short durations, were recorded on mechanical counters as soon as they occurred.

In the past several years Weiss has continued to refine the SOC to emphasize the value that each behavior holds for its recipient. The initial SOC listing was expanded to approximately 400 items, each of which carries either an appetitive value (i.e., the sought-after goals of a relationship), an instrumental value (i.e., the mechanics of maintaining a relationship), or is a by-product of the relationship (i.e., the results of being in a relationship that are unrelated to the reasons for initiating the relationship) (Weiss, 1978). A panel of 12 judges assigned each of 400 items to 12 marital areas that represent the labels that spouses typically use to describe their relationship. These 12 areas fit into the appetitive-instrumental-by-product distinction in the following manner: Appetitive behaviors belong to the areas of companionship, affection, consideration, sex, communication process, and coupling activities. Instrumental behaviors include the areas of childcare, household management, financial decision-making, and employment-education. By-products of the relationship occur in the remaining two areas of personal habits-appearance and self-spouse independence. The link that the SOC provides between cognitive labels, such as affection, consideration, etc., and specific quantifiable behaviors makes this instrument a valuable introduction for couples to social learning theory.

The revised SOC is packaged in booklets that can be used for seven days of data collection. Spouses are instructed to complete the SOC at approximately the same hour each day. The task is made easier for spouses if they get into the habit of completing the SOC immediately before retiring for the night so that they do not need to recall events from the previous day. Once they are familiar with the SOC, filling it out should take no longer than 20 minutes per day. But, that alone, without any additional homework assignments, is a substantial time commitment for most couples. When couples begin to use the SOC, midweek phone calls are recommended to ameliorate any difficulties that the couple may be having with the instrument. Later on in the therapy the therapist can use these phone calls to affirm the importance of these data and to encourage consistent recordkeeping.

Although the revised SOC does not include ratings of "pleasantness" within its daily recording format, Weiss has developed a procedure for analyzing personalized values and costs attached to each pleasing SOC behavior. Weiss' cost-benefit system requires each spouse to rate self-benefits (how beneficial each item would be if it occurred) and self-costs (how costly it would be to provide each behavior to one's partner). Each spouse identifies the subset of pleasing items that would be a benefit to receive and rates these along a 5-point scale from 1 (Of No Benefit) to 5 (Extremely Beneficial). The partner then indicates the cost of giving those behaviors along a similar scale from 1 (No Cost) to 5 (Extremely Costly). These data are quite useful when it comes time to engineer behavioral exchanges between spouses.

Several studies have been conducted on the psychometric properties of the original SOC. Normative data collected by Birchler, Weiss, and Vincent (1975) revealed that 12 distressed couples, as compared to 12 nondistressed couples, exchanged significantly fewer pleases and significantly more displeases; the Please:Displease ratios were 4:1 and 30:1 respectively for distressed and non-distressed couples. Wills, Weiss, and Patterson (1974) provided a reliability check on spouses' accuracy of reporting pleasing and displeasing behaviors by asking each husband, without the wife's knowledge, to double his demonstration of affectional pleases to his wife. Affectional pleases as reported by the wives significantly increased while other please and displease subtotals remained unchanged. There are as yet no studies that examine the reliability and validity of the revised SOC and provide normative data on that instrument.

What effect do specific marital behaviors, such as those contained in the SOC, have on overall marital adjustment? Herein lies the true value of this type of assessment. It is necessary to determine which specific behaviors actually affect relationship satisfaction if the eventual goal is to enhance that satisfaction. Significant associations between the Locke-Wallace and SOC have been found by correlating the Locke-Wallace with total frequencies of pleases (Margolin, 1978b) and with Please: Displease ratios (Weiss, Hops, & Patterson, 1973). Yet since neither relationship satisfaction nor behavioral frequency data are static measures, one method to understand the association between the two measures is to examine the similarities in their patterns of fluctuation. In filling out the SOC, spouses are also instructed to indicate their satisfaction with the relationship for that day by marking a 9-point scale from 1 (totally dissatisfied) to 9 (totally satisfied). Using this scale, Wills et al. (1974) attempted to determine the extent to which marital satisfaction ratings are related to both pleasing and displeasing affectional and instrumental behaviors and to the quality of non-relationship daily activities. They found that the five predictors, when examined together, accounted for 25% of the variance in marital satisfaction. Displeases accounted for a greater portion of the variance than pleases. In addition they found that husband's satisfaction depended more on instrumental behaviors than affectional behaviors; the opposite was found for wives.

However, the amount of variance accounted for by different categories of behaviors varies greatly from spouse to spouse. In a case reported by Margolin, Christensen, and Weiss (1975), the husband's marital satisfaction was much more dependent on affectional than instrumental behaviors. Affectional pleases and displeases respectively accounted for 20% and 29% of the fluctuation in his satisfaction; instrumental pleases and displeases respectively accounted for only 9% and 6% of the variance. Examining the relationship between each of the 12 categories and satisfaction on the revised SOC, Margolin has found that an individual category can account for as much as 50% of the total variance in marital satisfaction. The identification of these highly significant categories is extremely useful in planning therapeutic interventions.

Overall we judge the SOC to be one of the most valuable tools available to the behavioral marital therapist. It is useful as: (1) a measurement of therapy outcome; (2) an ongoing measurement to evaluate the effects and effectiveness of various therapeutic interventions, and (3) a tool to help plan and implement the intervention strategy. To some degree these multiple uses of the SOC can be at cross purposes with one another. Since the SOC provides ongoing feedback to the couple, it is reactive as an instrument to assess outcome. Even if it is used strictly for pre- and posttreatment assessment, participant observation on the SOC can create a situation approximating dyadic training. However, Weiss and Margolin (1977, p. 570) point out that any type of spouse observation "is reactive since it provides discrimination training to spouses as well as bringing observed responses under social control." This caution certainly applies to the SOC but the extent of the reactivity is not entirely clear. When couples used the SOC over a two week period without any therapeutic intervention, total please and displease frequencies did not change (Wills et al., 1974). Another sample of couples used the SOC for a four week period which included two weeks of a nondirective therapy to improve couples' communication. Over time, these couples continued to report the same number of SOC pleases but their frequency of displeases decreased significantly (Margolin & Weiss, 1978b). Even when the frequency of reported behaviors remains constant, the SOC may have a reactive influence on spouses' relationship perceptions. Mere recognition of the ratio of positive to negative behaviors provides couples with new input regarding their relationship exchange. Even distressed couples usually find that, in sheer numbers, the benefits of the relationship (pleases) outweigh the costs (displeases). Although the effect of this type of information is not known, when using the SOC it is critical to recognize its potential as an unintentional agent of change. Later on, in Chapter 6, we will explore reasons why the therapist may intentionally choose to employ the SOC as a method to induce behavioral and cognitive change.

It is also possible for outsiders to collect information about a couple's interactions in the home but these observations generally are limited to social exchanges and do not examine the couple's highly intimate interactions or their exchanges of service-oriented behaviors. Two recent observational systems were developed to collect data on a comparatively limited set of behaviors that frequently occur when spouses are together. Robinson and Price (1976) selected the following nine behaviors for home observation: attending, agreement, approval, positive physical interaction, concern, humor, laugh/smile, compliance and compromise. Follingstad, Sullivan, Ierace, Ferrara, and Haynes (1976) sampled both positive and negative behaviors, including smile, eye contact, positive physical contact, compliment, agreement, suggestion, criticism, interruption, and disagreement. The purpose of the observations made by these sets of investigators was to assess the rate at which each of the identified behaviors occurred during a couple's naturalistic interactions in their home. Observations were usually made during or immediately following the dinner hour. The only structure put on the couple was that the spouses were to remain within the viewing distance of the observers, were to avoid extensive interactions with their children, and were to curtail their television watching and phone calls.

Weiss et al. (1973) describe their application of the *Behavior Coding System* (BCS) (Patterson, Ray, Shaw, & Cobb, 1969), a 29-category coding system that has been widely used to code family interactions. Based on their limited findings when coding couples who had been seen for marital therapy, these researchers concluded that outside observers are not privy to many of the behaviors that are important to intimate adult relationships. This conclusion gained further support when both Robinson and Price (1976) and Follingstad et al. (1976) found that the behaviors in their coding systems generally yielded insignificant correlations with measurements of marital satisfaction. It seems as though collecting several hours of data in couples' homes does not provide much information on how the spouses manage their exchange of major reinforcers. At this stage of our technology, gains from such observations do not warrant the high costs of sending outside observers into the home.

What Factors Contribute to the Central Relationship Problems?

The objective in answering this assessment question is to gather information which can be used to formulate a behavioral analysis for the specific concerns that spouses bring to therapy. Whenever this question cannot be answered through more standardized assessment methods, the information must be collected through self- or spouse-monitoring procedures. Although behavioral assessors have developed several methods for observing one's own behavior, there are no definitive guidelines by which to collect these data. The therapist, in consultation with the clients, must decide how each target behavior can best be recorded. Compared to other assessment procedures which strive for standardization, the format for these monitoring procedures is very much dependent on the therapist's ingenuity in designing instruments that can be applied to the assessment of idiosyncratic couple problems.

Marital assessment has the unique advantage of being able to rely on two participant observers: Both spouses can provide information about themselves and each other. Self-observation for the purposes of marital assessment resembles self-observation procedures used in other types of behavior therapy (see Ciminero, Nelson & Lipinski, 1977). Spouse observation has been preferred over self-observation in behavioral marital assessment since it focuses attention on the marital dyad rather than on spouses as separate individuals. Having both partners monitor the same observational target provides the therapist with a measurement of perceptual accuracy between partners; this can be one of the most instructive uses of spouse monitoring since it alerts the therapist to the differences between spouses in the ways that they view specific behaviors.

In identifying appropriate self- or spouse-monitoring procedures, the therapist must decide upon: (1) the behaviors to observe; (2) the unit of measurement, and (3) the method of recording observations. To facilitate the first step of monitoring, which is discriminating whether or not the behavior has occurred, it is best that target behaviors be easily recognizable and relatively discrete. For example, a couple that is to monitor their expressions of affection must first define affection: Are both verbal and nonverbal expressions of affection included? How do affectionate behaviors differ from sexual gestures? The therapist and couple must also determine a reasonable time frame for observing the behavior and a method for recording its occurrence. The alternatives in this regard include: (1) frequency of occurrences (e.g., number of times the wife compliments the husband); (2) total length of time spent in the behavior (e.g., amount of time that husband spent with the children each day); or (3) percentage of times that the behavior occurred in the presence of a specific antecedent (e.g., each time the husband agreed to help out around the house in response to a specific request from the wife). To observe behaviors that are high in frequency or that "run together" such that there is no clear onset or termination, it is useful to employ time-sampling procedures (Mahoney & Thoresen, 1974). The spouse then indicates whether or not the target behavior has occurred during a predetermined interval of time. Stuart (1969), for example, employed time-sampling procedures as part of his assessment and intervention strategies in counseling four distressed couples. Each of the four wives had requested that her husband "converse with her more fully" (p. 503). After considerable discussion to identify the level of conversation that was positively reinforcing to each wife, she kept track of her husband's conversational performance by deciding, at one hour intervals, whether or not he had met the criterion level of conversation. The ringing of a kitchen timer functioned to remind the wife, at regular intervals, that it was time to assess whether her husband had met the behavioral criterion for the preceding interval. This type of coding procedure guaranteed that the wife maintained a predetermined rate of coding. When Stuart then introduced his intervention procedures, the time-sampling procedure assured that husbands would receive feedback on their performance at regular intervals.

In general, when the purpose of the assessment is to observe the incidence of specific behaviors or cognitions, the method of recording must be chosen on the basis of how accurately spouses will be able to recall these events over time. The premise behind the SOC, for instance, is that spouses will be able to remember those events for a 24-hour time span and, therefore, can limit their recording of behaviors to once per day. For events that are difficult to remember from one moment to the next, self-monitoring cards or mechanical event records are the preferred methods of recording. Devices of this nature, which spouses must keep accessible for coding at any time, should be inconspicuous enough that they are not cumbersome or embarrassing for the user. Once the exact recording procedures have been decided upon, it is necessary to provide spouses with a structured form that clearly identifies the behaviors to be observed and that provides a graph or some other format for recording data at the desired intervals. The therapist increases the probability of receiving usable information by being as explicit as possible in specifying the type of data that is needed.

The *behavioral diary* is the procedure most commonly used when the primary purpose of the assessment is to obtain information about the environmental variables that control a specific behavior in addition to data on the strength of that particular behavior. Generally, spouses are asked to indicate, in a narrative description, what events immediately preceded and followed the target behavior. For spouses who are unaccustomed to writing accounts of their experiences, it is best to design recording forms that contain specific questions which are pertinent to the assessment problem: What was the sequence of events? Who was present? Where did it occur? What was the outcome? We have learned that spouses who have difficulty expressing themselves during the therapy sessions often encounter equal difficulty when asked to express themselves on paper.

The *Anger Checklist* (Margolin, Olkin, & Baum, 1977) is an example of an instrument that was developed on the basis of many persons' behavioral diaries and that functions towards the same objective of providing a thorough accounting of angry interchanges between spouses. While this instrument lacks the sequential aspect that a diary provides, the checklist tends to elicit much greater detail than the diary and is a less demanding task for clients. The purpose of this checklist is: (1) to describe the types of angry responses that spouses exchange during a disagreement and (2) to measure whether spouses learn through therapy to express their anger more constructively and to limit themselves to anger expressions that are neither physically nor emotionally harmful. The Anger Checklist contains 79 anger reactions which span the following categories: Somatic Cues (e.g., clenched jaw, tightened forearm, quickened pulse), Emotional Cues (e.g., hurt, out-of-control, frustrated), Angry Actions (e.g., banging fists, pacing, slapping), Angry Thoughts (e.g., "You've got no right," "I want to be rid of this person") and Angry Words (e.g., accusations, threats, curses). Spouses record each incident of anger by checking each reaction that they observed in themselves or their partners. The list is interchangeable for self-monitoring or spouse-monitoring except for nonobservable somatic, cognitive, and emotional cues. This inventory is useful in making spouses aware of the multiple components of their anger and in increasing their recognition of early signs of anger. Therapy to help spouses control destructive expressions of anger should reduce items checked in the angry actions and words categories. It is assumed that angry thoughts and feelings will continue to be recorded but that the composition of items will signify a reduction in intensity. As yet there are no published data on this instrument.

While reports of assessing specific behavioral events through self- and spouse-monitoring procedures have frequented the behavioral literature, reports of assessing cognitive events have been infrequent. One exception is the assessment of *Pleasant Thoughts about the Spouse,* which was introduced by Patterson and Hops (1972) in an attempt to assess the cognitive correlates of specific behaviors. They found that changes in spouses' reports of pleasant thoughts about one another were associated with fewer aversive interactions in the home, as noted by trained observers. Instructing clients to record both the pleasant thoughts about the spouse and the concomitant behavior of the spouse can also provide valuable diagnostic information regarding the types of behaviors that are indeed pleasing for the respondent. In general, the monitoring of self-statements is an unexplored area in behavioral marital therapy. Such monitoring could provide an important outcome measure for spouses who enter therapy with high rates of derogatory statements about the partner or high rates of self deprecatory statements about their own abilities to function in the relationship. It is recommended that clients be instructed to record positive thoughts, rather than negative thoughts, since the mere recognition of such thoughts will draw attention to these positive, rather than negative, aspects of the relationship. Thus, the husband who labels himself as an incompetent lover can benefit from keeping track of the times that he views himself as an adequate or better lover, and recording the specific events that lead to his more favorable evaluation. Positive behavioral changes tend to be most persistent when spouses' self-perceptions keep pace with the behavioral changes.

The same methodological precautions that we enumerated in regard to the SOC also apply to the self-and-spouse observational instruments described in this section. These procedures are potentially reactive, particularly when the target behaviors are perceived by the observer as having a positive or negative valence (Kazdin, 1974). There is also the problem of sustaining reliable coding (Lipinski & Nelson, 1974) in that over time, the procedures can lose their initial interest for the client and become quite tedious. In addition, spouses do not necessarily maintain the same coding standards from day to day. A pat on the behind could be viewed as an affectional gesture during a moment of playfulness or as an annoyance during a time of seriousness or concentration. Similarly, a husband's offer of "Can I get you something at the store" might sometimes be greatly appreciated but at other times may provoke annoyance if the wife wants the husband to stay home and babysit the kids so that she can take a nap. The only means that the therapist has to stabilize spouses' observational thresholds is to specify behaviors as precisely and objectively as possible. Coding of some types of behaviors can be rehearsed during the therapy session to obtain a sampling of spouses' accuracy and to remedy any questions of behavioral definition. In addition, it is important to convey to spouses how their data enhance the value of their treatment. The importance of these data can be underscored by paying attention to the data and by actively employing the data to plan future interventions.

How Do Spouses Attempt to Bring about Change in Their Relationship?

This assessment question is based on the premise that change is a natural component of marital relationships and that, through the course of a relationship, spouses will develop a variety of ways to effect marital change. Measurements that answer this question explore the extent to which spouses employ aversive rather than rewarding change mechanisms. The most commonly used method to assess their change-inducing interactions has been for spouses to engage in problem-solving discussions that are then coded by trained observers or by the spouses themselves.

Coding systems used by others trained to assess couples' negotiation skills have been limited to laboratory-based investigations. These are in contrast to the home observations, described earlier, in which couples are to interact naturally rather than to resolve a problem. The original laboratory-based marital assessments were designed to evoke spouses' decision-making patterns when resolving therapist induced differences on tasks having built-in conflicts. The purpose of these tasks was to measure existing levels of agreement between spouses and spouses' power vis-a-vis each other. The assessment tasks introduced by social learning theorists were designed to produce samples of behavior that are highly related to naturalistic problem-solving. That is, couples engage in time-limited discussions to resolve differences of opinion on problems that truly exist in their relationship. Scoring of these discussions is more concerned with the process by which spouses resolve conflict than the actual outcome or final decision. The problem-solving discussions are audiotaped or videotaped and then coded for specific behaviors that the researchers have judged a priori to be either facilitative or destructive to the negotiation process. Thomas, Walter, and O'Flaherty (1974), for example, present a comprehensive listing of 49 unproductive verbal behaviors that, when coded from a tape-recorded discussion, provide direction for the ensuing therapy.

The Marital Interaction Coding System (MICS) developed by the Oregon project (Hops, Wills, Patterson, & Weiss, 1972) presents an intricate analysis of couples' problem-solving discussions. This 29-category coding system provides data on both verbal and nonverbal behaviors in the sequential patterns in which they occur. The 29 MICS codes have been a priori classified into the following categories: Problem Solving (accept responsibility, compromise, problem solution), Positive Verbal (agree, approval, humor), Positive Nonverbal (assent, laugh, positive physical contact, smile), Negative Verbal (complaint, criticize, deny responsibility, excuse, put down) and Negative Nonverbal (no response, not tracking, turn off). The MICS has gained most recognition as a pre- to postintervention comparison measure. However, preintervention MICS data are useful in developing a profile of each spouse's problem-solving skills as well as a compendium of how each spouse immediately responds to the partner's previous behavior.

Although the MICS can be used to code a wide range of situations, it has been applied primarily to 10-minute videotaped samples during which spouses strive to come to a resolution on each of two predetermined problem areas. Topics for these discussions are chosen so that both a major and minor conflict area are represented. It is often necessary for the therapist to assist the spouses in choosing topics that are couple issues, e.g., "how we express anger" rather than one spouse's personal gripe, e.g., "husband's temper." Once both topics have been defined the therapist leaves the room to simulate a more naturalistic discussion with-

	H		QU/PD		AT	QU/PD	QU/PD
	W	PD		PD		LA/PU	
	H	QU/PD		AT------------	------------	---IN/PD	QU/PD
	W		PU	NS	PS	CR	

FIGURE 1. One minute sample coding using the Marital Interaction Coding System. (From Weiss, R. L. Marital Interaction Coding System Manual, 1975).

out the intrusion of a third party. The two 10-minute discussions run consecutively with the therapist indicating, through a knock on the wall, when to begin and end each one. While the majority of couples report that this situation elicits behaviors that are similar to what they do at home, the possible effects created by this stimulus situation cannot be ignored: Spouses are committed to remaining in the room for the full 10 minutes, they must stop abruptly at the end of the 10-minute period, and they are aware of being observed and/or videotaped.

Figure 1 presents a 1-minute sample of MICS coding that was taken from the Marital Interaction Coding System Manual-Revised (Weiss, 1975, p. 5-6). Each of the two numbered bands of data represents 30-seconds of sequential coding. The 30-second intervals contain separate lines for husband's (H) and wife's (W) behaviors, which are indicated by the abbreviated codes (e.g., PD, QU). Observers code horizontally across the page within the 30-second intervals, alternating their focus between husband and wife. A new 30-second interval is indicated by a prerecorded beeping sound which signals the coders to move to the next line and to begin by recording a verbal code for the speaker and a nonverbal code for the listener. The topic of the sample displayed above is each spouse's dissatisfaction with the kinds of clothing selected by the other.

> "Mr. H. was of the opinion that Mrs. H spent too much time and money making herself presentable, while Mrs. H. felt that her husband was not sufficiently concerned with his appearance. At the end of the interview, the therapist asked the couple to discuss this problem for approximately 10 minutes, attempting to arrive at a resolution . . ."

The dialogue between spouses is presented below. MICS codes which are in parentheses correspond to the abbrevations in Figure 1.

She: And you wear clothes with holes in them. (*Problem Description*)

He: Why not? (*Question*) I don't think that really matters. (*Problem Description*)

She: (*neutral tone of voice*) Well, I think, I feel like it's a bit of a reflection on me. It bothers me to have you going around looking like that, wearing "holey" Levis. (*Problem Description*) (*he has been maintaining contact*) (*Attention*)

He: Why does it bother you? (*Question/Problem Description*)

She: (*said while giggling*) Because I don't think everyone in the world wants to look at your crotch. (*Laugh/Put Down*)

He: Well, ah, what about a hole in my knee? (*Question/Problem

Description) (*Beep sounds, indicating end of a 30-second interval*) Why does it bother you? (*Question/Problem Description*)

She: (*hostile tone of voice*) You just look like something the cat dragged in, or something. (*Put Down*) (*neutral tone of voice*) I'm not asking you to wear a suit, you know. (*Negative Solution*) I just want you to look clean, and . . . (*Positive Solution*) (*he has been attending*) (*Attention*)

He: (*interrupting*) I hope I do look clean. (*Interrupt/Problem Description*)

She: (*hostile tone*) Yeah, when you've got holes and old, faded cruddy, rotten "holey" Levis on. (*Criticize*)

He: What difference does that make? (*Question*) I don't think that makes any difference, no difference at all . . . (*Problem/Description*) (*beep sounds indicating end of 30-second interval*)

The MICS is the most widely used instrument for evaluating couple interactions and has been adapted to meet the needs of a variety of investigators (Follingstad et al., 1976; Heath, Kerns, Myskowski, & Haynes, 1977; Klier & Rothberg, 1977). Examination of the psychometric properties of the MICS reveals a somewhat mixed picture. Interobserver reliability has been reported to exceed minimum criterion levels of 70% agreement (Weiss et al., 1973) when coders are trained to that level and then continue to meet in weekly training sessions to maintain their high performance. Test-retest reliability measures between the two 10-minute samples have also been high (Margolin, 1978b). However, there have been no data reported on the reliability of individual codes. Validity studies on the MICS have shown that distressed couples, compared to nondistressed couples, engage in significantly fewer problem-solving statements and significantly more aversive behaviors (Vincent, Weiss, & Birchler, 1975). Pre- to postintervention comparisons using the MICS have indicated that couples increase their use of constructive problem-solving statements and reduce argumentative responses through the course of treatment (Patterson, Hops, & Weiss, 1974). However, in a recent investigation by O'Leary and Turkewitz (1978) the MICS did not prove to be a sensitive index of couples' improvement in therapy. In general, it is important to remember that MICS codes were not derived empirically; the relationship between MICS codes and effective problem-solving is still to be demonstrated.

Gottman has developed a coding system that was based in part on the MICS and is of equal complexity to that system (Gottman, Notarius, Gonso, & Markman, 1976). Gottman's system was designed to code both the content of each message and the nonverbal behavior that accompanies the message. The 22 content categories, which are coded from verbatim transcripts, have been a priori classified into eight summary codes: Agreement, Disagreement, Mind Reading, Problem Solving, Problem Talk/Feeling, Communication Talk, Summarizing Self, and Summarizing Other. To code nonverbal behaviors, the coders jointly scan the transcripts and videotapes for positive or negative facial expressions, positive or negative voice tone cues, and positive or negative body position and movements. Gottman et al. (1976, p. xix-xx) illustrated their dual coding with this example: "In the following sequence the wife's statement would usually be coded as a disagreement in the context following the husband's proposal because it apparently functions to disagree with the husband's idea of how to spend the vacation.

H: Let's spend Christmas at your mother's.
W: You always get tense at my mother's.

We code that message as a mind-reading statement (MR) by which we mean she is attributing feelings (or thoughts, motive, and actions) to her husband. We have found that all couples mind-read but that the nonverbal delivery of the mind-reading statement determines whether it gets seen as a sensitive feeling probe or as a criticism." Gottman's system, which attempts to determine the function of a statement within its context, differs from MICS coding, which does not presume knowledge of spouses' intentions. Interobserver reliabilities with the Gottman system are 85% for nonverbal behaviors and 91% for content codes. Interestingly, Gottman reported that, except for the agreement category, content codes alone do not discriminate well between distressed and nondistressed couples. But combining nonverbal codes with the content codes produces a powerful discrimination.

Overall, the coding of negotiation samples holds a great deal of appeal for clinicians who regard communication process as very important in couple interactions. It is necessary to note, however, that the coding systems are based primarily on assumptions of the clinician/researcher as to what constitutes effective communication. Assumptions of this sort are finally beginning to be explored more systematically through comparisons of distressed and nondistressed couples and through explorations of the association between problem-solving skills and marital adjustment.

As previously mentioned, MICS summary scores discriminate distressed and nondistressed couples (Vincent et al., 1975), but individual codes have not been examined for this. The Gottman, Markman, and Notarius (1977) findings reveal significant differences between distressed and nondistressed couples in rate of agreement, regardless of affect, and in rates of feeling expression, mind-reading, and disagreements, all with negative affect. However, no differences were found for problem-solving statements or metacommunicative statements. A recent study by Klier and Rothberg (1977) found that distressed, compared to nondistressed, couples make more references to unrelated issues, emit more nonfacilitative behaviors (complaint, criticism, and disagree) and express emotions less frequently. Contrary to expectations, there were no differences between the samples in frequencies of trait descriptions, specific behavioral descriptions, or general facilitative behaviors (approval, accept responsibility, problem solution, and humor). In one other exploration, out of the seven behaviors expected to discriminate conflict and accord, only volume, criticism, disagreement and sarcasm were accurate discriminants; swearing, rate of speech and gestures were not (Resnick, Sweet, Kieffer, Barr, & Ruby, 1977). These studies, which represent initial steps in the empirical exploration of what constitutes effective problem-solving, indicate that only a portion of the behaviors assumed important to communication effectiveness do indeed discriminate distressed and nondistressed samples.

Studies that examine the relationship between problem-solving skills and overall marital adjustment are even more unsettling. These studies have not demonstrated a strong correlation between specific behaviors coded by an outside observer and subjective impressions of marital satisfaction (Heath et al., 1977; Follingstad et al., 1976; Margolin, 1978b; Robinson & Price, 1976).

However, these findings do not necessarily mean that the assessment of communication skills is a misguided endeavor. Even if problem-solving and other communication skills are not always the identifying feature for marital discord, effective communication may be an important factor in the distressed couple's attempts to remedy their situation. To work successfully on their problems, distressed couples may need to utilize skills that are beyond the repertoire of the average couple. The assessment of problem-solving samples informs the clinician of the behavioral excesses and deficits that might impede a couple's attempts to resolve relationship issues.

The same types of negotiation samples that have been coded by trained others have also been coded by the spouses themselves. While the spouses could be trained in the same observational procedures that the outside observers employ, there would be few gains in training spouses to provide the same data that can be retrieved more profitably by trained coders. Thus, the rationale for spouse coding is to assess the nuances of meaning that spouses assign to their own interchanges that may be uninterpretable to an outside observer. Spouse coding of negotiation samples is based on the possibility that the perceived valence of an interaction may be idiosyncratic to a couple and not based on researchers' stereotypes of effective communication.

Gottman, Notarius, Markman, Bank, Yoppi, and Rubin (1976) built a "talk table" which allowed spouses to code ongoing communication along a 5-point Likert scale (1-supernegative; 5-superpositive). Spouses coded the valence of both the Impact of the behavior received and the Intent of the behavior exhibited. The Gottman et al. results suggest that it is possible to discriminate distressed from nondistressed couples on the basis of the impact but not the intent of spouses' statements. That is, although both distressed and nondistressed spouses had intended to send the same number of positive statements, distressed, compared to nondistressed, spouses reported that they received fewer positive messages. Margolin (1978a) also built an electromechanical system for the purpose of having spouses code their own and their partners' communication positiveness. Observations were made during videotaped playbacks of ten minute negotiation sessions so that the spouses did not have to code their behavior while simultaneously participating in the conversation. Data on a sample of distressed couples revealed very low agreement between spouses on the total frequency of positive behaviors exhibited by either partner. This perceptual inconsistency between partners could be the result of: (1) spouses' different views of what constitutes communication helpfulness (e.g., husband views his question as information-seeking while wife views it as a way for him to avoid giving a straight answer to her question) or (2) spouses' difficulties in observing the process versus the content of communication (i.e., they become emotionally involved in the content of their discussions and forget to make process observations).

In evaluating the utility of having spouses code their own negotiation sessions, we must assume that spouses' observations are colored by subjective impressions since each observer has more than a cursory interest in the outcome. Similar to the types of self and spouse coding we discussed previously, these assessment procedures, which also involve participant observation, are subject to reliability and reactivity problems. Yet these procedures were purposefully designed to sacrifice coding accuracy to gain access to spouses' judgmental evaluations regarding their attempts to negotiate change. The perceptual inaccuracies between spouses that surface within the context of these assessment procedures are indicative of the divergent expectations that the partners hold regarding how they should negotiate change. Armed with data from these assessment procedures, the therapist has an index of the work to be done to help spouses develop mutually acceptable negotiation skills. It is our impression that spouse coding procedures hold a great deal of promise as a method for developing intervention goals on the basis of the couple's perceptions of their own problem-solving needs. However, the ability of these procedures to generate useful outcome data is greatly compromised by their methodological shortcomings. In planning an overall assessment strategy, it is best to combine spouses' coding of their own and their partners' negotiation skills with more objective coding procedures.

RECOMMENDATIONS

From this review of specific assessment instruments, it is evident that there are numerous procedures available to assess marital functioning. The recent proliferation of behavioral marital assessment instruments has been a natural accompaniment to the rapid development of behavioral marital treatment programs. At the same time that we see the need for still additional assessment procedures, we hope that these are not developed at the expense of the procedures that already exist. There is a strong need for further data regarding the reliability, validity, and reactivity of measures currently in use; the ultimate capacities of many of these instruments are simply not known. It is also necessary for assessment procedures to be tested on broader population samples. The true merit of these procedures will be evidenced only after they are further tested by persons other than their originators and with populations other than those upon which they were initially evaluated.

Future Directions

Earlier in this chapter we alluded to the fact that several of the possible options for assessing marriages have received no attention. Let us examine two of these options more closely. As you may recall, our list of observer sources included significant others who are close to but outside of the marital partnership. Possible observers in this category include other members of a couple's household, neighbors, friends, or work associates. There are obvious ethical considerations with this suggestion and the observations could only be made with full knowledge and consent of the couple. The therapist would need to discuss fully the potential liabilities associated with "airing one's dirty laundry" to public inspection. Yet, marital problems are rarely well concealed. It is not uncommon for friends and relatives to find they are unintentional witnesses to a couple's problems. It is likely that these observers could make a valuable contribution to the assessment picture, particularly if their observations were systematically communicated to the therapist. If the couple agreed to this type of observation, feedback from these persons could become a meaningful source of support and reinforcement for the couple's effort in therapy.

The assessment question of how spouses attempt to bring about change in one another has also received somewhat limited attention. Although this information is critical to the social learning approach, assessment of this question has been restricted to brief, staged negotiation discussions. Yet the evolution of a couple's patterns of relationship change spans a much broader time frame and involves a wider range of behaviors than these assessment situations permit. An adequate description would necessitate information regarding: (1) who makes what requests, demands, threats, etc., and (2) what is the partner's immediate and eventual response. These types of information could only be obtained through data collection that is of long duration and that occurs in the home. However, the home observations conducted thus far have been for brief time periods, and have sampled only limited periods of the day. In addition, it is likely that the observers' presence acted as an obtrusive influence for the couples. To alleviate these problems, Patterson et al. (1976) recommended the use of tape recorders in the home that would automatically activate at certain decibel levels or at timed intervals, or that could be mechanically activated by the couple. The advantages of these methods is their capability to collect data at frequent intervals, for indeterminate time lengths, at varied time periods and without having to introduce a stranger in the couple's house. Although these procedures have not yet been used for marital assessment, they have been used by family therapists to assess parent-child interactions (cf. Bernal, Gibson, Williams, & Pesses, 1971; Christensen, in press; Johnson, Christensen & Bellamy, 1976).

Choosing an Assessment Strategy

In light of the large number of available assessment instruments, the clinician faces the task of choosing a subset of these to use. We recommend approaching this decision from the perspective of formulating an overall assessment strategy and choosing instruments that complement each other. This overall strategy should contain an array of instruments that provide some information on each of the four basic assessment questions and that sample a variety of assessment methodologies. This strategy should include formalized instruments to obtain reliable data on the basis of standardized norms, as well as tailor-made procedures to measure progress on couples' idiosyncratic concerns. While the therapist's strongest evidence for therapeutic change comes from the formalized procedures, couples' evaluations of treatment effectiveness rest upon the individualized measurements.

The clinician's ultimate choice of which procedures to adopt hinges on the practical issues of cost and utility. Unfortunately, there is somewhat of a trade-off between procedures that are methodologically desirable and procedures that are efficient to administer. Procedures that necessitate a corps of trained observers and elaborate recording equipment are very time-consuming and expensive to implement. However, some of these procedures can be redesigned for greater practicality. For example, audiotaping a couple's negotiation sessions either in the counseling session or at home requires a minimum of effort. Even without the benefit of a formal coding system, observations of actual samples of interaction are more informative than asking couples to recreate the situation in their own words. Samples of behavior that can be directly viewed or heard by the therapist provide the opportunity for assessment of specific skill deficits. While spouses may recognize their lack of success in problem-solving discussions, they are often unable to articulate the missing skills. Thus, even informal observations of actual behavior samples are a useful adjunct to spouses' own descriptions.

Despite the methodological limitations of spouses' observations of themselves and their partners, these are the most frequently used data collection procedures in marital assessment. A benefit of these procedures is their flexibility in terms of setting. They are applicable in any setting where the spouses can directly observe one another's behavior (e.g., at parties, in the store) or where they are knowledgeable about the partner's actions without having directly observed them (e.g., the husband knows that his wife did the laundry even though he did not see her do it). Administration and interpretation of these measurements are relatively straightforward. Compared to questionnaires or interview information, these data have direct applicability to a behavioral treatment and provide a constant mechanism for feedback on therapy effectiveness.

However, these data collection procedures are only of use when measurements are made at frequent intervals and repeated over time. Since there are no norms, each datum point derives meaning only in comparison to other data points by the same individual. By observing these data points for trends over time, one can discern whether behavior change is related to specific therapeutic interventions or to factors that are extraneous to therapy. This type of repeated measurement can also determine whether improvement maintains beyond the specific intervention or whether the behaviors return to their preintervention rates. A precise method for measuring the correspondence between change in a particular behavior and the application of a specific intervention is the multiple baseline approach (cf. Hersen & Barlow, 1976). In the multiple baseline approach, several behaviors that have been identified for change are simultaneously observed over time. The clinician then applies an intervention that is intended to change only one of these behaviors and notes the effect on all the behaviors. This sequence is repeated until the intervention has been applied to all behaviors. At each stage the one behavior intended for change should show that effect while all the others remain constant. It is only then that the therapist can attribute change to the specific therapeutic intervention. To the clinician whose primary goal is the couple's improvement, these procedures may appear superfluous. What is the importance of knowing the specific point at which change occurred as long as improvement can be verified? There are two reasons. It is valuable for the therapist to learn what specific procedures marked the onset of change; this knowledge can function to make that person's work with that couple and other couples more effective. Secondly, the knowledge of what specific procedures worked provides the couple with a strategy for resolving similar situations that arise in the future.

Relative to observations by an outside observer or by the spouses, questionnaires and interviews offer the least objective and specific information. When compared at pre- and postintervention periods, they furnish a subjective index of spouses' perceptions of improvement but do not reveal what accounts for the change. Preintervention data collected through these methods provide the therapist with many clues about what is troubling a particular couple and what would be a satisfactory treatment outcome. These clues direct the therapist to the marital areas that require further exploration through more objective measurement procedures.

An additional consideration in choosing among assessment procedures is the specific abilities that spouses bring to the therapy session. Basic literacy skills are, of course, essential to pencil and paper measurements. A fluent reader who is familiar with the SOC can complete that inventory in less than fifteen minutes. For a slower reader who requires an hour to complete that same task, the SOC will soon become highly aversive.

In designing assessment procedures to suit a particular couple, the capabilities of both spouses must be considered. For example, the assessment of specific cognitive events works well for some couples but not for others. Spouses who are introspective about their marital relationship may find it both easy and therapeutic to record their relationship thoughts. Once they record a thought on paper they may no longer need to ruminate about it. However, other spouses who are less aware of discrete thoughts find it difficult to record cognitions and do not follow through on such tasks. It is important for the therapist to know enough about a couple to judge whether a particular assessment procedure will be unduly difficult or discouraging to the persons.

There is one final guideline in choosing an assessment strategy. Our strong emphasis on assessment is based on an important premise: Assessment procedures should be used only if they are benign or beneficial to the couple. Assessment should not put the clients in a situation that will cause them additional emotional pain or result in an intensification of their marital problems.

How to Elicit Cooperation Regarding Assessment

Some of the assessment procedures of choice from the therapist's point of view require a substantial commitment on the part of the couple. Spouses' reactions to the assessment procedures are largely dependent on the therapist's attitudes towards assessment and how these are conveyed to the clients. The two therapist dimensions, enthusiasm and confidence, which are important in the initial stages of therapy are equally important in eliciting cooperation in regard to assessment. The therapist must be enthusiastic about each assessment task, stressing its utility and its intrinsic interest to the participant. The therapist must also feel confident that what is being requested of the clients is, indeed, essential to the treatment process. The following statement is an example of how to communicate the purpose of assessment to clients:

> I need to learn as much as possible about you, and about your lives together so that I can plan a treatment that will meet your specific needs. As soon as I've collected the information necessary to plan effective treatment, I will share my perceptions with you as well as the ways that I think we can resolve some of these problems.

Even with a full explanation, clients may not differentiate between assessment and treatment. This distinction is necessary only so that couples do not get discouraged when two weeks of assessment have elapsed and there has been minimal or no change.

In presenting a couple with an explanation of the preintervention assessment procedures, it is best to be realistic and empathetic about the amount of effort required, but firm about needing the information as a prerequisite to the next stage of therapy. Making the contingency clear that therapy will continue only after the preintervention data have been collected will increase the probability of receiving that information. The therapist's firmness in this regard functions to reassure clients about the therapist's expertise and increases the clients' commitment to produce accurate data.

Therapist firmness in requiring participation during the assessment can also function as a precedent for the therapist control that will follow during treatment. By retreating from a request for assessment data, the therapist diminishes the impact of his/her future requests. We encountered one couple who suddenly refused to choose topics for their ten minute negotiation sessions. Although these discussions had been described as problem-solving sessions, the couple heard the instructions for this task as an invitation for conflict. Indeed, this couple had such a high frequency of arguments that they had called a moratorium on the discussion of any problem areas. However, knowing this was a controlled situation that could be discontinued if it became destructive for the couple, the therapists held firm. They stressed that the purpose of these discussions was for the couple to do everything in their power to avoid arguments and strive towards problem resolution. In addition, the couple was encouraged to choose topics on which they could profit by a brief discussion. The couple did engage in the negotiation sessions. Although they showed high rates of coercive behaviors, they completed these sessions feeling that they had accomplished more during that talk than they had during discussions that occurred in the past several years. Insisting upon the negotiation discussions with this couple was necessary for baseline data as well as for establishing the expectation that therapy requires new, sometimes risky, interactions.

When it is finally time for postintervention assessment, the therapist must present a rationale that differs from the one used at preintervention. Posttreatment assessment is beneficial as feedback to the therapist but less necessary from the couple's perspective. In requesting clients to repeat the preintervention assessment tasks, the therapist should offer to hold an additional session with the couple to review the assessment findings. Feedback to the couple that compares their pre- and posttest data can be quite valuable in reinforcing their progress.

Summary

Assessment is equally important to both the therapist and the couple since it functions to chart the course of the therapeutic intervention. Although the necessity for assessment may be clear to the therapist, the couple who is uninitiated to therapy procedures cannot be expected to understand its function. Thus, it is important for the therapist to communicate his/her intentions regarding assessment and to establish some realistic expectations about this aspect of treatment. It is equally important for the therapist to reinforce the clients for their efforts. The couple will come to view assessment as a necessary and integral part of their therapy if the data are indeed treated that way by the therapist. Therapist actions convey this message more forcefully than words or explanations. The forthcoming chapters on specific treatment procedures illustrate how assessment information is used to shape the formulation of a treatment strategy.

CHAPTER 5

Persuasion, Influence, and the Collaborative Set: The Nonspecifics of Marital Therapy

CONTRIBUTIONS to the behavioral marital therapy literature have been oriented toward a description of the technology of behavior change. A number of papers have discussed communication training and problem-solving (Jacobson, 1977c, 1977d; O'Leary & Turkewitz, 1978), contingency contracting (Weiss, Birchler, & Vincent, 1974), or have provided summaries of behavior change technology (Eisler & Hersen, 1973; Liberman, 1976; Liberman et al., 1976; Rappaport & Harrell, 1972; Weiss et al., 1973). Recently, Thomas (1977) has devoted an entire book to the technology of training couples in communication and decision-making skills. We will also elaborate extensively on the technological aspects of various behavior change procedures (Chapters 6-9). Indeed, the ability of behavior therapists to describe their clinical strategies in clear, discrete, specific terms is one of its supreme advantages. This capacity for specification greatly facilitates communication between therapists, simplifies the training of new clinicians, and minimizes the difficulty of replicating the outcome research of others. The assertion that technology has served behavior therapy well is indisputable.

However, technology must be delivered in some context, and it is the description of context that is lost between the lines of publications about technology. The presentation of direct behavior change procedures is only a portion of what transpires during a therapy session. As Goldfried and Davison (1976) explained, "We're continually impressed by the distance between written descriptions of behavior therapy and what occurs in practice" (p. vii). The nontechnological transactions between therapist and couple will in large part determine whether or not couples respond favorably to the technology. How services are delivered, when they are delivered, and what transpires during therapy sessions *in addition* to this delivery will collectively mediate the couple's response to a treatment program. *Our guess is that the most common determinants of treatment failures are not the inappropriate or ineffectual use of technology, but the inability on the part of the therapist to provide a context conducive to the clients' reception of his intervention.* To begin with, the behavior therapist's task is exceedingly difficult if the couple does not accept the validity of a behavioral exchange framework for their particular relationship problems. Since this model is not one that is typically adopted by people in our culture to explain relationships, it cannot be assumed that the framework will be accepted without a strategic effort by the therapist to encourage it. At the very least a couple must be willing to behave *as if* the model were appropriate for them.

A consideration related to these perceptions is the clients' willingness to commit themselves to a course of therapy: behaving in accordance with the therapist's instructions, collecting data at home, engaging in a variety of practice exercises between therapy sessions, and the like. An initial commitment to this rather arduous endeavor will greatly facilitate subsequent tolerance of costly expenditures in time and effort.

Both the adoption of the therapist's perspective and the willingness to render a commitment to intensive therapy can be related to a more general construct which is often bandied about among clinical theoreticians: *client expectancies.* To the extent that clients *expect* to be helped, the probability that they *will be* helped is greatly enhanced. For one thing, positive expectancies can alleviate early session anxiety, an outcome which is therapeutic in and of itself. In addition, positive expectancies affect the process of therapy, and thereby exert an indirect influence on outcome. For example, compliance with homework assignments is more likely if the couple is optimistic regarding the potential benefits of therapy.

Positive client expectancies are related not only to the perceived credibility of the treatment paradigm, but also to client perceptions of the therapist as a competent expert who is capable of helping them. Furthermore, the therapist must be perceived as someone who cares about the future of both the relationship and the two individuals who have entered into the relationship. The first section of this chapter discusses various clinical strategies for inducing and maintaining positive expectancies, by influencing couples' confidence in the treatment strategy and their trust in the person delivering the treatment approach to them.

Much of the technology used by the behavior therapist in marital therapy assumes that the couple has adopted a *collaborative set.* By this we mean that both spouses must conduct themselves as if they viewed their relationship difficulties as a common problem which can be solved only if they work together. Couples seldom enter therapy with this set. Instead they typically view therapy as a way to demonstrate to the partner and to themselves that they are blameless, and that the other is at fault; or at best, they view unilateral change on the other's part as the primary prerequisite to an improved relationship. A collaborative set will usually not emerge without the therapist's direct efforts to induce it. The second major section of this chapter is devoted to a consideration of strategies for establishing a collaborative set.

Although the emphasis throughout the entire book is on modifying relationship *behavior,* the alteration of couples' thoughts and attitudes also plays an important, if less easily specified, role in therapy. The creation of a collaborative set is one example of desirable cognitive changes which can facilitate behavior change. Others include helping couples relabel the causes of relationship problems, and altering their unrealistic expectations about the relationship. The third section of this chapter discusses cognitive restructuring as a tool in behavioral marital therapy, and also considers the advantages and disadvantages of devoting considerable time in therapy to modifying belief systems rather than overt behavior.

In the final section of the chapter, we discuss the use of "paradox" in marital therapy from a behavioral perspective. Paradoxical or strategic interventions (Haley, 1963; Haley, 1976; Sluzki, 1978) are widely publicized, and used as the primary therapeutic tactics by communication-systems therapists. Certain types of strategic intervention are consistent with a behavioral perspective, and our discussion will include examples of situations where paradoxical interventions can be facilitative within a broad-spectrum behavioral approach.

Underlying this chapter is a theme regarding the importance of therapist qualities even in a structured technological approach: The therapist actively orchestrates and directs the change process in behavioral marital therapy, and it is through his/her influence that technology has an effect. The therapist is in an almost unique position to influence the future of a relationship, and to quote, in a slightly distorted way, a basic dictum of communication theory, "A therapist cannot *not* influence." It is our belief that successful therapy requires the effective use of direct influence, and that the therapist who is unwilling to accept this legacy will be unsuccessful in helping couples. Moreover, the therapist must exude enthusiasm and confidence in his/her approach, or he/she cannot expect an enthusiastic response from the clients. In this sense, therapist expectancies are as important as client expectancies, since the former are important mediators of the latter.

Of all the chapters in this volume, this one is the most speculative. The suggestions we make and the strategies we recommend are largely unsupported by any experimental research. Thus, we remind the reader that she/he must be cautious in accepting the validity of these suggestions. However, we have found these tactics to be helpful in our clinical work with couples, and continue to note the unsuccessful endeavors of therapists who expect technology to work in a vacuum.

THE CREATION AND MAINTENANCE OF POSITIVE EXPECTANCIES

By asserting that a client's expectations regarding the likelihood of a positive therapy outcome influence actual outcome, we imply nothing magical. It is not as if a couple somehow interacts more positively or enjoys sexual activity to greater degrees as a direct consequence of confidence in the therapist or the therapy program. However, positive outcome expectancies may increase the likelihood of other events which do exert a direct influence on outcome. First, for spouses who are considering whether the investment of therapy is worthwhile, surely their predictions regarding the likelihood that substantial benefits will accrue influence whether or not the decision will be affirmative. Second, outcome expectations may affect the couple's tendency to comply with the therapist's instructions. Again, the investment inherent in costly behavior changes and engaging in difficult homework assignments between therapy sessions is more likely to occur if, from the vantage point of the investor, the potential benefits outweigh the costs. Third, as long as outcome expectancies remain high, persistence in the face of adverse circumstances remains likely. Often progress in marital therapy is nonlinear, and evidence to contradict both therapist's and couple's optimism occurs periodically. Clients who continue to experience positive expectations will not be as easily dissuaded by such unfortunate downswings. In all of these cases, expectancies seem to act as cues for responding in a way which is necessary for therapy to be successful; thus, expectancies mediate improvement in an indirect way. Moreover, as we briefly mentioned earlier, positive expectancies can reduce anxiety in both partners, and thereby provide direct therapeutic benefit. Anxiety about the future of the relationship, anxiety about possible separation from the mate, and feelings of hopelessness are ubiquitous concomitants of a distressed relationship. To the extent that positive expectancies in early stages of therapy mitigate these reactions, some immediate benefit has been provided. This anxiety reduction in turn often leads to an even more optimistic stance regarding the ultimate outcome of therapy.

In discussing ways to desirably affect couple expectancies, we will begin by looking at the earlier stages of therapy, and the opportunities for the therapist to sell the couple on the treatment and its potential benefits. The client who buys into the paradigm invests more in therapy. Then we will examine some more general ways to maintain expectancies during subsequent stages.

Establishing the Credibility of the Treatment Program

Couples who enter a therapist's office for the first contact almost always experience at least a moderate amount of anxiety and disorientation. The prospect of confiding in a stranger is sufficient to elicit apprehension, particularly in those rather common instances where the couple has habitually hidden their problems from their friends and relatives, indeed often from each other. Added to this apprehension is anxiety generated by the unknown territory of the therapist's office: What is this person going to be like? What are we going to have to do? How long will it take? At times couples enter therapy with expectations based on their own previous experiences in therapy, knowledge they have acquired from the media, and experiences that their friends have had. Often, the expectations are dominated by misconceptions. Other couples enter with minimal expectations and therefore with even more uncertainty. In essence, it is generally unpleasant to be on the brink of this odyssey of marital therapy, and couples are prone to developing strong impressions, rendering early judgments as to the desirability of engagement in the endeavor crucial.

Couples are, in other words, very tentative when the initial contact begins. They are certainly not committed to therapy; for this reason most couples do not respond positively to immediate, unexplained therapeutic intervention. We recommend that the therapist immediately reassure the client that, despite their presence at this intake interview, they have not committed themselves to a therapy regimen; as we suggest in Chapter 3, by delineating a period of time reserved for "evaluation," and by presenting them with an overview of the assessment process, the therapist helps the couple relax, because their tentativeness has been endorsed, indeed it has been reciprocated, by the therapist. By presenting a summary of the evaluation procedures to be occurring during the next two-three weeks, he alleviates much of the initial disorientation. The couple now knows what to expect at least in the immediate future. Thus, the couple can be made to feel better almost instantly, and their first reaction to therapy and to the therapist can be an exceedingly positive one. If the therapist then conducts an initial interview which follows the guidelines suggested in Chapter 3, thereby encouraging some "positive tracking," the couple is likely to leave the initial encounter more committed to therapy than when they entered the office.

A noteworthy consequence of behavioral assessment is that couples are often impressed by it as a thorough, exhaustive undertaking. As couples learn that they will be assessed from a myriad of vantage points, and that the assessment will be systematic, marital therapy is likely to be initially perceived as credible. When this initial demonstration of professional sophistication is combined with anxiety reduction associated with the factors mentioned above, therapy has made an auspicious debut.

Within the process of assessment, precautions should be taken to minimize stress. By grading the intrusiveness of the assessment procedures, the therapist allows them to confront the important issues in their relationship gradually. It is generally true that self-report inventories produce less stress than live communication assessment, especially if videotape is used. Therefore, we usually reserve the assessment of a couple's communication skills for the last phase of evaluation. As we have already mentioned in Chapters 2-4, couples often receive some additional benefits from the completion of self-report inventories that encourage positive tracking and foster the acknowledgment of relationship strengths as well as the identification of problem areas.

The interpretive meeting which follows the assessment phase is critical to the establishment of positive expectancies. Couples should leave that session with a clear understanding of how the therapists view their relationship, a reasonable overview of the structure of therapy, and feelings of optimism about the potential benefits to be derived from therapy. Finally, they should have verbally committed themselves to the program of therapy.

We have found it useful to structure this session by presenting a couple with a formulation of their relationship, based on all of the assessment data collected. Then, after delineating our view of both the strengths and problem areas of the relationship, and suggesting some of the possible antecedents for the latter, we present the couple with our proposed treatment plan for helping them improve their relationship, including an estimate of the length of therapy. Finally, the session ends with a mutual decision as to whether marital therapy will be pursued.

In presenting the structure of this session, we wish to emphasize three important themes which are consistent with the goals of establishing treatment credibility and generating positive expectancies. First, couples' strengths should be emphasized, along with their problems. We discuss relationship strengths *first*. Again, couples' tendency to notice only the problems in the relationship creates the risk that when these problems are enumerated in therapy, an improved relationship will seem a hopeless task. An equally thorough enumeration of strengths will aid them in maintaining a realistic perspective on the current state of the relationship, and may even remind them of positive dimensions which they had been ignoring. Second, the therapist should express, both by the content of his/her speech and in the style of presentation, confidence regarding the possibilities for improvement, without encouraging the perception that the therapist will do it for them. *That is, the therapist is encouraging them to be optimistic while at the same time emphasizing that an improved relationship is ultimately their responsibility, and will require an intensive and sustained effort on their part.* Third, in the presentation of both relationship analysis and treatment plan, it is incumbent upon the therapist to adapt the theoretical framework to the couple's situation, rather than fitting the couple into a rigid theoretical framework. A treatment plan is much more credible if it follows logically from the couple's problems than if the model assumes primacy, and it appears that the couple's problems are being adapted to it. Each of these themes will now be discussed in detail.

I. *The emphasis on relationship strengths.* Below, the transcript of a portion of a first therapy session is reproduced, to illustrate the integration of relationship strengths with marital problems.

T: One thing that I want to emphasize is that in many ways you two have, in my view, a very strong relationship. It may not feel that way to you now, but you are paying attention mostly to the problems. From my perspective you have a basically positive and loving marriage, and our task will be to build from this solid foundation. And that is exciting for me, and it should be to you, because it gives us a lot of room for optimism.

W: I'm not feeling very positive about it right now.

T: Of course you're not. You're both unhappy and angry at each other, and your problems are real and significant. But I think it's also important to recognize that you have a lot going for you. For example, on the forms you were both able to list 10 things the other person does that please you. Coming up with ten things is no easy task even for happy couples.

W: It wasn't easy (*laughs*).

T: Have you looked at each other's lists yet?

W: No (*husband shakes head*).

T: Let me read Helen's list of things that John does that please her. John, Helen said that you are a good father, that you help around the house, that you make a good living, that you are gentle, that you can be a good lover when you want to be, that you are good-looking, intelligent, that you are careful not to awaken her in the morning, that you walk the dog. I guess that was where you started having trouble thinking of things—(*both John and Helen laugh*), and that John pays the bills on time.

(Then the therapist reads John's list of things Helen does that please him.)

T: You also were able to mention a number of common interests, which shows that there are still a number of things you like to do, such as sailing, going out to eat, going to the theater, and so on. You still enjoy each other's company, at least sometimes. And you sleep together at least three times a week, with no complaints, right?

H: No, we used to have sex problems, but we've pretty much worked them out. Sex is not a major bone of contention.

T: OK, and when I sent you home last week to collect data, you brought me back mostly good days. There was really only one bad day last week. That day was terrible, and we'll get to that, but the rest of the days were all at least average, and some of them are good.

H: Yeah, I guess that our problem isn't that we constantly fight, but that when we fight we really destroy each other.

T: Yes, you do, you fight destructively with each other. And we're going to talk about that. But again, let's take your communication. Except on those rare occasions when you're mad at each other, you have some nice things going. You're seldom abusive, and even when you disagree you're usually kind to each other. So, all in all, I think there is a lot of good stuff going on, more good stuff than bad. Helen, are you surprised that I'm saying this?

W: Yeah, I am. I've been thinking that it's hopeless for two months. I don't know. I'm going to have to think about what you've said but it's true that I have been ignoring all of John's nice qualities. You really are a wonderful person. Everyone else thinks so. And I always used to think so. And he's great with Jason (3 year old son). And I guess we still have a lot going for us. But Dr. X., why not just find someone whom you don't have to go through all this shit with? Why bother working hard like this, when there are probably people out there who could more easily give us what we want. We're just so different . . .

H: That's her new thing, now. She never used to say we're different. In fact, she used to talk about how much alike we were.

T: Well, I just want you both to realize that there is some reason to be optimistic. You seem to be asking an important question. You could be rid of all of these problems. You could just get out. And you have to decide whether improving things is worth the struggle. I see some indication that it is. And I think you do too.

H: Well, I've always felt that way. I think Helen's just seeing the grass is always greener on the other side.

W: Just coming here is showing me that all is not bad. The forms helped me think about things a different way. So yeah, that's why we're here. It's just that sometimes I wonder. And if this doesn't work I don't think we'll have any questions, or at least I won't.

In a great majority of cases, there are significant areas of strength in a relationship, in addition to the problems that brought the couple into therapy. These should be enumerated, and the enumeration should be precise and specific. In the above example, the therapist specifically asked for a reaction from the wife, because her response to his elaboration of strengths was more questionable, since she was less committed to the relationship at that point. *Also, it is important not to imply that the couple's perception of their problems is invalid; the reality of their suffering must be acknowledged, even as their strengths are being emphasized.*

The therapist must remain flexible, however, since this type of introduction is not applicable to all couples. For example, a couple in their mid-fifties who had been married for 27 years exhibited few notable relationship strengths. Their severe difficulties had existed since the beginning of their marriage, and had continued unabated for its entire duration. Rather than negative tracking, this couple exhibited a relative complacency about their problems, as if to say, "miserable as we are, this is what life is like." The wife in particular had been extremely tentative about marital therapy, and the referral came about primarily as the result of a severe depressive reaction on her part. Instead of emphasizing the strengths of the relationship (which were virtually nonexistent), this couple needed to be jolted out of their complacency. The therapist's introductory remarks in the interpretive session are indicative of the differences between this session and the one described above:

T: We've been spending time putting together a lot of information, and I am very concerned about both of you. You have some very serious problems as a couple, and for many years now these problems have made it difficult for either of you to lead normal, happy lives. Now you've reached a critical point in your lives. You have a unique opportunity to do something about your situation. If you decide to do nothing, it's a good bet that you will both continue to be unhappy for the rest of your lives. I strongly urge you not to choose doing nothing. You could also break up as you've (*directed to the husband*) been suggesting. That would give both of you a chance, although it would be difficult for you, and it would be lonely at least for awhile. Or you can both say to yourselves, "Dammit I am going to do something about this relationship," and you can commit all of the energy you can muster to changing things. And believe me, it will take more work than anything you've ever done before. And even then I don't know if I can help you. It is hard to change after 27 years. But in my judgment there is a reasonable chance for the relationship if you both work your tails off to change things. I'm talking about hard, intense work. Working hard during sessions, working hard between sessions, devoting your lives for a few months to improving the relationship.

W: But Dr., we have seen positively the worst marriages in captivity, and everyone has thought of us as a happy couple for most of our marriage. We know we have problems but we've been able to tolerate them all this time, and I've seen so much worse. Do you really think it's worth it to try to teach two old dogs new tricks?

H: It's always been this bad (*very uncharacteristic of the husband*). The Dr. is right. Pat just doesn't face reality. My bags are half-packed, that's the only reason she's here.

T: Pat, it is awfully scary to imagine something changing after 27 years. And it is even scarier to imagine the thing ending. I know that. It's terrifying. But I think Harold is right. You look through the relationship in rose colored glasses. You almost needed to be hospitalized last week. Your husband is depressed. Believe me, you are both good people. You deserve better than this relationship as it currently exists.

(The rest of the session was spent pinpointing the specific problem areas, and discussing the reciprocal nature of their aversive exchanges.)

The above example describes a fairly atypical situation, and is mentioned primarily to illustrate the dangers of a preprogrammed rationale which fails to take individual differences between couples into account. With a great majority of couples, an emphasis on strengths during the interpretive session is clinically indicated.

II. *Personalization of the theoretical rationale.* In presenting couples with an analysis of their relationship problems, and the proposals for treating those problems, it is important that the idiographic nature of the formulation be emphasized so that it is clear to the couple that the treatment plan is a function of their own personal needs. In contrast, by emphasizing the theoretical model rather than the couple, it appears to the couple that the therapists are adhering rigidly to a theory, and not altering the model to fit their needs. The treatment is likely to be perceived as less credible in the latter case. Consider the following explanation, presented to a couple near the beginning of the interpretive session:

> *T*: The treatment program for couples that we use here is based on the principles of social learning and behavior exchange. Research in other areas of psychology has pretty well convinced us that marital happiness can be best understood by looking at the daily exchanges of rewarding and punishing behavior between spouses. If a couple is unhappy, you find that they are not rewarding each other much, or they are punishing each other a lot in their day-to-day interaction. The best way to help them seems to be to help them learn more effective ways of rewarding each other and. . . .

In this example, the therapist's theory is determining the treatment approach and there is little reference to the specific relevance of this approach for the couple in question. The instructions could have been recorded and presented routinely to all couples who came through the marital therapy clinic. It seems to belie the intensive assessment which preceded it. Couples are likely to feel processed, and this may negatively alter their perceptions of the credibility of the treatment.

Certainly we *are* presenting a theoretical model of marital therapy, and we are suggesting that the model contains sufficient flexibility and comprehensiveness to be applicable to a wide variety of relationship problems. But it is also true that there is room for remarkable diversity in treatment plans, depending on the particular difficulties that a couple brings into therapy. Couples are likely to adopt a more committed posture when the extent to which the treatment plan follows directly from the evaluation is conveyed to them. The effectiveness with which this relationship between assessment and treatment is communicated depends on the points that are emphasized in the therapist's presentation. In the above example, the theory is emphasized, and the individualized nature of the treatment plan is not adequately conveyed. In the excerpts of a more desirable presentation in the paragraphs below, notice how the therapist conveys both the couple's problems and the proposals for treating those problems:

> *T*: There are a number of things which seem to be preventing you from enjoying each other at present. First of all, there are unsolved problems that have been around for a long time, and have taken their toll over the years. You have swept these problems under the rug until recently, and in the past few months

you have suddenly confronted them but have been unable to effectively deal with them. You know which problems I'm referring to, right? Sex is one. You've (*to wife*) been unhappy about Dennis' decision-making power over when and how to have sex for a long time. Second, you have not gotten together on how to manage the kids. You disagree on when they should watch TV, how polite they should have to be at the dinner table, how they should be punished, and who should punish them. But rather than adopt a consistent policy you simply hit them with your different standards. So the kids are confused, and you are mad at each other. Third, you (*husband*) have felt for years that Pam is overinvolved in activities outside the home, and that affects her functioning in the home, as you see it. Fourth, and possibly most important, your communication has been less than satisfactory. You (*to wife*) have been very unhappy about not enough conversation from Dennis when you're home together in the evening. So, I've mentioned sex, the kids, outside activities, and communication. And, of course, there are other things. But these are the major problem areas. Am I right?

The therapist begins by delineating the couple's major problem areas, without alluding to a theoretical model. Notice, however, that a model is being introduced implicitly in the specific delineation of problem areas: namely, that their manifest, observable complaints will be pinpointed as *the* problems, rather than as surface manifestations of other underlying problems. Notice also that, after listing the complaints, the therapist immediately elicits feedback from the couple as to the validity of his formulations. It is important for the therapist to track the couple's reactions to his remarks so that he can respond to any disagreements that they might be entertaining. In any problem formulation, the process must be a collaborative one between therapist and couple, and the couple's perceptions must be considered at all stages. In addition to the obvious relevance of the couple's perspective, the therapist must constantly track the couple's reaction to his remarks in order to respond to any confusion and concern on their part. Any unverbalized unanswered misgivings serve to detract from the credibility of the presentation.

W: I think that you've hit them. I just feel like my husband's not around even when we're home together. You know, he wants me to be there, but what for? I don't get any feedback. It's like talking to the wall. I don't know why it should matter to him whether I'm there at all.

T: But it does matter, doesn't it, Dennis?

H: (*after a long pause*) Yeah, it does (*he laughs*). I know that I should talk more. We have to find out what makes me talk less.

The therapist must counter any attempts by either spouse to blame the partner for causing the problems. Here the wife allegedly agrees with the therapist's previous remarks, yet shifts to an interpretation which places her husband at the center stage as primary causal agent. The therapist deflects her remark by eliciting a statement of "good intentions" from the husband, which mitigates the most ominous aspect of the wife's accusation, namely, that he does not care whether she is present.

T: Yeah, we have to find out what to do about that. We have to find out about what to do about all of these things. But none of these problems is unusual or uncommon in and of itself. The important point is that you haven't dealt with them effectively. Until recently, you haven't dealt with them at all. And looking at your attempts at problem-solving last week, it's not hard to see why these problems are still lingering. The fact is you don't have the skills to solve your problems. Your attempts don't work. And so you sweep them under the rug. Or you get more angry when you try to work on them. One of your biggest problems is that you can't sit down together and satisfactorily solve your problems. If you could deal with problems effectively as they came up, then none of these issues would seriously jeopardize your relationship because you would eliminate problems as they arose.

W: Well, Dr., I try to sit down with him, but he doesn't give me any feedback. And we don't get anywhere. I know what we need to do, but I can't get Dennis to do it.

T: I know you feel frustrated, Pam, because it feels like you are making an effort but it is not being reciprocated. I wonder though what it feels like from your point of view (*to Dennis*).

H: She always wants to talk about the relationship. I mean I don't mind talking about it sometimes, but that's all she wants to do. And when I express my opinion she gets mad when I disagree.

W: But you won't fight with me. It's OK if we disagree, Dennis. That doesn't mean that we shouldn't talk about it. What's wrong with a little anger? I think that's what the Dr. is saying.

T: Well, not exactly, Pam. I am saying that both of you find the other uncooperative. In fact, you're both being uncooperative. You (*to husband*) by being withdrawn and not giving feedback, and you (*to wife*) by punishing his attempts to respond to you. Neither of you tune in to your impact on the other. You're both so concerned about how you're being victimized and exploited by each other that you ignore your own role in making it difficult to solve your problems. And this is my second major point. The first was that you have a lot of problems because you're ineffective at problem-solving. *The second point is that each of you has a theory about the relationship which says that your problems are caused by your partner.* Pam, you think the marriage is in bad shape because Dennis is withdrawn and he doesn't talk to you. Dennis, you think the problems exist because Pam nags you and spends too much time in community activities. You both think that if the other would only change, things would be nice. You each see yourselves as poor innocent victims of the other person's bad behavior. Well, let me tell you, let me give you an expert opinion. I have seen this pattern before, and you are both right. But more importantly, you are both *dead wrong!* You are both responsible for the problems. Your (*to wife*) verbal intimidation and nagging lead him to not want to talk to you. And your (*husband*) withdrawal makes her feel rejected, and because of that she jumps down your throat. He keeps to himself at night because your behavior (*to wife*) gives him the impression that he's not important. And she leaves at night because when she sticks around she feels rejected by you (*to husband*). I doubt whether either of you believes me. But I hope I will have the opportunity to show you both that you only see one side of it, as many unhappy couples do. But I, as an objective observer, can see both sides of it, and if you would broaden your theory, and learn how the other person sees it, and become sensitive to them and see the wisdom of their point of view, you would be halfway home—even if we stopped there and did nothing else.

W: I can see what you're talking about now. But in the beginning I started leaving and being bitchy after not getting anything from Dennis. Now you're right. I'm sure I don't make it any better.

T: I have no way of knowing how this whole thing got started. We can't go back in time and figure it out. But we don't have to. Because how this pattern got started is irrelevant for us now. The present reality that has to change is that you are in a vicious cycle where you each continue to generate new undesirable behavior in your partner. And this is really the third point. That each of you underestimates your power over the other. You each have an incredibly powerful influence over the other. Probably the single most powerful cause of each of your behaviors is the other person's behavior. Here you are, puzzling over how to get the other person change, and you're ignoring your ace in the hole—your own behavior. The easiest way to get the other person to change is by rewarding them for changing their behavior with *your* behavior. . . .

In the above transcript, the therapist manages to convey essential principles of behavior exchange and reciprocity, but only as they are directly relevant to Dennis and Pam. The formulation never becomes a dry theoretical exposition; instead, the focus of discussion is always on the couple. It should also be noted that the therapist is able to exercise a great deal of license in being critical of each spouse's narrow view of the relationship problems. This license is accepted because it takes place within a context of empathy and support for each person's experience, as expressed at various points in the passage. In order to be free to criticize the clients without alienating them, the therapist must establish a foundation of support and understanding. Also, notice that the therapist carefully maintains a balance in directing comments to both members, and takes steps to equalize the contributions of both spouses to the discussion.

When shifting from a delineation of problem areas to a discussion of their deficits in problem-solving, the therapist again encounters the wife's attempt to blame the husband for the difficulties. Again, the therapist shifts to the husband so that his experience is included in the formulation. This serves as a transition into the therapist's emphasis on the "tunnel vision" exhibited by each of them in their biased analyses of their difficulties. The therapist must persistently negate all efforts by a particular spouse to redefine the relationship problems in a way which places the burden of change on one individual.

Later in this session, the therapist proposes a treatment plan. Notice how the treatment plan follows directly from the formulation of their difficulties:

T: It seems that we have four major tasks in therapy. First, you two need to learn some effective strategies for solving problems. And we should focus on that a lot, using videotape, practice, and some suggestions from me. That way, you will be able to deal with problems effectively as they arise, instead of having them continue to bug you for months and years at a time.

H: That sounds like what we need.

W: Can you really help us with that, do you think?

T: Sure, if you work hard. It will be a lot of work, but it's something that could be very helpful to you if you work hard at it. You'll have to practice the things we do in therapy at home between sessions.

H: How long is this going to take?

T: I would say we should probably agree to meet 11 more times after tonight. That should be enough time. If there is more work to be done at the end of three months, we can always do some more work when the time comes. But I haven't finished outlining the treatment plan. There's some important stuff still to come. We're also going to focus on putting you both in touch with your abilities to influence each other in a positive way. You both have the power to make each other much happier than you are currently, but you're holding back waiting for the other person to make you happy. So I am going to insist that each of you adopt my theory for now, and stop worrying about the changing other person, and start focusing on what you can do to please your partner and improve the relationship. You'll find, I think, that the most effective way to change your partner is to change yourself. And that is something you have complete control over.

W: That is going to be hard for me to do. I feel like I've done so much already. Frankly, I'm tired. I want you (*Dennis*) to do something.

T: I'm sure it does feel like you've done a lot already. But I'm going to try to help you, as well as Dennis, make your efforts more effective. It's important that we view today as the beginning of a new era in your relationship. The past doesn't count. You have to look at the future.

W: I'll try.

T: Now then, I think another important area of focus will be on your communication in situations other than the problem-solving situation. For your communication to improve, we need to help you both learn to bring out better communication in each other. Dennis, you need to become more responsive to Pam. You need to listen to her better, and learn how to show her that you're listening. She also needs to know that you understand her and above all, that you're interested. I'm sure you are interested, and that you do care. It's just that for her it's not enough unless you can show her that you care. She needs to see it and hear it in your behavior. Otherwise, as far as she knows it doesn't exist. And Pam, you need to show Dennis that he can feel free to express himself without getting stomped on by you. And this will take some work. Finally, I think you both need some child management guidance. We can talk in practical terms about how to work more effectively together in handling Chris and Mary Jane. So, how does that sound? Do you think if you learned how to communicate better, solve problems effectively, reward each other more, and develop a unified policy on handling the kids things would be better?

H: Sounds good to me.

W: Too good to be true. We're going to be a tough case.

T: It's never easy because old behaviors die hard. But I am confident that if you work hard you can get anything you want out of this.

The preceding excerpt illustrates one final effort on the part of the irrepressible wife to blame her husband. Again, the therapist acknowledges her feelings, but emphasizes the *reciprocal* nature of their difficulties.

The couple has received a treatment plan which is credible primarily because it follows logically from the specific problems as formulated by the therapist. Rather than trying to proselytize for the behavioral point of view and to sell the couple on an abstract model, the therapist has kept their current situation primary, and introduced principles subtly and always in conjunction with the idiographic emphasis. Despite the deemphasis on presenting abstract theoretical principles, consider all of the principles that have been introduced: (1) The treatment program focuses on changing future behavior, rather than understanding how the problem arose. (2) To change behaviors in a relationship, it pays to focus on the interpersonal reinforcers and punishers currently provided by the spouse. (3) Reciprocity is characteristic of married couples. (4) Behavior change or problem-solving skill deficits are important antecedents in the progressive accumulation of unsolved problems, etc.

In addition, a number of other relevant aspects of behavioral marital therapy are reflected in the above formulation: its use of homework assignments, its short-term, often time-limited nature, and its insistence that couples avoid inferring malevolent intentions or pejorative personality traits from undesirable behavior. Related to this latter point was the therapist's distinction between the husband's communicative behavior (interpreted by the wife as signifying a lack of love) and his feelings (which the therapist assumed did include love and caring). This also reflects the behavior therapist's tendency to accentuate the positive whenever possible: the husband had good intentions attributed to him despite unacceptable behavior, which the wife misinterpreted as a lack of caring.

III. *Expressing optimism about the outcome of marital therapy.* In the transcripts from the previous section, the therapist expresses confidence that the couple will improve, which is an important practice in the attempt to generate treatment credibility and positive outcome expectancies. At the same time, the therapist should neither guarantee positive changes nor imply that the changes will be produced by the therapist, independent of hard work and dedicated practice by the couple. The therapist's expressed optimism can be anxiety-reducing for a couple, and will usually result in increased persistence and a more sustained effort. Both the anxiety reduction and subsequent persistence on the part of the couple have obvious facilitative effects on the chances of improved relationship functioning. However, if the optimism is expressed in a way which implies that a miracle will take place, many clients will become skeptical. Moreover, remarks which imply that cure is in the therapist's rather than the clients' hands may have deleterious consequences for task persistence and effort. More importantly, they may become demoralized upon the inevitable realization during therapy that change involves sustained and single-minded effort.

The therapist's enthusiastic yet tempered optimism is an important component of this process of generating positive outcome expectancies. Statements such as "It will be easy," "There's little doubt that you will be helped by therapy," and "I wouldn't worry, this is going to help you" may have the effect of forming the impression in clients that the therapist underestimates the significance of their difficulties; feeling misunderstood can result in the opposite to the intended impact of the expressed optimism. Tempered yet enthusiastic optimism is reflected in the following examples:

> I think we can be of some help to you. It will take hard work on your part, but you should feel reasonably confident that you will receive considerable benefit if you make best use of therapy. You have some significant problems, make no mistake about that. But in our clinic, we find that couples who work hard usually improve things considerably.
>
> We are not going to offer you a pill that will magically turn you two into a happy, problem-free couple. But I think I can say that there is every reason to be optimistic. With 2-3 months of hard work from your end and from mine, there's a very good chance that you will walk out of here feeling much better about your marriage.

Such statements of optimism are often more effective if supplemented by supporting evidence, either in the form of statistics derived from your clinic, or data from published research. We typically include summaries of outcome research in the explanation of treatment:

> My optimism is not coming out of the blue. The type of therapy we will be engaged in has been studied in a number of scientific investigations, and the results have been extremely positive. Generally, between ¾ and ⅘ of all couples who receive this type of therapy improve substantially. Not all couples get better, but most do. The approaches we use are the best supported of any approach to marital therapy. So, I think you can be optimistic not only on the basis of your own relationship strengths, which are considerable, but also on the track record of our model, which suggests that a majority of couples are helped by it.

By emphasizing the use of a broad, theoretical model which has been successful in helping other couples, the earlier personalization of the treatment rationale is complemented. By now the couple should understand that there are some overriding principles which guide the therapist in the formation of a treatment plan; yet the principles allow for considerable flexibility in the formation of a treatment plan, which is ultimately a joint function of the model and a couple's particular needs and presenting problems. Note also that a couple's basis for optimism should never be presented as *simply* a function of the nomothetic statistics presented to them. The specific strengths of the relationship, as outlined earlier in the session, should be emphasized as the basis for their optimism. The ultimate effect of the therapist's presentation, combining an exhaustive enumeration of couple's strengths as well as evidence from outcome statistics, presented in a self-assured yet tempered style, should create positive expectancies and a firm commitment to therapy.

To finalize the couple's commitment to improving their relationship, it is often helpful for both therapist and clients to sign a written contract, specifying the nature of the obligation on both sides. Not only does a written agreement prepare couples for their upcoming formation of behavior change agreements (Chapters 6, 7, and 8) but it provides a ritual which symbolizes the commitment on the part of both partners to the process of change. If they agree in writing to complete their homework assignments, follow the therapist's instructions, and collaborate toward the common goal of an improved relationship, they are more likely to persevere in these endeavors once therapy commences. Contracts should be adapted to the individual couple. A typical treatment contract is presented below:

TREATMENT CONTRACT:
JOHN AND MARY G. AND DR. S. 9/3/76

John G. and Mary G. agree to participate in eight weekly two-hour therapy sessions, designed to improve their relationship. They agree to work hard and collaborate toward this common goal. They will complete all homework assignments, follow all of the therapist's instructions, including the collection of data at home.

The therapist, *Steven S.*, agrees to use all of his expertise to help John and Mary achieve these ends. He will also explain the logic of all therapeutic techniques, instructions, and homework assignments. Progress will be evaluated continuously, and at the end of eight sessions the therapist will present a complete evaluation of all gains achieved, along with his assessment of what still needs to be done in order to improve the relationship further.

Signed

.... John G.

.... Mary G.

.... Steven S.

SPECIAL PROBLEMS DURING THE INITIAL PHASE OF EVALUATION-THERAPY

The Reluctant Spouse

Every experienced marital therapist has faced the difficulty created by a spouse who is initially unwilling to participate in therapy. Often, the reluctant spouse denies either the existence or the primacy of marital problems, and insists that the problems reside within the partner, who is likely to have a history of wearing the label "identified patient." In these instances the spouse is likely to equate participation with the assumption of his/her own psychiatric label. Or the reluctant spouse may feel threatened by the possibility of being cited as the cause of his/her partner's behavioral or emotional difficulties. Thus, the key to involving these spouses is to persuade them that their participation attributes neither a mental illness nor a causal role for the partner's problems to them. However, such persuasion presupposes that the spouse attends at least one assessment session.

Since the early meetings are clearly labeled as evaluation meetings, the spouse's attendance during this phase is usually accomplished with minimal difficulty. Few spouses refuse the request to "help us with our evaluation." Therapists will have more trouble "hooking" a reluctant spouse when they make no clear distinction between evaluation and treatment phases (cf. Ables & Brandsma, 1977). Reluctant spouses are often made to feel overcommitted when they are forced into immediate therapy since they consider therapy *for them* unnecessary. This fact provides an added rationale for labeling the initial contacts as *evaluation sessions.*

Once each spouse has begun to participate in evaluation, the normal process, especially the interpretive session, usually convinces the spouse of the need to define the problem in terms of the relationship. Most reluctant spouses agree readily to participate, once they are assured that they are neither being blamed nor given a psychiatric label on the basis of their commitment to improve the marriage. *The reluctant spouse should not be manipulated into participation through the use of deception.* For example, to treat the couple for marital problems while at the same time continuing to define the reluctant spouse's role as distinct from the role of client sets a precedent of false pretenses. The events of therapy will quickly contradict the therapist's delineation of the reluctant spouse's role, and thus elicit mistrust, which neutralizes or reverses expectancies and greatly increases the risk of premature termination. If treatment is to focus on the relationship, this must be made explicit during the interpretive session. Most spouses realize by this time that participation is not the threatening prospect which they initially anticipated that it would be, and will readily agree to become involved.

The situation is quite different when a spouse is reluctant to participate in therapy because he/she has already decided to opt for separation or divorce. In our view any attempt to cajole such spouses into therapy should be undertaken cautiously if at all. For one thing, the therapist is placing himself in the position of acting as an advocate for the partner who has made contact with the therapist. Or, the therapist must be assuming, in requesting the reluctant spouse's presence despite his/her expressed decision to end the relationship, that coming to talk with the therapist is in the reluctant spouse's best interests, despite the latter's assertion to the contrary. There are some rather serious ethical problems inherent in a therapist's imposing his influence on one who has chosen not to be influenced, even if the decision is not in his or his partner's interest, in the view of the therapist. One could argue that this situation is no different than the prior example where we advocated encouraging the reluctant spouse's participation. However, we perceive an important difference between the two situations, namely that in this latter situation the reluctant spouse has taken a position which is in direct opposition to the goals of marital therapy, whereas in the former instance the spouse is aligned with the goals but has misconceptions regarding the relationship between his involvement and his partner's (as well as his own) increased satisfaction. We can qualify this admonishment to some degree by mentioning an important exception; in the service of facilitating a smooth separation, assuming that *both* spouses desire to separate, it seems acceptable to offer one's services in a straightforward manner to the reluctant spouse. But even in this situation it is probably preferable for the spouses to be seen separately rather than together, as we will explain in Chapter 9. In summary, the question of how to involve a reluctant spouse is often less problematic than the question of *should* one involve a reluctant spouse? When the situation warrants an affirmative response to the "should" question, the "how" question can usually be handled with relative ease.

Compliance with Data Collection Instructions

During the assessment phase as well as in subsequent treatment phases, behavior therapy requires that couples collect information at home; this information is vital during both periods. Here we are focusing primarily on facilitating compliance during evaluation and assessment, since the strategies for facilitation are similar from one phase to another. Often, an imprinting phenomenon occurs during assessment, where the precedent that is set for compliance determines whether it becomes a problem in the future. Couples from whom compliance can be induced during assessment are likely to persist, but it is difficult to overcome initially erratic or uncooperative responses to these instructions in later phases. In addition to the importance of having the information provided by couples, an important message is conveyed in the therapist's ability to enforce his directives and instructions. The therapist who insists on and effectively induces compliance is in control of therapy; the therapist whose suggestions are not followed is allowing the clients to restructure treatment according to their own short-term wishes, few of which are therapeutic.

Ongoing monitoring of target behaviors at home, from baseline assessment to treatment termination, is *the* primary data collection task for couples. Seldom is the daily tabulation experienced as enjoyable, once the novelty has ebbed. The key to attaining and maintaining compliance with data collection instructions is a consistent presentation and rationale which not only emphasizes their importance, but also introduces and utilizes them as an integral part of therapy. That is, if the home data are simply used to measure the ongoing impact of therapy, spouses' tendency to continue the recording is likely to wane. If, on the other hand, the data are used, discussed regularly, and in other ways integrated into the therapy program, the probability of continued compliance is greatly enhanced.

Here is a typical example of how we introduce the spouses to data collection using the Spouse Observation Checklist (SOC):

> Now I'm going to give you some instructions which are very important. As a part of the evaluation procedure, you will begin to record some of the events that take place between the two of you every day. This will give us some information which we can't get in any other way: namely, the patterns of interaction and exchanges that go on at home. You will be doing this from now until the end of therapy, if we should decide to pursue that. So, later we will be using this information to begin working on some of the problems. We'll also look at it every week and see how we're doing. So, we will be making a lot of use of this information, and I find that it functions like a seeing-eye dog for me. I am blind without it. So, it is necessary for you to do the work every day, and do it carefully.

With this preface, the therapist can then explain the mechanics of the assignment to couples. In closing, the therapist might emphasize the following points:

> Let me warn you, although this will be somewhat interesting to you at the beginning, you will also experience it as difficult. The easier it gets, the more boring and tedious it will become. In short, this will be a pain in the ass. I wish there was some way around it, but like anything else, change is hard work. And surprisingly, some couples find the monitoring and data collection so useful that they continue it on their own, even after therapy is over!
>
> We are going to call you every night this week at 11:00 p.m. to collect that day's data. This way we will have it as part of our initial formulation, which we want to present you next week. Any questions?

It should be apparent to a couple receiving this type of introduction that the data collection is important. The therapist's anticipation of couples' aversive reaction often has the effect of moderating the actual reaction somewhat, since the anticipation is often worse than the reality. The phone calls act as icing on the cake, and nip procrastination in the bud. Knowing that they will receive a nightly phone call, couples are unlikely to underestimate the importance of the assignment. If, on the night of a phone call, one or both spouses have failed to complete the assignment, the therapist must reiterate the necessity of completion: "We really need to have this data every day." The phone calls can be gradually faded as the couple demonstrates a consistent performance. However, all through therapy periodic, random phone calls should be maintained at least once a week.

In addition to the steps already taken, compliance is more likely if the couple is shown specifically how their data are being used in the overall treatment strategy. For example, the data should receive a great deal of attention during treatment phases which focus on increasing positive relationship behavior (see Chapter 6). Moreover, often we begin treatment sessions with a graphic presentation of data collected so far with respect to salient target behaviors. No matter what areas of the relationship are serving as the primary focus at a particular point in time, data can and should be used on a weekly basis to closely monitor on-going process. If all of the above steps are taken, compliance is rarely a major obstacle.

If data collection becomes erratic or inconsistent during therapy, the therapist may have to institute contingencies which will ensure consistent performance from the couple. The therapist's stance in this regard should not be punitive, but rather should emphasize the delays in progress which are the inevitable result of inconsistent data collection.

Since treatment strategies will be based, at least in part, on this information, treatment planning and modification cannot be undertaken without it. Occasionally, it may be necessary to postpone therapy sessions if the requisite data collection assignment has not been carried out. The setting of such a contingency clearly puts couples in control of their own rate of progress. If they recognize that the data comprise their ticket to the next session, it will be difficult for them to avoid collecting them since their avoidance will be explicitly postponing the benefits they can derive from therapy. Seldom will couples renege on data collection or other homework assignments when the connection between the latter and therapeutic progress is spelled out so explicitly.

Seeing Spouses Individually

In conjoint marital therapy there is a common dilemma regarding the advisability of meeting with spouses individually, a dilemma which is particularly acute during the assessment phase. Despite the emphasis in therapy on open, honest communication, a particular spouse may be unwilling to reveal certain information to the partner, information which may be important for the therapist to be privy to. Current engagement in extramarital sexual relationships, unbeknownst to the partner, constitutes the most obvious type of secret which is more likely to be uncovered in an individual session with the spouse who is involved in the clandestine enterprise. Not to have access to such information leads to the therapist's operating in a partial state of ignorance. Weiss et al. (1973) have coined the term "illicit contract" to describe the therapeutic alliances which are formed devoid of such mutually shared information. In the absence of all relevant facts, the treatment plan may be derived from inappropriate premises. The following example illustrates how therapy can be irrevocably harmed by the therapist's not having access to all relevant information:

A couple in their early fifties entered therapy at the prodding of the husband, who insisted that the marriage was not jeopardy, but who nevertheless expressed the belief that the relationship could be significantly improved by therapy. The wife grudgingly accepted the husband's desire for therapy, although she remained ambivalent. During the early stages of therapy, the husband subtly resisted making any substantial changes, and in the process seemed to contradict his expressed desire to improve the relationship. The incongruities in his behavior aroused the therapist's suspicions, at which point, without warning, the husband suddenly announced that he had decided to terminate his marriage, having surreptitiously secured an apartment and contacted a lawyer. An individual session revealed that he had been involved in an affair with another woman, and his manuevering of the couple into therapy was a ploy to securely involve the wife in a healing environment so that he could leave her knowing that she was being taken care of. Although it is unclear whether or not this illicit contract would have been revealed during an individual session with the husband in the evaluation phase, it is certainly apparent that the plan was effectively concealed from the therapist in the protective exclusivity of the conjoint process.

Now consider the problems inherent in the conducting of individual sessions during the evaluation phase. First, individual sessions militate against the notion of a relationship focus. Since spouses are often predisposed to view the other partner as the one with *the* problem, the therapist often needs to exert considerable skill in altering this focus. However the rationale for individual sessions is presented, the idea that secrets are permissible is necessarily fostered. Individual sessions present the opportunity for each spouse to complain about the partner, and to enter into competition with one another for the therapist's sympathy. Now consider the consequences of a secret which is revealed by one spouse during a private sessions with the therapist. What are the therapist's options concerning how to deal with the situation? In order to elicit the information, it is necessary for the therapist to promise confidentiality. Thus, once the secret has been revealed, an alliance has been formed which excludes the naive partner. At the very least this pact is likely to affect the perceptions of the secretive spouse, who might justifiably view himself or herself as having a special relationship with the therapist. The therapist can urge the client to share the information with the uninformed partner during a conjoint session, but the therapist cannot force the client to do so. Nor is the sharing of such information always clinically indicated. If, through either clinical contraindication or, more problematically, due to the spouse's insistence on maintaining secrecy, the information is not to become mutual, the therapist must proceed under constraints which might seriously jeopardize his or her effectiveness. In addition to assuming a special relationship with the secretive spouse, at times the secret might reveal conditions which preclude the possibility of a viable therapy contract. We, for example, will not treat couples if one spouse is engaged in another sexual relationship during the therapy program (see Chapter 9). Faced with this information, a therapist taking our position must either initiate termination or convince the spouse to drop the new partner. When confronted with this choice, the secretive spouse is inevitably being coerced, in violation of the understanding which elicited the confession. Even if the spouse responds to this ultimatum by revealing the information to the partner and abandoning the affair, resentment toward the therapist is liable to hinder future collaboration on his or her part. If termination becomes the only recourse, this must be explained to the uninformed partner.

This is a very difficult clinical dilemma, for which there is no obvious solution. Each therapist must decide, on his own, resolution of this avoidance-avoidance conflict. The solution may vary with the idiosyncracies of each case. Whatever the therapist decides, the primary focus should always remain on the relationship. Thus, the first interview should always be a conjoint interview. If individual sessions are used at all, they should be used sparingly and only after careful consideration of the benefits and liabilities accruing as a result.

Maintenance of Positive Expectancies During Treatment Sessions

While initial expectancies can often produce tangible benefits for both the process and outcome of marital therapy, initial sets can be negated or reversed if subsequent contacts produce evidence which contradicts the basis for positive expectancies. Feedback from the experience of therapy must be consistent with the initial expectations or new, less optimistic, predictions will begin to be entertained. The most important determinant of whether or not these expectancies are maintained is the presence or absence of immediate benefits. Once actual treatment sessions begin, the immediate occurrence of positive behavior changes reinforces initial positive expectancies. Such reinforcement should have a powerful impact on future expectancies, and should fortify couples against subsequent disconfirming experiences. If benefits are not immediately forthcoming, on the other hand, the momentum created by evaluation and interpretive sessions will be vitiated rather precipitously. Mileage produced by pretherapy strategies requires tangible benefits for sustenance. The section below on creating the collaborative set will elaborate on techniques for attaining initial benefits. Chapter 6 is also devoted to strategies for achieving this end.

In addition to the acquisition of rather quick positive behavior changes, other factors in the therapy milieu are important in the maintenance of positive expectancies. Therapist *control* is particularly germane. Throughout therapy, the therapist must be in charge. She/he must determine what happens during the therapy sessions, affect what transpires between sessions, and demonstrate his/her competence in anticipating subsequent events.

By control we mean nothing insidious or diabolical. We are simply referring to the importance of the therapist's maintaining his/her complementary relationship with the couple as an expert who acts as the architect of the process of relationship enhancement. The therapist's credibility and the couple's resultant confidence in his/her ability to help them are best maintained by a clear delineation of this vertical arrangement. A strong, authoritative therapist who enforces his/her directives will be more likely to successfully counter a couple's tendency to circumvent their responsibility for changing their behavior. Since, as we have already emphasized, couples often find behavior change to be a difficult proposition, the control issue can make a crucial difference.

Structure is an important manifestation of therapist control. In behavioral marital therapy, each session has an agenda, and each agenda bears a direct relationship to a clearly specified treatment goal. Clients are seldom unclear as to why a therapist structures a particular session the way she/he does. From session to session, there is continuity, coherence, progression, and predictability. The structure follows from the theoretical model as well as from the use of a behavioral technology; in addition it serendipitously fosters confidence and credibility. The marital therapist must often struggle to maintain the structure and direction provided by the treatment program. Couples often attempt to alter the agenda. The therapist can and must resist couples' efforts to control or redirect the content of a therapy session. The most difficult challenge to the therapist's attempts to follow-through on a preplanned agenda is the occurrence of "crises" during the week. The couple enters the therapist's office asking him/her to referee a major fight or become involved in a dispute. Although these events can and should be discussed in the process of perusing the previous week's data, they should not assume preeminence. In the excerpt below, a couple brings an argument into the therapist's office. He deals with it in a way consistent with our beliefs:

W: So, John spoiled the whole weekend by acting like a creep. All my friends were uncomfortable.
T: It sounds like you were not only angry but also embarrassed.
W: You bet I was embarrassed.
T: It's clear from your data, as well as from what you're saying now, that it was a bad day. I also notice that you bounced back rather remarkably the next day. John, how did you change your behavior on Sunday to make Helen feel better?

(Here the therapist attempts to place the negative event in proper perspective, by emphasizing the positive elements in the week rather than dwelling on the negative. He also finds a positive component in a displeasing interaction, namely the resilience manifested by the couple the next day.)

H: We had an orgy that night, that's what did it (*laughs*).
W: That had nothing to do with it. I think we need to talk about why this keeps happening when we're around other people.
T: That is an area that we will focus on. Right now I'm interested in finding out about the rest of the week. The next day was a very good day. Can either of you help me understand how that came about so easily?

The wife attempted to alter the preplanned agenda for the session, but the therapist prevented her from doing so by focusing on the remainder of their data as he would normally do. Notice that behavior therapy does stress the importance of the therapist's learning of the past week's events; the on-going data which couples collect, and which the therapist peruses at the beginning of every therapy session, serve that purpose. However, it is seldom advisable or necessary to digress from the dictates of a treatment plan in order to discuss in detail a displeasing event which occurred during the week.

An additional factor which influences a couple's perception that the therapist is in control is the extent to which events that transpire in therapy seem to correspond to the therapist's predictions. Unexpected backslides contribute to pessimism to the extent that couples anticipate smooth sailing. Positive expectancies are not synonymous with magical expectations, and a therapist maintains his credibility only by accurately anticipating these almost inevitable regressions. In addition to expressing continued optimism and confidence in the ultimate effects of therapy, the therapist should predict valleys as well as peaks. This way, even a reversal of positive therapeutic changes seems to be under therapist control, and while such a reversal may be unpleasant, it is far from a catastrophe. On the other hand, if a reversal of therapeutic progress occurs in the wake of cavalier optimism on the therapist's part, not only will it be upsetting to the couple, but it will also detract from the therapist's credibility.

During the two weeks following the first therapy session (interpretive), a couple manifested substantial increases in both their exchange of positive behaviors and subjective feelings of satisfaction with the relationship. These improvements were reflected in the data which both spouses were collecting in the home, which indicated a virtual elimination of all recorded "displeasing" behavior, along with substantial increases in the frequency of "pleasing" behavior. During Therapy Session #3, after discussing the data and the encouragement felt by both partners, the therapist remarked as follows:

"Of course, not every week is going to be like this past week. Change is a long, hard struggle, and you aren't always going to be successful in providing benefits to one another. The biggest danger is that you will start to expect your spouse to be perfect all of the time from now on; then, when one of you screws up, as you inevitably will, you will conclude that the changes are not real, and that it is all hopeless. Don't let that happen. Transgressions will occur, and all it means is that you're human."

It is important that the therapist issue this reminder while things are progressing well; otherwise, it is a post hoc response, and is less powerful as a countervailing force. If the therapist's warning accurately predicts subsequent transgressions and reversals of progress, the prediction mitigates the negative impact of the temporary regression. If the therapist is wrong, and the couple simply continues to improve, then no harm has been done. The prediction of temporary interruptions or reversals of progress is also used by systems-oriented therapists in order to overcome couples' efforts to control the therapy situation and resist the therapist's attempts at social influence (Haley, 1976). If the therapist predicts or at times even directs couples to become worse, couples can remain free of therapist control only by getting better. Thus, the therapist and the couple win either way.

COLLABORATIVE SET

Much of the technology described in Chapters 6-9, and especially communication and problem-solving training, can not be effective unless couples collaborate. Regardless of how dissatisfied they are, they must work together to learn the skills on which the treatment program focuses. A therapeutic emphasis on the shaping of relationship skills presupposes that both spouses accept a perspective which attributes their current difficulties to *mutual* behavioral deficits and excesses, and that both accept a prescription requiring that they *both change* together. Perhaps the paradox in all of this is that this rather sophisticated, rational perspective on marital interaction is most likely to be found in happy couples, and least likely to exist in relationships that seek therapeutic assistance.

In other words, it is rather unlikely that couples who enter therapy will spontaneously entertain a perspective consistent with a model stressing reciprocal causation and prescribing mutual change. As earlier discussions in this chapter have already indicated, endemic to marital distress is an inability on the part of each spouse to perceive his/her own contributions to the problems. Most commonly, at least one spouse views himself as blameless, and consequently views change as a unilateral venture for the partner. Therapy, for these spouses, is viewed as an opportunity for the therapist to help convince their reticent partners that they are correct. In cases where each spouse views himself as blameless and, therefore, as not needing to change, it is frequently hoped that the therapist will vindicate his (her) point of view. The therapist is seen as a judge, who will pronounce one of them guilty, after hearing complaints and countercomplaints from both sides.

The therapist usually has to induce collaboration in couples, since they seldom enter therapy with an inclination to collaborate. A *collaborative set* is a generalized tendency to respond to the tasks of therapy in a collaborative manner; it is the antithesis of the response set which most distressed spouses bring into therapy. In order for intervention strategies such as communication training and contingency contracting to be effective, couples must be persuaded to behave in the spirit of collaboration, that is, to adopt a collaborative set. Let us first consider the conditions under which one might expect couples to alter their perspective from one of competition and recrimination to one of collaboration, and then suggest some maneuvers to bring about these conditions in therapy.

In theory spouses might adopt a collaborative set in response to the exhortations of the therapist. If the therapist's theory, which emphasizes reciprocal causality and the necessity of mutual change, is sufficiently persuasive, couples might be convinced to alter their own theories, and thereby adopt the perspective of the therapist, from which will follow collaborative behavior. This transition would require highly developed skills in persuasion on the therapist's part, and is an unlikely possibility, although one that should not be ruled out. More realistic is the possibility that the therapist can persuade them to enact collaborative behavior, while adhering to their old theories. That is, if the therapist can simply persuade the couple to behave *as if* they held a collaborative theory, therapy could proceed; presumably collaborative behavior, if consistently exhibited, would produce a desirable response to the behavior change procedures, which would, in turn, alter the intransigent belief systems, thus creating a set which is consistent with and conducive to subsequent collaborative behavior. Next, the power of the therapist's persuasive abilities is accentuated if each spouse is convinced that it is in his/her self-interest to behave collaboratively. Since spouses seldom enter therapy driven by a desire to increase their partners' satisfaction, moral appeals to the desirability of making the partner happy will be much less potent than a convincing argument that collaborative behavior is in each spouse's best interest.

Finally, an increase in satisfaction during the initial phases of therapy will often foster collaborative behavior in subsequent phases. Not only do immediate benefits enhance the therapist's credibility, and thereby render each spouse's adoption of the therapist's model more likely, but early improvement generally increases the likelihood of the emission of pleasing behavior by each partner, a prospect which will affect collaboration in a positive way. Put simply, couples who like each other are more likely to collaborate.

Four strategies for fostering a collaboration have been suggested. Let us now consider each one.

Persuasion During the Interpretive Session

Earlier in the chapter the transcript of Dennis and Pam receiving a formulation of their difficulties from the therapist emphasizes the explicit statement of the reciprocal nature of their difficulties. By pointing out examples of how each spouse contributes to and reinforces the current problem behavior, the therapist strengthens his case. Of course, the ability to point to specific examples of reciprocal causation depends on the success in uncovering them during the assessment phase. The persuasiveness of the therapist's formulation will be a joint function of additional factors, such as his level of competence and expertise as perceived by couples, and his ability to anticipate their reservations and objections to his formulation (e.g., "You probably don't believe what I'm telling you now").

Although the presentation of a persuasive formulation emphasizing reciprocity and mutuality can contribute to the acceptance of such a notion by spouses, it is unlikely in and of itself to convince them to abandon their earlier notions. For this reason, the suggestion by the therapist that couples assume a temporary *as if* posture can be an effective adjunct to the beginning of a collaborative set.

Enacting Collaborative Behavior

In the transcript below, the therapist convinces a skeptical spouse to behave in a collaborative manner.

T: So, you need to stop worrying about the other person and start paying attention to your own behavior. Steve, how does all of this strike you?
H: It doesn't seem true to me. I find myself developing points to dispute with you. My experience doesn't correspond to what you're saying. Maybe you will prove me wrong.
T: I can understand how it feels different to each of you. And I can't expect you to disregard your experience and simply accept the fact that I'm right. But how about if we reserve judgment for awhile and simply adopt my theory as a hypothesis. I'm going to ask you to act in therapy as if I'm right. Can you do that?
W: I can.
H: Sure, it should be interesting to see what happens.
T: I predict that if you behave as if my formulation is correct, you will begin to experience some benefits. If I'm wrong then nothing will change. You have little to lose. Clearly your old beliefs were not helping the two of you much.

The encouragement for couples to behave in a certain way, regardless of their attitudes and feelings, is often uttered by behavior therapists, and it has led to criticism from some quarters. The essence of the criticism is that we are encouraging couples to behave in a way which is discordant with their feelings and thereby prompting phony, deceptive behavior between members of a relationship. Such criticism is misguided, since *the encouragement of collaborative behavior here is put forth for its strategic value, as a temporary expedient whose ultimate goal is attitude change as well as behavior change.* If one were to suspend therapy until the perspective justifying cooperative and collaborative behavior emerged spontaneously in each spouse, suspension would be permanent—there would be no therapy. We are encouraging adaptive behavior on the assumption that cooperation will lead to positive changes in the relationship, which will foster attitudes and feelings consistent with cooperative behavior. If increased satisfaction does not result, couples will not continue to collaborate, as a behavioral exchange model predicts. Thus, we are relying primarily on reinforcement produced by the cooperative behavior to maintain that behavior. Our proddings only serve as initial prompts. By urging couples to do what we tell them despite the dictates of their beliefs, we are generating the beginning of a reciprocal change which in many instances will bring about cognitive as well as behavior change.

Appealing to Self-interest

Spouses usually enter therapy because they are suffering, in their view, at the hands of the partner. In light of this coincidence of hurt and blame, any attempt to induce them to be *nicer* to their partner during therapy must be accompanied by an emphasis on the benefits that will accrue to them as a result of such an endeavor. Telling them to try being nice because "it is nice to be nice," or because being nice will "make your spouse happy" is unlikely to be successful, because spouses do not care to make their partner happier until they have become happier. What they fail to realize, and what an effective therapist must show them, is how they can help *themselves* by changing their behavior. As the transcript of Pam and David illustrates, that couple exhibited a common tendency for each to underestimate his/her ability to modify the other's behavior. In the formulation of the couple's problems, the therapist should stress the potential for behavior influence in marriage. In many cases the most expedient way to induce one's spouse to change is by reinforcing desirable behavior through the enactment of positive behavior oneself. Thus, collaborative behaviors in therapy can be urged as a means to the end of increased benefits for the spouses who provide them.

Collaboration Following Positive Changes

Perhaps the safest and most prudent path to the induction of a collaborative set is to produce positive changes at the beginning of therapy, changes which do not in themselves depend on collaboration. These initial positive changes will make later collaboration more likely (cf. Margolin et al., 1975; Jacobson, 1977d; Weiss, 1978; Weiss et al., 1973). The desirability of delaying procedures, such as communication and problem-solving training, which depend heavily on collaboration between partners, until some positive change has occurred is one of the reasons that therapy often begins with a general focus on increasing positive behavior.

Instructions to increase positive behavior can be given in such a way as to require minimal collaboration. For example, each spouse can be directed to study the partner's data each night and alter his own behavior, on the basis of what the partner has been recording, in an attempt to increase the partner's daily satisfaction rating. The next night they each look again to see whether or not their manipulation has had any effect. The procedure consists of an ongoing process of studying the partner's data, altering one's own behavior and monitoring the effect of the new behavior on the partner's data. Collaboration is not a prerequisite to the completion of such an assignment.

This procedure can be taken one step further, and the therapist can actually capitalize on the couple's competitiveness as they enter therapy. In the following transcript, the therapist is instructing a couple in how to systematically please one another, using the data that they are collecting at home:

T: Your task is to study the relationship between your behavior and the other person's daily satisfaction rating. You may be surprised to find that the things you think make the other person happy really don't make much of a difference. I wonder if you know how to please each other on a day-to-day basis. Many people think they do, and find out that the things they think are important don't really make much of a difference.

In this assignment both partners are given the challenge of demonstrating that they can control the other person's satisfaction through his behavior. Neither spouse wants to be shown up in this assignment. Both want to show the therapist that they are knowledgeable regarding how to please the partner; thus, they enter into competition for who can be the most effective spouse in emitting pleasing behavior. However, in spite of their competitiveness, they will usually improve the relationship if they persevere with the assignment. As each makes a concerted effort to become more pleasing, each receives more pleasing behavior from the other, and what begins as competition ends, often within a week, with a substantial increase in relationship satisfaction. Suddenly, a collaborative spirit emerges.

There is much that the therapist can do to foster the early inclinations toward collaboration. In reviewing the data which couples collected during the previous week, the therapist can have each spouse focus on himself, rather than asking each spouse to critique his/her partner's performance. This way the point is driven home that each spouse should focus on changing his/her own behavior in a way which will increase its reinforcing potency in the relationship; the partner's change will take care of itself. This focus on one's own behavior is, after all, the essence of what we mean by a collaborative set. The following excerpt occurs during the third therapy session, after a couple has had a week to try to increase positive behavior:

T: Gary, tell me what you did to increase Marsha's satisfaction with the relationship this week.

H: I didn't really do anything in particular. Just tried to be nicer, not get on her case so much.

T: Her data show that you made some specific changes. Do you want to take a look at it?
H: Yeah. . . . Well, I called her on Wednesday to tell her I would be late.
T: Right, I noticed that. What else?
(long pause)
W: He didn't do the weekend babysitting.
T: Wait a minute. Marsha, we're talking now about the good things that Gary did to please. Can you help us?
W: He was pretty good, but I can't think of anything specific.
T: Why don't you take a look at your data.
W: He dressed nice when we went out.
T: Yeah, that was something you talked about last week. What else?
W: He didn't drink.
H: That's right. Only one beer all week.
T: How about that! I noticed that affectionate behavior went way up this week too.
H: Yeah, that's what I was saying. There again I was trying to be nicer.
W: You also listened to me when I talked to you even when the T.V. was on *(they both laugh).*
T: My God, you were working awfully hard this week Gary. Was it hard?
H: No, not really. I just had to concentrate a little harder. See I always knew that she liked these things, but I didn't think they were that important.
T: Well, they obviously are important. Look at the daily satisfaction ratings. They're all high, except for this one day when none of the things we just mentioned happened.
H: Yeah, I was in a bad mood that day, and that was a slip up.
T: And look at what difference it made. How about Marsha? What did she do differently?
H: She didn't yell as much. Except one day when I could've killed her.
T: OK, I'm more interested now in hearing about her accomplishments. You say she didn't yell as much? What did she do?
H: She shut up *(they both laugh)*. She was nicer.
T: Is he forgetting anything, Marsha?
W: No, I tried mainly not to nag or yell.

The therapist's strategy was to direct each spouse to focus on his/her own behavior, or to focus on the other's behavior only to give compliments. Often spouses are also asked to be critical of themselves, but seldom are they encouraged to criticize one another during this period of reflection on the previous week's data. *Self-scrutiny and self-criticism are tacitly put forth as the optimal way to improve the relationship.* Once this focus on self begins to pay dividends, a collaborative set in each partner should be strengthened.

The therapist must pay attention to the maintenance of a collaborative set, once it has been formed. Not only must she/he remain alert to its erosion throughout therapy, but she/he must behave in an exemplary manner himself/herself, that is, in a manner which reinforces the emphasis in therapy on reciprocity and mutuality.

For example, the therapist must remain neutral, and resist efforts by each spouse to acquire him/her as an ally. This does not prohibit temporary alliances, but rather consistent partnerships between therapist and one client.

When couples drift back into old competitive patterns, the therapist must stop them and present feedback which reminds them that their goal is an improved relationship rather than an individual triumph. Drifting back and forth between collaborative and competitive behavior is particularly noticeable during communication training (see Chapter 7). At certain times, the goal becomes winning the discussion rather than solving the problem. By persistently labeling such self-defeating behavior, couples gradually master the distinction between the two stances.

W: You did the same thing when your parents came to visit. You didn't want them to know that we were sleeping together.

H: I did not. I didn't care whether they knew or not.

T: Notice what's going on. You're arguing about the occurrence of an obscure past event. Who's right matters in terms of winning the argument, but it's irrelevant from the standpoint of problem-solving. I'm not saying you shouldn't ever try to beat each other. Tennis, ping-pong, swimming, arguing about whose memory is better—those things we all do. Just don't do them while you're problem-solving.

COGNITIVE RESTRUCTURING

Behavior therapy has gone "cognitive" in recent years, as evidenced by recent books attempting to integrate behavior modification with mediational accounts of human behavior (Mahoney, 1974; Meichenbaum, 1977). The new emphasis on cognitions as targets for therapeutic change is also reflected in the growing popularity of cognitive psychotherapists such as Beck (1976) and Ellis (1962) among behavior therapists (e.g., Goldfried & Davison, 1976). Despite the rather fundamental difficulties inherent in operationalizing and measuring cognitive change, and the theoretical impurities introduced by mediational models, the cognitive resurrection appears irrepressible.

It is interesting to note, in light of the current cognitive fixation among behavior therapists, that cognitive restructuring has been an important part of behavioral marital therapy from the latter's inception. Early papers by Stuart (1969) and the Oregon Marital Studies Group (Weiss et al., 1973) discussed the importance of relabeling faulty attributions on the part of distressed spouses. These early papers also specified "satisfaction" as a fundamental goal of marital therapy, despite the focus on behavior change as a *means* to achieve increments in satisfaction. It is also noteworthy that social psychological exchange theory, from which much of the behavioral exchange model is derived, is largely a cognitive model in that the *standard* for judging the adequacy of rewards received from a partner is an internal one, based on a combination of past experience and the spouse's *perception* of gratification obtainable from alternative relationships or the state of nonrelatedness. In our book, we have mentioned cognitive restructuring as an important component of therapy in a number of contexts. Particularly in this chapter, we have discussed the importance of maintaining clients' "positive expectancies" regarding the outcome of therapy, and the need for inducing a "collaborative set." In our discussion of contingency contracting (Chapter 8), we caution that spouses' "attributions" are likely to be adversely affected by behavior changes that occur following their specification in a contract.

We feel strongly that an awareness of cognitive states benefits the marital therapist. Without intervening to alter faulty perceptions, unrealistic expectations, and the like, behavior therapy is likely to have little impact on a distressed couple (Margolin & Weiss, 1978b). In this section we will enumerate some of the more common uses of cognitive restructuring, followed by an attempt to temper the zeal of cognitive therapists by emphasizing the need for maintaining a behavioral perspective despite the adjunctive value of cognitive intervention strategies.

Faulty attributions often need to be corrected before spouses will enthusiastically engage in a collaborative effort to modify undesirable relationship behavior. Of particular salience are inferences based on undesirable behavior. For example, during the early stages of therapy, one wife discussed her husband's lack of expressiveness as follows:

> *W*: You don't open up to me, I never know how you're feeling. I can't stand that, it makes me feel unwanted, like I'm living with a stranger. If you don't trust me enough to share yourself with me, then I'll have to find someone who will.

This woman's husband seldom offered his wife unsolicited expressions of feeling, either in regard to her or in regard to other facets of his life.

From the absence of expressive behavior, the wife inferred that her husband neither *trusted* her nor *loved* her. While her request for expressions of positive feeling from her husband (particularly toward her) is perfectly legitimate and understandable, her inferences were unwarranted. The husband's lack of expressiveness in this case was more accurately construed as a *skill deficit* which in turn was partially due to his being punished by his mother for such feeling expression in the past. Because feeling expression was discouraged in his family, he never developed skills in formulating such remarks, and anticipatory anxiety regarding the consequences of such expression prevented him from doing so with his wife.

The therapist must acknowledge the distress that this behavior is generating in the wife, but at the same time challenge her inferences. If she is challenged effectively and consistently, both spouses should experience considerable relief, although the request for change should remain, since *verbalizations* of love and caring demonstrate *feelings* of love and caring, and therefore serve important reinforcing functions in marriage:

T: Mark is awfully quiet about his feelings, and that is very troubling to you. Mark, can you understand this? Telling her is the only direct way she knows that you care about her.
H: But I do care about her.
T: Do you?
H: Yeah, very much.
T: How much?
H: I don't know (*laugh*). Ten on a ten-point scale (*they both laugh*).
T: (*To wife*) You are the most important person in the world to Mark. There is no question in my mind about that. He loves you and trusts you; I sense that and it is touching to me. But you see, he doesn't know how to tell you. We have to teach him.
W: If you love someone, the words should come.
T: Now Valerie, I can't let you get away with that. That's very easy for you to think, because of your gift at feeling expression. But it's simply not true for Mark. He hasn't had any practice. His feelings are no different from yours, but we have to help him behave in a way that shows you what his feelings are.

When spouses infer a lack of caring from a behavioral deficit, they are likely to be demoralized; however, if they view the behavioral deficit as behavior which is inconsistent with the underlying feelings, the deficit is likely to remain a problem but no longer will be viewed as a catastrophe.

Another misattribution common to distressed couples will be discussed at length in the chapter on communication training. This is the tendency to attribute behavior either to underlying personality traits or malevolent intentions. This type of labeling can occur at any stage of therapy, and it is certainly not always a misattribution. However, spouses often do misinterpret the causes of their partners' behavior. The therapist must tenaciously correct those faulty attributions. On other occasions where the basis for the behavior in question is unclear, the therapist can strategically reinterpret the attribution in a way that casts the behavior in a more positive light. In the following excerpt, the couple is discussing the husband's tendency to conceal certain things from his wife; here they are discussing a bounced check which the husband intercepted before the wife discovered it.

W: You can't accept responsibility for your behavior. Whenever you do something wrong, you lie, deceive me. I can't stand your dishonesty.

T: It seems like her approval is very important to you (*to husband*). You care so much about what she thinks that you can't get yourself to tell her when you screw something up.

Here the therapist chooses to interpret the husband's behavior as indicating that he cares very much about his wife's opinion of him, a much more positive, and not any less accurate, outlook than the wife's perspective, which attributes her husband's behavior to the trait of "dishonesty." Again, it should be emphasized that the reattribution does not justify the husband's abdication of behavior change responsibilities. However, it does offer a more affirmative perspective on the relationship, and restricts the issue to one of faulty behavior, rather than the more elusive and fundamental question of negative personality traits. A personality trait is very difficult to change, and implies something defective about the *person*. Behavior, on the other hand, can be changed, and an isolated behavior in need of change carries with it no global judgment as to the person's nature.

Another common focus for cognitive restructuring centers around spouses' conceptions of love. Some couples are perplexed about the question of whether they still love one another. They view this question as a global, all-or-none proposition, and assume that therapy will help them to decide definitely whether this love still exists. During the course of therapy, they tend to be perplexed as their feelings vary from week to week, which they interpret as vacillation regarding the question of love. They view this lability as evidence of an unstable relationship. The lack of constancy in their feelings can accentuate their pessimism about the relationship, and impede their effort in therapy.

This preoccupation with the presence or absence of love stems from cultural beliefs that romantic love is a qualitative state which either exists or does not exist. The historical development of this conception is eloquently described by Lederer and Jackson (1968). What spouses fail to realize is the dependence of their feelings about their partner on their partner's behavior. Once the relationship between their subjective feelings and their partner's behavior is elucidated, the lability is likely to become less puzzling and less threatening.

One wife became demoralized after four therapy sessions as a result of a backslide which followed three weeks of basically positive, loving interaction between the couple. She began the next therapy session concerned that she no longer loved her husband. It was obvious to the therapist that this woman was happy and "in love" with her husband when his behavior suggested that he loved her. Although this behavior had been present during the three weeks of progress, he had slipped during the past week, a rather common occurrence in marital therapy following an initial period of substantial progress. The therapist decided to intervene in a way which would demonstrate to the wife that she had lost her perspective. Luckily, the last session had been videotaped. The therapist replayed an excerpt from the session which showed a tender exchange between them: The husband had been discussing his difficulty in dealing with the pressures of his job, and his feeling that without his wife's support and love he would have found it impossible to face those pressures every day. His wife was extremely touched by his admission, and she left her chair and hugged him. The therapist stopped the tape and replayed the physical exchange. He then turned the tape off and spoke to the couple:

T: The woman in that tape loves her husband!
(There was a long pause, during which time both spouses looked at each other, the wife with tears in her eyes and the husband successfully fighting the tears although his face was flushed and he gazed at her tenderly.)

W: (*While weeping*) But why do I lose those feelings the way I did this week?

T: (*To husband*) Maybe you can answer that.

H: Because I'm not always good to you. This week I ignored you. I stopped trying. I'm sorry.

W: You know, it's not very hard to make me happy.

H: I know. I've been working at it, and it hasn't been that hard. But this week I fucked it up.

T: You see, love is a funny sort of thing. You love John but you don't love everything about him. So when you don't get much from him, those feelings don't come out. But just because you don't love all of his behaviors doesn't mean you don't love him.

W: Yeah.

T: You see, John, you have to work to maintain her love. Sometimes you'll fail. But lately you've learned that you can do it most of the time.

Couples often enter therapy with unrealistic expectations stemming from utopian views on the ramifications of being in an intimate relationship. The therapist must help couples identify the myths inherent in these expectations so that their demands are not excessive or perfectionistic. For example, the following excerpt illustrates a rather common myth which our culture imposes on marriage, and the therapist's attempt to debunk the myth:

H: If two people love each other, they should know instinctively what the other person wants and needs. I shouldn't have to tell her what to do or how to make me happy. If she doesn't know by now, that says something about us.

T: So you're saying that married couples should have ESP.

H: No, but they should be able to sense the other person's needs.

T: It sure would be nice if you could read each other's minds. But you are putting your finger on a very common myth about marriage, that love means you should be able to read each other's mind. Those are famous last words for many couples. That point of view is getting both of you into trouble. The only way you can know what the other person wants from you is by his telling you. The only way! You can't expect him to guess. It's much easier and more efficient to tell each other. You're going to have to take my word about that.

W: Are you saying that we can't expect each other to be sensitive enough to anticipate what the other person needs?

T: I'm saying that belief is pure and utter horseshit. And it is responsible for more divorces down through the ages than you can imagine. You're going to have to give up that hope or you might as well kiss the relationship goodbye. If the only kind of marriage you're willing to accept is a dream world marriage, you might as well divorce each other now and spend your time fantasizing about the relationship based on ESP.

The therapist in the above excerpt was direct and even harsh on this issue because of the tenacity with which this couple clung to this myth. By taking a categorical stand on these unrealistic expectations early in therapy, he forces the couple to choose between a real relationship which requires verbalization and discussion of desires, and an unattainable ideal which, if not relinquished, will seriously jeopardize the value to be placed on substantial, albeit less sublime, changes. In the excerpt below, the wife's nostalgia for the past elicits another common, unrealistic expectation of long-term intimate relationships:

W: What I really want is to recapture the times we used to have. We were very much in love once. It was romantic. We didn't have a care in the world as long as we had each other.

T: I'm not sure I can help you do that. You seldom run into couples who can maintain the romance long past the honeymoon. Don't forget that there was a lot of mystery back then, everything was new, you were discovering each other. Now you know each other, there is not as much to discover. The honeymoon ends in the best of marriages. What you can give each other now is a great deal of satisfaction and fulfillment, and occasional romance. But what you're talking about is going back to an era that is over, an era that is part and parcel of early courtship and the process of getting to know each other.

Finally, many couples express the conviction that in order for legitimate behavior change to occur in marriage, feelings must change *first*. They would prefer to wait for their partner to *want* to change his/her behavior before demanding that she/he do so. Therapy, if these couples were to construct the treatment plan, would focus on inducing a change in feelings, following which they assume that behavior would automatically change in the desired direction. Similarly, they may expect an insight-oriented approach, which would attempt to uncover the underlying causes of their partner's undesirable behavior. They would view such insight as a prerequisite to behavior change.

In responding to such predilections in couples, the therapist should not be critical of the couple's world view regarding behavior change. Such beliefs can be quite impervious to verbal exhortation, and there is no need to challenge these suppositions. Rather, the response should emphasize the practical advantages of focusing on overt behavior, and the reciprocal relationship between feelings (or insight) and behavior. If the correlational nature of the relationship between feelings and behavior is emphasized, and the causal sequence is viewed as irrelevant, then the decision regarding intervention can be made on the basis of practicality and efficiency. Our technology for changing behavior is considerably more developed than our technology for changing feelings and attitudes. Happily, the effectiveness of a behavioral approach suggests that if couples can be induced to behave more positively and engage in predominantly pleasing behavior, attitudes and feelings can be expected to change (although not always) in a direction which is consistent with the new, desirable behavior. Here is an illustration of how one behavior therapist conveyed this message to a somewhat reticent couple:

> *W*: I don't want him to be considerate of me unless he wants to.
>
> *T*: Part of being married is learning that you sometimes have to do things for your partner that you would rather not do, simply to please your partner. I am not concerned that you feel reluctant about changing. Our experience has been that once you start putting yourselves out for one another again, you begin to get more, and you don't feel like you're being put out anymore. So what I'm saying is you may ask each other to do certain things that you don't want to do *in the short run;* but eventually you will be reaping the benefits of your giving, and by then you *will want to.*

We have enumerated a number of examples of attempts to restructure cognitions which seem either maladaptive, unrealistic, or simply inconvenient from the standpoint of therapeutic progress. Since faulty attributions and self-defeating thoughts seem to be so prevalent in distressed couples, why not use an essentially cognitive approach to treating couples, rather than relegating it to an adjunctive status? After all, cognitive therapy seems to be effective for a variety of self-defeating emotional and behavioral problems (Beck, 1976; Ellis, 1962; Meichenbaum, 1977). Often the behavior about which spouses complain does not seem inherently undesirable or displeasing; conceivably in such instances it may be appropriate to focus exclusively on the attributions, irrational ideas, and the "meaning" of the behavior for spouses, and attempt to modify the irrational thought processes.

Despite the ostensible cogency of this argument, an exclusive cognitive approach has sufficient limitations to justify confining its status to that of a subordinate and supportive role. First, it is our belief that in many instances these self-defeating cognitions are artifacts or consequences of the partner's behavior. When a wife interprets her husband's behavior as evidence of a lack of love, more often than not the behavior (or lack of behavior) produced the inference. Even if the inference has generalized to the point where it obfuscates the spouse's ability to accurately interpret more neutral behavior, it makes more sense to focus on modifying the behavior which served as the antecedent and *raison d'etre* for the attributions, while simultaneously discussing the attributions in ways suggested above. When a spouse exhibits a pathological tendency to make sweeping interpretations of virtually all aspects of his/her partner's behavior, and it seems that these interpretations reflect predisposing *schemata* which the interpreter brought into the relationship, that person may require individual therapy to correct these faulty cognitive predispositions. For example, some depressed people may tend to interpret all aspects of their spouse's behavior as evidence that they are regarded as, and therefore are, worthless. Consequently, because they view themselves as unlovable, relationship behavior delivered by the partner is likely to be viewed as rejecting or unloving. When cognitive distortions attain this level of severity, it is doubtful that an exclusively dyadic approach can remedy the situation.

An additional consideration favoring a primary focus on overt behavior has already been alluded to, namely the relative ease of changing overt behavior. Assuming that attributional phenomena interact with behavioral phenomena in a circular, self-strengthening fashion, clinical strategy may often be reduced to a question of expediency. Whereas thoughts are often automatic and difficult to modify, behavior is voluntary. Moreover, the ability to validate the presence or absence of behavior change allows for a constant monitoring of progress. If, on the other hand, the therapist's focus were exclusively cognitive, the effectiveness of treatment at any given point in time would be more problematic and potentially ambiguous.

The task of modifying thought processes is nothing about which to be cavalier. Approaches that emphasize cognitive change tend to utilize behavioral procedures along with the heavily-emphasized cognitive instructions, and to the extent that such procedures are effective, the mechanisms of change are very much in doubt.

In closing this section, let us emphasize that there are exceptions to every rule. Behavior therapists might at times find a cognitive emphasis advantageous. Consider the case of a couple whose primary complaint was the wife's irrational jealousy. Although the husband was quite innocent, even to the point of lacking "lust in his heart," the wife would engage in jealous tantrums whenever they were in the presence of other couples. Her tantrums included crying, saying "I hate you!" to her husband, and insisting that the evening be terminated prematurely. This behavior precluded much contact with other people, and severely constrained the husband's initiations of friendship and fulfillment outside of the home. The therapist ventured the following interpretation of the woman's jealousy during one of the early therapy sessions:

> You unconsciously believe that your jealousy is the only thing that prevents him from leaving you. You're afraid that unless you con-

> stantly act suspicious and remind him that he's being watched, he will get involved with another woman. And since you never stop being jealous, you can never test your hypothesis. Well, let's test it. I predict that if you stop displaying your jealous rituals, he will remain faithful to you. Then you will know that you don't have to be jealous to keep him in the relationship, and you will stop feeling jealous.

Although the wife reported no awareness of the theory which the therapist attributed to her, she accepted the formulation and agreed to refrain from her jealous behavior. They pinpointed the behavior in question, and then arranged for a series of interpersonal contacts with other women. The wife successfully behaved in a non-jealous manner. He did not engage in any extramarital liaisons. And gradually, her jealous *feelings* disappeared.

The therapist's formulation was plausible, but its real utility lay in its strategic value. Since the wife "accepted" it, she acquired a rationale to change her behavior. The cognitive restructuring intervention was necessary to justify her behavior change to her, which in turn led to an elimination of her jealous feelings. The case illustrates the usefulness of presenting new belief systems to clients as a way of producing discriminative stimuli for new behavior. A new belief system is at times necessary to justify behavior change to a spouse.

THE USE OF PARADOX IN BEHAVIORAL MARITAL THERAPY

This chapter closes with a discussion of another intervention strategy not derived from a strictly behavioral perspective. It has become popular in marital and family therapy circles to attempt the production of behavior change by presenting clients with *paradoxical* instructions: Although there are a number of ways to define paradoxical instructions, essentially they consist of instructing clients to engage in the very behavior that has been identified as a target for elimination in therapy. One common example is to suggest to a couple (or family) that they have a relapse. Another is to encourage a verbally abusive couple to argue or fight at a frequency which exceeds their base rate. Paradoxical instructions were popularized by the writings of Milton H. Erickson, and more recently Jay Haley and Victor Frankl (Haley, 1973, 1976; Frankl, 1975).

Although various rationales have been presented for the use of paradox in marital and family therapy, the most widely accepted explanation is based on the belief that couples and families often resist the therapist's efforts to change their behavior. These families will disobey the therapist's instructions and thereby frustrate both themselves and the therapist. Resistance is viewed as a largely unconscious process, based on the homeostatic functioning of a family system, which exerts force to maintain the status quo whenever an external change agent (the therapist) attempts to interfere with its stability. Since the family's collusive defensiveness leads to the adoption of a stance which resists outside attempts to influence it, when the therapist instructs them to behave pathologically, the only way to resist the influence attempt is by changing for the better. Once such instructions are conveyed, the therapist has improved his/her position regardless of how the family responds. If they resist his attempts to influence them, they must improve. If they "obey" the therapist and engage in pathological behavior, they have established a precedent for following the therapist's instructions, and will be more likely to do so later when the therapist instructs them to improve.

Underlying the philosophy of paradoxical instructions is a view of therapy as a struggle for control between therapist and client(s) (Haley, 1963; Sluzki, 1978). Clients, according to this perspective, do not relish surrendering the control over their lives to a therapist, and will consequently avoid behaving pathologically if the therapist tells them to engage in pathological behavior. Two assumptions which are basic to the general systems approach are necessary to justify paradoxical instructions as an intervention strategy. First, there is an assumed discrepancy between the family's claim that the target behaviors are *involuntary,* and the reality of the situation, which is that the behaviors are *voluntary*. Behavior therapists also accept this assumption for most target problems reported by couples. Second, and even more central to the system's perspective, is the notion that maladaptive behavior in a marriage or family exists primarily for its communicative function. That is, undesirable behavior is seen as a metaphor, as a statement about the current power relationships among family members and a symbol which defines the terms of family interrelationships.

It is this latter assumption which generally restricts the use of paradox to eclectic practitioners who believe in its efficacy and to advocates of a systems perspective. *A behavioral exchange model does not accept the assumption that most target behaviors presented by couples can be best understood as metaphors serving a communicative and relationship defining function. Rather, behavior is seen as primarily a function of its environmental consequences for the individual engaging in that behavior, and the topography of particular relationship responses is viewed literally rather than symbolically.* Whereas communication theorists assume an unconscious agreement between family members which ultimately *ap-*

proves of the target behaviors despite their conscious protestations, behaviorists adopt the more parsimonious view that *apparently* aversive behavior is *actually* aversive to family members. Moreover, rather than adhering to the homeostatic conception of a family as striving for maintenance of maladaptive behavior patterns and resisting change, behavior therapists assume that couples who ask for help generally wish to be helped. When the change process is a struggle, and it often is, behavior therapists assume that the manifest ambivalence on the part of spouses reflects the short-term aversiveness of behavior change, rather than ambivalence about the goal of an improved relationship. It is difficult and costly to discard habitual behavior patterns, despite the long-term benefits, just as it is difficult for the alcoholic to cease his/her alcohol consumption, despite the long-term benefits. In sum, couples often find the *means* difficult, but that does not imply that they are resisting the *end*, which is an improved relationship.

Thus, paradox as a general strategy of marital therapy is inconsistent with a behavioral perspective. In order to enhance the likelihood of compliance with therapist directives, the behavior therapist stresses tactics to directly enhance the persuasiveness of instructions, such as those emphasized in this chapter. However, at times paradoxical instructions can be viewed as consistent with and facilitative within a behavioral exchange framework. What follows is a discussion of clinical situations where strategies similar to paradoxical instructions seem indicated.

A young couple entered therapy in a state of crisis and fought frequently between sessions. Their fights were extremely destructive, and often included physical violence. The fights threatened to compel a separation before therapy could begin to reverse the coercive chain. The therapist needed to temporarily suspend these altercations in order to allow the therapeutic process time to exert a positive effect on the relationship. The following transaction took place during an early therapy session:

T: You know, it's amazing to me that you two have such vicious fights at home. In here you both are so polite and subdued.
W: It gets very ugly to be around us when we're fighting.
T: But it does present a problem for my evaluation. I can't really get an analysis of you two and how things get destructive unless I can see and hear the two of you acting destructively.
H: You want to come for dinner? (*All laugh.*)
T: How about if the two of you fight for me right here?
H: Now?
T: Yeah, I'll leave and watch through the one-way mirror.
W: We can't do it now. I'm too inhibited.

H: She has to get mad at me first. Then nothing stops her.
T: Couldn't you say something to get her mad?
H: You want to try it?
W: OK.

The couple was unable to fight, and the episode led to amusement and laughter.

T: Well, this is really a dilemma. Somehow I have to get this information. I have an idea. I'll give you a portable cassette recorder to take home, and a tape. Whenever you start to fight, go into the living room, turn on the tape, and fight in the living room. Then at least I can hear how it sounds.
W: You're suggesting that we fight and tape it?
T: Yeah, I can't think of any other way to get the information. And since you're fighting every week anyway . . .

The therapist convinced the couple to comply with the plan. When they returned the following week reporting that, for the first time in months, they had not engaged in one argument, the therapist appeared bewildered and his response was punitive. He insisted that they fight at least once the following week; otherwise, progress would be retarded. Alas, the fighting was over between this couple, and therapy had to proceed without this invaluable assessment information. Therapy proceeded smoothly and successfully subsequent to the ceasefire induced by the instructions to fight "on the air."

Although this intervention might be viewed as paradoxical, it is also consistent with a model which emphasizes the environmental control of behavior. By giving the couple the cassette recorder, the therapist was capitalizing on his own value as a discriminative stimulus for polite, rational behavior. Handing them the cassette was akin to "coming over for dinner." Now, any time the couple fought, they would be fighting in front of the therapist. Thus, despite his instructions that they tape their fights, the real purpose of the intervention was to stop the fights. If the therapist had presented the instructions by saying, "Here is a cassette tape recorder. Take it home and record all fights. Perhaps knowing I am going to listen to them will get you to stop fighting," the couple would probably not have bothered to turn on the recorder, and fighting would not have decreased. By using deception, the therapist convinced them that he needed the information for assessment, and they would have felt obliged to record all arguments. But since the therapist was an SΔ for fighting, the fighting stopped.

Another couple entered therapy with the primary complaint being the husband's premature ejaculation. The couple was in their early twenties, and had been married for about one year. Neither had prior experience with other lovers. The husband ejaculated about five seconds after intromission, and this pattern had existed from the beginning. He reported a tremendous amount of anxiety in the sexual situation, which had again been present from their first sexual encounter. Just prior to their consummation, he had read Masters and Johnson's *Human Sexual Inadequacy* (1970) and recalled fearing that he would be impotent. They had tried the "squeeze technique," Masters and Johnson's very successful approach to the treatment of premature ejaculation, on their own, and it failed because the husband was unable to recognize the premonitory cues preceding ejaculation, and the squeeze could not be applied in time to block ejaculation.

It quickly became apparent that this man was so anxious in the sexual situation that he was insensitive to sexual sensations. And of course the key to ejaculatory control is sensitivity to and recognition of the body's response to sexual stimuli. He expressed hopelessness about the problem, and entered therapy to discover whether he was biologically defective, an explanation which he felt was likely. At the end of the initial interview, the therapist presented the couple with a homework assignment:

> *T*: I need to know exactly how long it takes you to ejaculate, in the worst possible instance. So here's what I want you to do. I'm going to give you a stopwatch. I want you to time yourself making love. Start timing when you penetrate, and let's see how long it takes you to ejaculate. *Try and ejaculate as fast as you can.* Let's see how bad the problem is at its worst.

The couple reluctantly agreed to take the stopwatch to bed, and to their utter delight, the husband endured without ejaculating for six minutes, by far the longest sexual encounter they had ever experienced together. Try as they might, they could not induce an episode of premature ejaculation that week. The therapist reclaimed his stopwatch, and sent them home, with weekly phone calls corroborating elimination of the problem.

Here was a couple who had never experienced a successful period of intercourse together. The therapist guessed that a demand for as quick an ejaculation as possible would provide them with their first opportunity to make love without performance anxiety. The initial success eliminated the hopelessness, ruled out the biological interpretation, and demonstrated to both partners that satisfying sex was a possibility for them. Just in case distractibility because of the stopwatch was responsible, the therapist quickly removed that source of distraction, and the improvement remained. Since the couple had already employed the Masters and Johnson approach without success, a recapitulation of that program would not have had much credibility. Moreover, if the opportunity for a mastery experience presents itself in therapy, and the mastery experience has the potential for a self-generating, curative effect, it is preferable to provide that experience than to rely on an intensive, technology-based treatment program. The former leads to the attribution that "we did it on our own." Just as in the previous example, a straightforward rationale, such as "I want you to have a mastery experience," would have failed; the paradoxical instructions were needed to remove the performance fears from the sexual situation. If premature ejaculation had continued, little would have been lost, since the couple had no expectation that the data collection would be curative.

A final example of the effective use of paradox in marital therapy involved a young couple crippled by "differential interest." The husband was desperately trying to please his wife, while she remained bored and indifferent to his solicitations. His constant approach behavior and noncontingent availability had lead to satiation, and the more reinforcement he delivered, the more she withheld. It seemed as if an intervention was necessary which would reverse this pattern. In contrast to the other examples, the therapist was straightforward in presenting these paradoxical instructions:

T: In light of all this (*the wife's lack of responsiveness to her husband, and his continuous attempts to please her*), I think the best thing for your marriage would be for you to have an affair with another woman (*to husband*).

(Both of them reacted with astonishment and perfunctory dismissal of the idea.)

T: I think it's the only way she's going to stop taking you for granted.
H: I don't have any interest in other women.
T: I don't believe you. Don't you have sexual fantasies about other women?
H: Sure, occasionally.
T: Are they about women you know?
H: Some of them.
T: Are any of them single?
H: Yeah.

As the husband began to discuss the subject with increasing animation, his wife listened avidly but passively. She expressed doubt that his sexual involvement with another woman would have a major impact on her, but gave her blessing to the idea, if that was what the husband wanted. At the end of the session the therapist presented a second option as an alternative to a sexual liaison: the husband could cultivate platonic relationships with other women, exclusive of sexual involvement. He instructed the couple to arrive at a consensus on which alternative would be most appropriate, and inform him at the beginning of the following session.

With most couples this would have been a very risky intervention, sufficiently so to contraindicate it. However, the therapist was virtually certain that a) the husband would not actually do it; b) the mere preoccupation with the idea would sever him from his obsessive giving to his wife; and c) any withdrawal of attention from her and redirected attention toward other women would renew her interest in him, at least to some degree. The following week they reported a preference for the latter alternative, the cultivation of platonic relationships. They also reported a considerable increment in time together, and the first positive sexual experience they had had since therapy began. The therapist expressed disappointment with the decision, but expressed willingness to help them maximize this "clearly inferior" option. The remainder of the session was spent planning the social contacts with other women, with the wife remaining a bystander. The husband began, in subsequent weeks, to broaden his interpersonal contacts. He derived a substantial amount of social reinforcement from these contacts, and not only became more "contingent" in his responsiveness to his wife, but also began to demand some behavior changes from her. She began to report increased satisfaction in the relationship. The husband learned a very important lesson from this new life-style, a lesson which is valuable to keep in mind when working with couples where spouses seem to differ in their preferred amount and degree of intimate contact. It is sometimes desirable to withhold from one's partner. In order to maintain a satisfactory balance between two individuals differing in their desire for affiliation, the more affiliative person can be encouraged to become less affiliative and more independent. The paradoxical instructions were instrumental in conveying that message to this couple.

Paradoxical interventions are not for the inexperienced clinician. Their consequences can be disastrous if they fail. It is necessary to pay attention to a number of guidelines when using the techniques of paradox (cf. Haley, 1976). *First, paradoxical directives must be embedded in a context of obvious caring and concern for the couple.* It should be clear to the couple that the therapist's ultimate concern is that they achieve a more satisfying relationship. If the latter is not communicated to the couple, they are likely to be insulted or feel bewildered. *Second, the therapist must simultaneously employ a sense of humor and a legitimate recognition of the significance and severity of the couple's problems.* Again, even though the therapist is suggesting the couple behave in a way inconsistent with the ultimate goals of therapy, it must be clear to the couple that their problems are being taken seriously, that the therapist is not simply playing with them. *Third, the therapist must present a credible rationale for the paradoxical instructions, such as the necessity of the task for evaluation purposes. Fourth, when the couple reports improvement after being instructed to deteriorate, the therapist must not "debrief" them.* Debriefing can undercut the potency of the intervention by leading to couples' feeling tricked or manipulated; it can also redirect their attention to the therapist as the one responsible for change. *Finally, paradox should be used rarely, and never capriciously.* In two of the three examples presented here, neither outcome (compliance or noncompliance) would have seriously jeopardized therapy; in the third example, the therapist was quite certain how the couple would respond. When in doubt, avoid paradox.

SUMMARY

This chapter could be subtitled "behavior therapy and beyond." The discussion focused on aspects of therapy which have been discussed rarely by behavior therapists, but which are instrumental in determining whether or not therapy is successful. The therapist does a great deal more than teach skills and encourage the use of positive control. She/he is constantly laying the groundwork for change. She/he is behaving in a way that will either enhance the potency of the technology, or negate it. From the initial interview to termination and even beyond, the therapist relentlessly attempts to produce a therapeutic milieu which is optimal for couples' receptivity to his attempts at influence. Perhaps the best way to summarize the chapter is that, in order to be an effective marital therapist, the therapist must convince the couple that he believes in what he is doing, that what he is doing is reasonable, and that he cares about the people that he is doing it for.

CHAPTER 6

Increasing Couples' Positive Exchanges

THIS CHAPTER describes our opening strategy for relationship improvement. We focus during this beginning stage on desirable relationship behaviors that are relatively easy to enact. Although couples often view therapy as a means to rid themselves of irritating aspects of their relationship, our initial strategy is to identify and accelerate those behaviors that would enhance the relationship and to pay little heed to the undesirable behaviors. This strategy contradicts clients' expectations that therapy will immediately confront the major reasons why the relationship is faltering. Since spouses rarely enter therapy ready to collaborate on the major issues, focusing on them at this time simply perpetuates the already familiar experience of frustration and failure. Our goal is to effect positive growth on nonconflictual issues so that the spouses experience success in therapy and learn that relationship improvement is within their reach. This has the immediate effect of increasing the couple's commitment and caring as well as the long-range effect of setting the stage for changes of greater consequence.

Until this time, spouses have demonstrated their commitment to therapy by fulfilling the assessment tasks but they have not yet invested in improving the relationship: In other words, they have not put forth efforts that bear a direct impact upon their partners. At this stage, spouses are directed to emit behaviors that "please" the other person and increase his/her overall relationship satisfaction. Although this step is less threatening than dealing with the major issues, it still involves risks for a distressed couple. Before discussing strategies for prompting increases in positive behavior, let us examine the rationale for choosing this therapeutic step as our initial intervention.

The rationale for focusing on positive behaviors comes from both empirical data and clinical experience. There is evidence that positive and negative relationship events are independent (Orden & Bradburn, 1968; Wills et al., 1974). That is, simply removing behaviors that cause marital tensions does not automatically lead to an increment in positive couple interactions. Weiss (1978) described the state produced by an absence of relationship pollutants in the following manner: "If all annoyances fell to zero rate/hour, one would be quiescent but not necessarily satisfied; soporific drugs might accomplish the same end" (p. 50). Although it is important that therapy lessens or eliminates undesirable marital behaviors, that alone is not a sufficient outcome. Indeed, if that were our primary purpose, we could best accomplish it by instructing spouses to refrain from interacting with one another. As marriage therapists we must set our sights higher than the removal of maladaptive symptoms and strive towards the actual improvement of relationship functioning. The acceleration of positive behaviors is a beginning step toward that objective.

A second empirical reason for our emphasis on positive rather than negative spouse behaviors is that undesirable relationship behaviors tend to diminish even if they are not the primary target of an intervention (Follingstad, Haynes, & Sullivan, 1976; Margolin & Weiss, 1978b). When Margolin and Weiss compared the effectiveness of three marital treatment conditions, they found that all conditions produced a reduction of negative behaviors although none had been designed with that specific intent. In comparison to the consistently significant finding of reductions in negative behaviors, positive behavior changes occurred only in those treatment conditions that included training directed specifically at increasing desirable relationship behaviors. These results indicate the importance of choosing treatment procedures that focus directly on the escalation of couples' positive exchanges.

A third reason for the focus on spouses' positive exchange is to address directly the general problem of reinforcement erosion. As mentioned in Chapter 1, habituation to one's partner is usually accompanied by a reduction in that person's reinforcement potential. Couples need to expand their repertoires of reinforcing behaviors to counter such effects. Yet, it is unlikely that distressed spouses are putting much effort into seeking new ways to reinforce one another. Unfortunately, this problem is self-perpetuating. Spouses become satiated after many repetitions of the same behaviors. Once the events have lost their reinforcing quality, it is easy to conclude that the wrong person is performing the activities. Spouses may then withdraw from the relationship rather than renew their efforts to find effective reinforcers.

An alternate way to view this situation is that the enjoyment from habitual activities has worn thin but there are other enjoyable events still to be experienced. The obvious test for this assumption is to introduce new pleasures and evaluate whether they provide greater satisfaction. Unfortunately, couples who experience this problem rarely have a list of potential reinforcers at their fingertips. This was keenly exemplified for us by a husband who, when asked to name ten rewards that his wife could supply for him, listed only food-related and sex-related items, all of which he was receiving regularly. With some couples, the tedium is so great that arguments are a welcome diversion: Allowing these couples to spend therapy time in arguments provides them with further evidence that conflict is the most rousing force in their marriage.

The intervention procedures described below relieve reinforcement satiation by having spouses monitor their rewarding potential and expand their range of available reinforcers. By discovering which behaviors are or are not reinforcing, spouses gain control over the quality of their relationship. If spouses exercise that control, they find their relationship problems to be less overwhelming.

Why is the acceleration of positive behaviors the entry point for the entire therapeutic intervention? One of the primary functions of accelerating the rate at which spouses exchange positive behaviors is to maneuver the couple into a position of readiness for more demanding changes. Upon entering therapy, spouses often feel deprived by the partner of gratification, depleted in their reservoirs of relationship energy, and unappreciated for the efforts they do expend. Before these spouses are ready to negotiate and resolve major issues, they must first be convinced that the relationship is worth their additional efforts and that they, in fact, can be on the receiving end of relationship benefits. This initial intervention is designed to provide spouses with an immediate "shot in the arm" of marital pleasures to revitalize their debilitated stores of relationship energy. If successful, this intervention makes spouses aware of the inherent worth of their relationship and encourages them to persevere through the remainder of therapy.

A final reason for beginning treatment with the exchange of positive events is the comparative ease of implementing this particular intervention. While some aspects of treatment require the mastery of unfamiliar behaviors (e.g., communication training) or an already established basis of trust (e.g., contracting), this therapeutic step has no such prerequisites. This intervention is designed to engage spouses in behaviors that they are already capable of performing and that they are not opposed to enacting. Since the benefits can be accrued immediately, this intervention can function to offset the more painstaking therapeutic procedures that require a certain level of competence before they render any gains.

Before describing how this intervention is actually implemented, permit us to attach a qualification to the general rule that therapy begins with an intervention to increase positive behaviors. In certain situations, there are immediate concerns that take precedence. When a couple's relationship is deteriorating rapidly and there are precipitating conditions that can be altered to halt the downward trend, modification of those conditions is the preferred course of action. The proposed strategy is also ill-advised when a particular problem is bound to worsen if it is not dealt with at once. Jan and Dave, for example, were in conflict over the impending visit of Dave's son, who would be staying with them for the summer. Dave wanted Jan to quit her job during that time but she was unwilling to do this. Since the visit was to occur only two weeks after therapy began, the therapist focused first on basic problem-solving techniques that the couple could apply to this immediate dilemma. Another more extreme example is the couple who seeks help for the problem of spouse abuse. As described in Chapter 9, the therapist must immediately attend to the issue of what it takes to terminate the abuse.

Another consideration for the therapist is whether or not the couple's data support the utility of an intervention to accelerate positive behaviors. On the basis of the couple's precounseling data, the therapist must decide if such an intervention is warranted. Research findings we have already summarized, that compare distressed and nondistressed couples (e.g., Birchler et al., 1975), suggest that the majority of distressed couples can benefit from this type of intervention. However, one does not blindly pursue this or any other strategy.

GENERAL STRATEGIES TO INCREASE POSITIVE BEHAVIORS

In this chapter we describe several types of interventions to increase positive behaviors that vary in terms of who chooses the behavior to be accelerated—the giver, the recipient, or both spouses together. The described interventions differ in format but share the aim of engineering an exchange that maximizes rewards to the recipient and minimizes costs of the giver. The interventions are designed to help each spouse emit behaviors that are already within that person's response repertoire. Thus, the target behaviors are those that require no new learning but that, for whatever reason, the person has not been emitting at a satisfactory rate.

Another common element is that each intervention elicits behaviors that have no negative emotional history for either the giver or the recipient. It is often the case that couples focus so much attention on the major, seemingly unsolvable issues that they ignore smaller, yet still significant, changes that are indeed attainable. The interventions described here redirect spouses' attention to those smaller issues and promote whatever change is possible without use of the more laborious problem-solving procedures.

The Spouse Observation Checklist (SOC) can serve as a convenient foundation for any of the interventions to accelerate spouses' positive exchanges. Using a procedure similar to Weiss' cost-benefit system (Weiss & Birchler, 1978) spouses modify their lists by assigning a value between −3 (extremely undesirable to receive) to +3 (extremely desirable to receive) to designate their liking of each item. The lists can then be pared down by eliminating all items that are neutral (zero).

Once the partners have indicated their preferences for certain behaviors, the SOC's are exchanged, as described in Chapter 5. Each spouse studies the other partner's data to formulate hypotheses about what she/he is doing that has an impact on the partner's daily satisfaction. Through such inspection of the partner's SOC, each spouse has access to the following types of information: (1) what behaviors she/he emits that the partner notices and records; (2) what impact that behavior has on the receiver, and (3) which behaviors the receiver marked as highly desirable but is not now receiving. At this stage of sharing information, it is helpful to forewarn the couple that they should not expect to agree on their selection of pleasing items. Otherwise, the spouses may react negatively to the fact that they have marked only a few of the same items, interpreting the lack of consensus as an indication of incompatibility. After a week of studying one another's SOC data, spouses are to set aside a short period of time each evening to review and discuss their data. If the therapist foresees that a couple will focus their discussion on the occurrence of displeases or on the absence of pleases, it is useful to structure the discussion by having spouses discuss the most important pleases of that day. The tape recording of these discussions fosters compliance with the instructions and also provides instructive feedback to the therapist.

Through the assignments to review and discuss SOC data, spouses learn how their efforts are best spent. For example, Peter and Pam had very different ideas about how much effort they should spend keeping their house clean. Since a tidy house was very important to Pamela, she was appreciative of Peter's efforts to complete his household tasks. Instances when Peter did not carry out his household responsibilities were recorded by Pam as major displeases. Peter, on the other hand, was lackadaisical about housekeeping and rarely noticed when Pam cleaned the house. Although Peter and Pam were aware of these differences, they each still expected the other to respond in a manner consonant with their own positions. Pam expected appreciation from Peter for doing housework and was disappointed when this was not forthcoming. Peter repeatedly acted surprised when Pam became upset at him for not completing his agreed upon tasks: After all, he would not become angry if Pam were delinquent in her responsibilities. In discussing their SOC data, it became evident that Pam could not rely upon Peter's response to sustain her efforts around the house. The efforts that she put into cleaning were to meet her own standards for a clean house. If appreciation from Peter was what she sought, she needed to emit behaviors that were important to him, which were more along the lines of affection and companionship. Peter, in return, came to realize the importance of his efforts around the house even though they afforded him little personal satisfaction. Regardless of whether or not he was affected by the dirty dishes in the sink, ignoring the dishes when he had agreed to do them produced a negative reaction in Pam.

It is an important and powerful lesson for partners to recognize the impact that they have upon one another. Having partners exchange and study the SOC conveys the message that each spouse is responsible for learning about and responding to the desires and preferences of the partner. Each spouse is also to avoid making assumptions that the partner's preferences are similar to one's own. Furthermore, through the described procedures, spouses learn how to identify important reinforcers by monitoring the effects of their behaviors on the partner. Initially, the spouses may be disappointed to realize that certain efforts to be pleasing are going unnoticed or unappreciated. Yet, often there is also the relief of finally learning what it takes to be pleasing to the partner.

Occasionally, partners put this information to use on their own accord and begin to emit more of the behaviors that the partner desires. However, the therapist can also provide a structure for partners to become more effective givers and receivers of relationship pleasure. Below we describe several procedures that have been used to enhance the positive exchange between partners. For the most part, responsibility lies with the therapist to recommend an intervention that provides a discernible and valuable improvement but, at the same time, minimizes the prospect of failure. The therapist also helps the couple plan for the intervention so that it is implemented with relative ease and spouses experience the anticipated benefits. Each intervention we will describe is most effective if it is presented in graduated steps. Accordingly, the goal of accelerating spouses' exchange of positive behaviors often prevails through several therapy sessions, consuming a portion of each of those sessions.

POSITIVE EXCHANGES DETERMINED BY THE GIVER

A strategy described in Chapter 5 to enhance the spouses' collaborative set involved having each spouse generate hypotheses of how to increase the partner's daily satisfaction with the relationship. Each spouse then tests those hypotheses by emitting the behaviors she/he hypothesized to be pleasing and examining the effect on daily satisfaction. The key factor when debriefing this assignment in the following session is that each spouse critiques his/her own behavior and avoids criticizing the partner. In addition to enhancing spouses' collaborative set, this assignment also fosters a more robust exchange of pleasing behaviors. If, however, the spouses themselves do not generate and test suitable hypotheses, the therapist can prompt this type of activity.

Production Targets

One strategy for couples whose low rates of pleases extend across many areas is to work towards a general escalation of positive behaviors, disregarding the types of behavior exchanges. This strategy arranges for a percentage increase over baseline rates of pleasing behaviors by setting a target number of pleasing behaviors that each spouse is to emit *each day*. A daily target is particularly useful for spouses who are highly reinforcing upon occasion but are generally quite lazy in their production of pleases. The daily target serves as a reminder to devote a certain amount of energy to the relationship on a consistent basis.

To implement the general increases in spouses' outputs of pleases, each spouse needs to be aware of his/her current rates of pleasing behaviors. This rate is examined in respect to whatever target rate of pleases is needed to boost the partner's satisfaction rating to an acceptable level. Weekly targets are then set so that the spouse shows an incremental change from week to week towards the designated end goal. It is essential in setting a production target of pleases that the target number be individualized according to base rates and the amount of time that spouses spend together. Whatever the target rate, the changes should be gradual enough so that they maintain from week to week. Midweek telephone calls from the therapist can be quite helpful in encouraging the spouses to keep working towards their goal, and, if they are having difficulty, to assess whether their goal is realistic.

A situation that can become problematic is the discovery of large discrepancies between spouses in their baseline rates of pleasing behaviors, i.e., one spouse appears to be putting out substantially more pleasing behaviors than the other. If the spouses are not already aware of this discrepancy, it is immediately obvious upon discussing the current rates at which they receive pleasing behaviors. Straightforward discussion of this issue is helpful to head off a spouse's protest of "Why should I work to put out more pleases? I'm already doing more than my share." An important factor to consider in this discussion is that the rates of pleasing behaviors are not absolute but are rates as perceived by the recipient of those behaviors. Thus, there is no way to sort out whether discrepant rates are a function of true differences in the givers' activity levels, differences in the perceptual thresholds of the receivers, or a combination of these two factors. The therapist can utilize the ambiguity in this situation by suggesting that the one partner's lower rates reflect an inadequacy in both partners—the giver's insufficiency as a supplier of pleases and recipient's deficiency as a careful observer and reinforcer of pleases that do occur.

Love Days

A widely advocated method of encouraging spouses to give more pleasures to one another is the use of love days (Weiss et al., 1973; Wills et al., 1974) or caring days (Stuart, 1976). This strategy is similar to previously described procedures in that each person is to increase his/her output of pleasant events. However, rather than producing a small increase in pleases that is consistent across days, love days evoke spurts of pleases on one or two days during the week. The effect tends to be more dramatic, since on the assigned day the giver of a love day is to double his/her output of pleasing behaviors. Spouses are assigned separate love days. On that day, the person giving the love day attempts to be exceptionally pleasing, independent of the actions of the partner. A peak in the recipient's satisfaction rating for that day validates its successful implementation.

It should be recognized, however, that the anticipation of a love day greatly heightens the recipient's expectations of relationship pleasures. To meet these demands, the giver needs to be armed with an extensive menu of pleasing events to include in the love day and to make it a success. Even then, miscommunication can irreparably mar a love day so that both spouses end up feeling frustrated or disillusioned, with the recipient wondering "How could she/he act that way on my love day!" and the giver thinking "There's nothing I can do to please him/her!" Love hours or love evenings, which bear fewer expectations and demands, can be used to test a couple's readiness for love days. A full love day can then be assigned after the couple has experienced success with the briefer assignments.

POSITIVE EXCHANGES THAT THE RECIPIENT REQUESTS

In the two strategies discussed thus far for accelerating positive behaviors, the person who is emitting the behaviors decides how she/he will be more pleasing. That person becomes familiar with the partner's preferences and is encouraged to sample from among those behaviors that the partner wants. However, the main goal is to generate an increase in total pleases. In this section we discuss the exchange of specific targeted behaviors that the spouses request of one another. The end product of this strategy is for each spouse to be able to formulate requests and for the other to agree to and fulfill whatever part of the request she/he can or will.

Specific Requests

A common roadblock in the exchange of pleasing behaviors is spouses' inexperience in making assertive, nondemanding requests of one another. The exchange of pleasing behaviors rests only in part upon the willingness of each partner to give pleasing behaviors. The other, equally important component, is the prospective recipient's ability to specify what she/he wants. Often this requires training in how to make requests.

A common problem that arises is spouses' reticence to take responsibility for requesting specific events that would be pleasing to receive. Consider the following comments:

> "Why should I tell her what would please me? Where she's been for the past 19 years?"
>
> "My husband knows what I want and he'd do those things if only he cared enough for me!"

The positions reflected in these statements pose real problems for relationships. They contain the implicit assumption that simply by living with a spouse, one learns the full range of that person's preferences, regardless of whether or not they have been clearly stated. There is also the suggestion that the partner possesses the power of a mindreader and can divine the changing needs and delights of his/her mate.

Another form of spouses' reticence to specify requests takes the following form: "I don't want to ask him for that. Then he'll do it out of obligation." This statement indicates that having to ask for something detracts from the rewarding nature of the behavior when it is received. After all, one never knows the partner's true motivation for engaging in the behavior. The therapist must counter this attitude. The above example typifies a common disservice performed by marital partners to one another. The present situation puts the accused spouse in the no-win situation of being blamed for not being a good husband but never being told how to improve as a spouse. Even if the wife has specified what she would like from him, the husband still has the power to decide how much he cares to do. At least then he can direct his efforts into behaviors that matter to the wife and stop wasting effort guessing what might please her.

Most couples benefit from training in the articulation of requests. Spouses do of course express their preferences but they may not communicate them effectively. Recommended formats for beginning requests include "I would appreciate it if you . . ." or "I would like you to . . ." or simply "Would you please. . . ." The second clause of the request must be stated in specific and neutral language so that the listener knows exactly what is being asked of him/her. For example, a wife's request that her husband spend more time with their daughter might be camouflaged with a criticism, such as "How come you're never home when I need you" or a vague injunction, such as "I want you to take more responsibility for raising our daughter." Framing the request in nonthreatening and precise terms not only clarifies the meaning but also reduces the pressure incurred by more global requests. An example of this would be "I would like you to spend from noon until three on Saturdays taking responsibility for our daughter." The husband learns that he does not need to modify every parenting action but merely needs to babysit once a week on Saturday afternoons.

To simplify the process of teaching spouses to make requests we may begin by having the couple refer once again to the SOC. From that list they can select a behavior that is already identified as something they would like very much to receive. The chosen behavior can then be restated in the format of a request.

There are several guidelines for spouses to follow when choosing their requests. It is at this time that we differentiate between requests and problem-solving issues. Spouses are to confine their requests to behaviors that have no negative emotional history and, in their estimation, can be performed by the partner at minimal cost. Any behavior that has been the subject of repeated discussions or has been the source of previous disappointments is not appropriate for this type of request. Those behaviors are to be earmarked as issues to be saved for problem-solving, which is described in the next chapter. Requests should also focus on behaviors which, if enacted, would actually increase the partner's pleasure rather than just removing irritation. Finally, the behavior chosen must be one that can be completed within the upcoming week.

Requests are not negotiated at this stage. The person of whom the request is made should simply agree to what she/he is willing to do. It is often useful to have that person state the probability that she/he will carry out the request. If the probability is low, a new request should be formulated.

At the beginning of the next session, the therapist should find out whether the requests were carried out. Therapist reinforcement is important for the spouse who has fulfilled his/her request. Enthusiasm on the part of the recipient spouse should also be encouraged. Unfortunately, sometimes the recipient is dissatisfied even though the request has been met. In those instances, the recipient must examine his/her own role in what has occurred: Did the person request a behavior that she/he did not really care about? What could she/he have done differently to have facilitated the other person's accomplishment of the request? Requests that are not fulfilled often signal that there is a conflictual issue underlying the request that may not have been immediately apparent. Rather than renewing these unmet requests for a second week, the couple should table them until a later problem-solving discussion.

Exchange Contracts

Writing down behavior exchange agreements is optional but it does serve to enhance the likelihood of the request being met. Although contracting is usually discussed as the last phase of problem-solving (see Chapter 7), requests can also be formalized through a written contract. When a request is put into writing, it is stated in the affirmative that partner A will complete behavior Y with X frequency. Consider the following:

> I, Eric, agree to tuck the children in bed on Tuesday, Thursday, and Sunday evenings.
>
> I, Tobi, agree to give Eric a hug and kiss each morning before getting out of bed.

Recording these agreements in writing serves several purposes. Spouses are more likely to state the agreement in precise and specific language if it is put in writing. The person who is to do the behavior is unlikely to agree in writing to a request that is unfeasible. In the service of implementation, written agreements serve both a mediating and a discriminative function. Contracts obviate the necessity to rely on memory, and thus provide a check for the self-serving distortions of spouses. Also, written agreements act as cues, reminding partners of the agreement and thereby increasing the likelihood of implementation. The discriminative power of a written contract is enhanced if it is clearly visible, e.g., by being posted at some convenient location (night table, refrigerator, bathroom mirror). Written agreements also serve as reminders in a more general sense, by signifying a couple's commitment to improving their relationship.

Even after behavior exchange contracts have been met, a spouse sometimes discredits his/her partner by expressing doubts about that person's motivation for emitting the behavior. Frequently, the spouse's skepticism reflects what he/she perceives as a lack of spontaneity in this situation (e.g., "How can I believe the nice things he said about me if he had an assignment to say at least one nice thing a day?"). The therapist cannot deny the deliberate efforts by each partner to carry out his/her request but that does not make the efforts any less worthy. If anything, the partner's desire to fulfill the contract is further evidence of that person's commitment to the relationship. It must also be noted that a signed contract facilitates fulfillment of the desired activities by identifying the importance of these behaviors. Yet, contracts of this type hold no real power over what each partner chooses to do.

There is, in addition, one therapeutic procedure that circumvents this concern by arranging for the *unscheduled* giving of gifts. The Oregon Marital Studies Program (Weiss & Birchler, 1978) originated a program known as the *Cookie Jar* in which each partner develops a pool of desired events that could be given by the partner at relatively minimal notice (e.g., a bouquet of flowers, cleaning up the back porch, a mutual sauna). Spouses write their items on color-coded slips of paper that are stored in the "cookie jar." Whenever one partner wishes to do something nice for the other, she/he simply draws the appropriately colored slip from the "cookie jar" and follows the instruction. It may be useful to review requests that spouses write, at least initially, to eliminate those that ask for global personality changes or the deceleration of behaviors. "Stop smoking," "Don't yell at the kids," and "Be more sociable" are all unacceptable requests.

The "cookie jar" differs from the previously mentioned procedures in that spouses are not required to engage in a predetermined number of pleasing acts by a particular point in time. When dipping into the "cookie jar" the partner is not fulfilling a therapeutic assignment but is spontaneously responding to his/her own impulse to be pleasing. Thus, simply the knowledge that the partner has drawn a request can be reinforcing to the recipient.

The "cookie jar" can be used at the end of therapy to fade out the therapist's input and still maintain the couple's exchange of pleasing events. The fact that there is a visible object, such as a cookie jar, serves as a discriminative stimulus reminding the partners to engage in positive exchanges. Once the procedure is set up, i.e., the cookie jar is filled, the requests are available for the spouses' use. In order for these procedures to be maintained, partners must periodically draw from the "cookie jar" and carry out the request.

MUTUAL SPECIFICATION OF A MORE PLEASING EXCHANGE

Sometimes it is most advisable to direct the couple's energies towards pleasing activities they both desire and can participate in together. Rather than the "giver-recipient" distinction we have previously referred to, this strategy involves both partners in identifying mutually pleasing events or considering how to approach certain situations in a more mutually pleasing way.

Couple Pleases

A variation of the general approach for accelerating individual production rates of pleasing behaviors is to increase "couple pleases," i.e., that subset of behaviors that both spouses mutually identify as beneficial to the relationship. Working as a team to increase the rate at which spouses exchange mutual relationship pleasures circumvents the problems that arise when one spouse demands a change that the other is reluctant to make. To implement this strategy, spouses still identify pleases they want to receive. However, they then combine lists, creating a subset of "couple pleases," which is composed of only those behaviors that both spouses identified as desirable events, and unite their efforts towards a target output of "couple pleases." While this approach of using "couple pleases" limits the variety of pleasing behaviors, some couples respond more favorably to these procedures, compared to individual pleases, since they clearly communicate that spouses are working *with* rather than *for* one another.

Companionship Activities

An intervention strategy that can be relatively easy to implement and can have far-reaching effects is that of increasing the frequency at which a couple engages in companionship activities. The purpose of this intervention is to involve spouses in enjoyable activities so that they come to view one another as discriminative stimuli for pleasure and enjoyment. It is not uncommon for distressed couples to experience deterioration in the quality or quantity of their shared recreational activities. Couples often assume that this situation will be remedied as soon as they have more time to be together or they resolve their more weighty problems. However, even if the absence of companionship activities has occurred secondarily to other relationship problems, the lack of such activities is, in itself, detrimental.

Good candidates for this intervention include those couples who, due to divergent interests, busy schedules, or wishes to avoid conflict, have developed a pattern of spending minimal recreational time together. While these couples might be concerned about their low frequency of companionship activities, they hesitate to suggest new ideas for fear that the partner would not be interested or, worse yet, might feel forced to do something that she/he does not enjoy. Poor candidates for this intervention are those couples who do not enjoy each other's company, either because communication has deteriorated or because they continue to be resentful over previous displeases. For these couples, companionship activities may be punishing.

Although one might imagine that the planning of companionship activities would be a relatively uncomplicated communication between spouses, that is not always true for a distressed couple. For example, some couples quickly agree to the first idea that is suggested and later discover that neither was particularly excited about that suggestion. They each agreed on the assumption that the other really wanted to do the activity. Other couples develop a pattern in which only one spouse is in charge of all social planning. Even if the planner grows tired of that responsibility and the other partner wants to have more input in these decisions, the pattern tends to be maintained unless the partners express their willingness for change.

When companionship events are the focus of the intervention to accelerate pleasing activities, the therapist must assist the couple in expanding their repertoires of these activities. The first step is for spouses to generate independent lists of enjoyable activities, thereby avoiding a situation in which one spouse is the lone planner while the other merely chimes in with "Yeah, let's do that" or "Any of those is fine with me." If ideas are generated verbally in the session, spouses should take turns identifying pleasing activities and should record those ideas so that they are not forgotten. Couples who have difficulty generating ideas on their own can accomplish the same objective by referring to the list of companionship events on the SOC. All couples should be encouraged to be as creative as possible and to produce as many suggestions as they can. Once ideas have been generated, the therapist and couple can then survey the lists, looking for activities that both spouses have indicated as possibilities. These procedures usually produce several activities that both partners view as potentially enjoyable.

The prudent therapist will not stop at this point but will then attend to the minute details of when and how specific activities can be integrated into the couple's schedule for the upcoming week. Even if a final decision is not reached regarding what the specific activity will be, i.e., the couple will either go to a ballgame or bowling, depending on the weather, what is important is that both partners have agreed upon a time that is set aside for their mutual recreation and enjoyment. Planning a Saturday afternoon activity may seem like a rather frivolous way to spend therapy time; yet, a highly distressed couple might never agree upon a time, disregard the entire idea, and return for their next session not having completed the activity if specific plans are not formulated in the therapist's presence. By planning the activity in the session, the therapist can actively monitor the discussion, reinforcing appropriate comments and discouraging comments that sidetrack the discussion. Since it is unimaginable for spouses to be talking about having a good time while they are upset with one another in the session, the therapist must quickly terminate and postpone conflict-laden material that could detract from a positive and supportive atmosphere. This material is frequently introduced out of long-standing negative habits and does not always represent a spouse's desire to pursue the conflictual issue. In many cases the tabling of negative discussions is helpful rather than detrimental to the therapeutic process.

One way to discourage remarks that detract from a positive focus is to emphasize that merely specifying what one partner wants does not commit the other partner to those activities. This message undermines the impression that the very mention of an idea by one's spouse obligates one to perform the behavior or to devise a good defense as to why it is not possible. It also limits the following type of crossfire comments: "You know we can't go to the mountains unless I get the car fixed and we can't afford to do that if you're still thinking about quitting your job." The therapist's job in monitoring these discussions is made easier by teaching spouses to separate the steps of generating ideas and discussing the feasibility of specific suggestions. The generation of ideas should be unimpeded by discussions about why a particular idea is or is not suitable. The optimal situation is for spouses to brainstorm until they have generated several suggestions, and then choose amongst those ideas.

There are two types of activities that are particularly suitable for an intervention to increase companionship events. A favorite activity that the couple has not engaged in for a long time but that reevokes the same anticipation as it did previously is definitely worth considering. The therapist should also direct the couple to novel, unfamiliar activities that will stimulate new patterns of interaction and avoid any repetition of past relationship failures. One of our favorite ideas came from Pete, a husband who originally had great difficulty verbalizing his ideas for enjoyable activities. After several weeks in therapy, during which time his wife's ideas dominated this couple's plans, the therapist handed each spouse a paper and asked them both to write down an idea. Pete's read as follows: "Let's have dinner on the floor with pillows, 10-15 candles all around. Eat only with toothpicks." Through this nonverbal means, Pete finally communicated one of his relationship fantasies. This suggestion was much to his wife's surprise and delight. The therapist in this case was quick to reinforce Pete for the creative idea that brought smiles of anticipation to both partners.

Even though companionship activities should be inherently rewarding and enjoyable, planning for these events must be regarded by the therapist and clients with the same degree of importance as any other homework assignment. The couple should be expected to have the assignment completed by the following session barring some highly unexpected circumstance. It is important that the therapist and couple consider whether the plan being discussed is realistic and manageable. One couple, for example, decided to splurge during their first week and go to an expensive restaurant that was well beyond their budgetary allotment for entertainment. In addition to their later regrets about spending that much money, the husband reported that he did not even enjoy the evening because of his concerns about whether he had enough money to pay the bill.

The therapist should not hesitate to exercise his/her option to discourage a plan that is not likely to succeed, even if the shortcomings of the plan are not immediately evident to the couple. One therapist encountered this situation when she recognized that the wife's suggestion of a walk on the beach was actually an indirect way of getting her husband in a situation where he would have to converse with her. This suggestion touched upon one of their major relationship problems since the wife constantly pressured the husband to open up to her and express his feelings. Although the husband was willing to accept the suggestion of a walk on the beach, perhaps not understanding the suggestion's ramifications, the therapist expressed her concern that the event might intensify relationship tensions. The therapist then directed the couple towards events they had previously suggested which involved more physical activity and less conversation. Initially we are advocating a very protective stance in working with a couple to explore all reasons why a plan might succeed or fail. This stance can then be abdicated as soon as the therapist is convinced that the couple will modify rather than abandon their plans if faced with an unforeseen obstacle.

Shared Avocations

The therapeutic strategy of developing common interests or avocations is similar to engaging in companionship activities in that each partner receives reinforcement from the activity itself as well as social reinforcement from the partner. However, shared avocations necessitate less intensive contact between partners and thus are more applicable for spouses who are hesitant to increase the amount of time they spend together as a couple. The rationale behind having spouses share a new interest is that this activity will offer them a focal point for interaction that is entirely divorced from the tensions of their past. Pursuit of the new interest may require taking a class, seeking information, or putting in hours of independent activity. None of these involves intimate interaction for the spouses. Yet, with both partners pursuing the same new interest, they have a positive context for interacting. For example, when both partners take tennis lessons, they may not be in the same class, and certainly do not always play together. What they can share is their enthusiasm for the sport. Then, when they do play together or discuss their separate matches, they may feel a new closeness based upon their common experiences. An added benefit is that the respect for one another's budding competence with the sport might increase the spouses' mutual attraction.

Shared avocations should also be considered for the problem of reinforcement erosion, when one or both spouses' effectiveness as a reinforcer has diminished after many repetitions of the same positive exchanges. Sheer increases in frequencies of pleasing events are not particularly helpful to these couples. What they need instead is novelty and variation, and the introduction of shared avocations can fulfill that need if the couple chooses the right activity. One couple who learned how to scuba dive found a great deal of pleasure in sharing their excitement over this activity. They were also comforted upon learning that they suffered some of the same fears about scuba diving. The shared avocation need not be a physical activity. Any situation that stimulates a new cognitive response or a strong emotional reaction provides a context for a rewarding exchange between the spouses.

Habitual Lowspots

Some couples report that there is a particular time of the day or week during which they repeatedly feel somewhat distant from one another. These times are not necessarily conflict ridden, but they are frustrating and disappointing for the couple. Frequently the lowspots are due to the couple's inability to structure this time to meet the separate needs of both partners. A common lowspot for couples is the period of time at the end of the day, when spouses reunite after their separate workdays. That tends to be a particularly busy time during which spouses experience many demands and have little time for one another. One spouse may want to converse about his/her day while the other has very different ideas, e.g., making dinner, reading the mail, taking care of the children, or spending time alone to unwind. Unless spouses have clearly specified what they would like from each other during this time period, their expectations are frequently unmet.

The reason for taking therapy time to restructure these relationship lowpoints is to help spouses communicate their requests to one another; then they can determine which of these requests can be readily integrated into that period of the day. Very often the partners are willing to fulfill each other's requests but heretofore have not known what they were. In working on increasing positive behaviors for this specific time period, the therapist must help each spouse identify what the partner could do to make the time more pleasant. Spouses sometimes find it helpful to consider several scenarios before they are able to identify specific behaviors, such as "greet me at the door," "offer me a beer," "take a shower," "sit down with me for five minutes," or "hold off dinner for a full half hour after I get home." When the couple is discussing these events, the therapist wants to make sure that the requested behaviors are carefully specified and that the partners are in accord about what is being requested. It is worthwhile to spend some time roleplaying an individualized request, such as a greeting that would express interest in the partner's day but not develop into a lengthy conversation, particularly if the request is not easily visualized. The extra time spent in illustrating or practicing these behaviors reduces the possibility that they will lead to conflict rather than pleasure.

Habitual lowspots usually signal that the couple is not exercising sufficient control over their relationship. When the lowspots occur at lengthy intervals (e.g., weekly, monthly) the couple experiences wide variations in their marital satisfaction but may not be aware of any particular pattern to the fluctuations. Viewed in light of each spouse's own good intentions, the rapid changes from good to bad have no obvious explanation: Spouses either blame their partners, or attribute the fluctuations to such uncontrollable factors as biorhythms, menstrual cycles, or the "irrefutable fact" that they simply cannot sustain more than three consecutive days of relationship harmony. While the patterns are a reality, they are usually a result of the couple's own doing. When the relationship begins to falter, one or both partners attempts to reverse the pattern by being an exceptionally attentive loving partner. This causes the relationship to stabilize temporarily, but unless the positive actions have been appropriately reinforced, they again taper off, setting in motion another negative cycle. Over time these cycles diminish spouses' good feelings about the relationship and their trust of the partner.

These cycles can be abated if spouses learn to maintain consistently high levels of pleasing behaviors. Sandy and Phil were a couple whose widely fluctuating frequencies of pleasing behaviors were first evidenced during the two weeks of pretreatment assessment. The initial intervention of assigning target production rates of pleases did not work; both spouses continued to record several days of extremely low rates of pleasing behaviors. However, it became evident at this point that the couple repeatedly reached their lowest exchange of pleasing events during the weekend. Based on that observation, the therapists decided to switch their strategy from accelerating pleasing events in general to increasing the pleasing exchange during the weekend in an effort to counteract additional downward trends. Continued analysis of this couple's problem revealed that Sandy typically waited for Phil to initiate weekend plans. When nothing happened, she became despondent, which was communicated to Phil as displeasure. By the time the spouses were finally together, which usually was on Sunday, the day was a disaster. Eventually Phil would apologize profusely for what had transpired between them and the disagreement would be temporarily forgotten until it was repeated the following week. This couple's difficulty was more a function of not knowing what they could expect from one another than of an incompatibility over what each spouse considered a good time. When they finally negotiated what to do with their time together, the spouses became excited over a variety of activities. However, differentiating individual versus mutual time and maximizing the quality of mutual time through preplanning continued to be important foci throughout the course of this couple's therapy.

Restructuring Relationship Rules

One further consideration in efforts to expand what is mutually acceptable in a couple's exchange is the role of relationship rules. Relationships are governed by rules which specify areas of appropriate and inappropriate behaviors for each partner. In most cases, these rules are not explicitly spelled out, but as Sager (1976) has shown, it is usually possible to derive a marriage contract from couples' covert expectations regarding appropriate and inappropriate behaviors. Spouses usually share some understanding regarding what kinds of friendships are allowed outside the relationship, who will initiate sex, and how that initiation will manifest itself, who is responsible for what household tasks, and the like. Each couple develops certain rules that are essential to the maintenance of a satisfactory relationship. However, other rules may limit the behaviors each partner engages in, thereby restraining the overall exchange of relationship pleasures. As part of the process of examining creative ways to increase a couple's exchange of relationship pleasures, it is often necessary to renegotiate restrictive or outdated relationship rules.

Relationship problems arise when some external change, either gradual or sudden, necessitates a need for changes in the rules governing the relationship, and these rule changes are not forthcoming. In Chapter 1 we mentioned that relationship dissatisfaction may be associated with a couple's failure to adjust to a major change in the relationship structure. Most long-term relationships pass through a number of stages: dating, beginning a sexual relationship, cohabitation, marriage, job changes, birth of children, departure of children from the home, aging, and so on. Each substantial change requires some behavioral adjustment on the part of the couple. Often, couples adapt flexibly to changing circumstances. At other times, however, couples fail to alter their behaviors adequately in response to a new era. In these instances, the new era can signal the beginnings of marital distress. Rule difficulties also manifest themselves in another general way in distressed relationships. If spouses have discrepant views as to what the rules are, each partner may act on his/her private expectations. The partners may then view one another as violating the nuptial agreement, when in fact the problem is actually one of communication. Neither partner has communicated his/her expectations to the other, and therefore reality-testing has not occurred. The therapeutic task in this case becomes one of expressing expectations, and then drawing up a single set of marital rules based on *shared* expectations. Even when spouses enter marriage with similar expectations, one partner may change his/her behavior at a later time due to influences or experiences outside the marriage. Because of these changes, old rules become anachronistic and new rules need to be formed.

Relationship problems also occur because of anarchy, the absence of any governing rules. For whatever reason, certain areas of mutual interest are not included in the marriage contract. As a result, whenever the couple interacts in this particular domain there is a power struggle, since no rules exist to make the decision for them. If couples enter therapy with such lacunae in their marriage contract, the therapist's task is to help create order out of chaos through a clear delineation of rules to cover the domain in question.

A written agreement to govern certain aspects of a couple's interpersonal behavior is the therapeutic strategy to compensate for an absence of relationship rules or a lack of resiliency in old rules. What follow are some case examples of transitional contracts; these cases illustrate the versatility of this therapeutic strategy.

After Bill and Dana had their first child, Dana became excessively burdened by her part-time job, her virtually exclusive responsibility for maintaining a clean house, and the added responsibilities of infant management. Bill, who was pursuing a Ph.D. degree in urban planning, continued to remain away from home 12-16 hours per day due to the requirements of his graduate education. Before the birth of the child Bill and Dana had been a well-functioning, happy couple. They would have remained happy were it not for their inability to shift their interpersonal patterns and responsibilities to accommodate the presence of a new family member. The resentment and insidiously progressive discord were neither discussed nor acknowledged until they reached the point where they argued and bickered constantly. The transitional contract which was constructed to accommodate to the new era read as follows:

> I, Bill S., recognizing that Dana has more work now than she can possibly handle, resolve to change my behavior in order to help her out and improve the marriage.
>
> A. I will assume certain household responsibilities that used to be hers: vacuuming, washing the dishes, cleaning the bathroom, and laundry.

B. On weekends, I will assume responsibility for Karen. This includes bathing, changing, feeding, and waking up with her.

C. On weekdays, I will always be home by 5:30 p.m., and if I have to work at night it will be at home rather than at the library.

I, Dana S., to reciprocate Bill's effort to help ease my burden at home promise to:

A. Assume all household and child-rearing responsibilities not allocated to Bill.
B. Help Bill out on weekends with his work by helping him with clerical tasks and going to the library for him when necessary.

* * *

Derrick and Pat had been married for two years, and experienced almost constant discord over their discrepant notions of what commitment to a long-term relationship meant. Unfortunately, rather than checking out their expectations with one other, they each quietly concluded that the partner had violated their unspoken agreement. Of course, since each entertained their own idiosyncratic views regarding the marital agreement, neither was in fact guilty of any violation at all. However, they were both guilty of not communicating their expectations to one another, and thereby perpetuating their discrepant versions of the marriage contract. Their new contract, negotiated in therapy, eliminated these discrepancies:

I, Derrick F., expect my wife to spend most of our week nights at home. I further expect her to have a part-time job rather than our living near poverty because of my having to carry the financial load. I expect her to share the disciplining of the children, rather than telling them "to wait till Daddy gets home."

I, Pat F., want to feel free to make a pass at my husband. Sexual initiation is not his exclusive right, and if I am horny on a given night, I expect to have the power to initiate sex. Furthermore, I expect major financial decisions between us to be mutual rather than dictated from above. I want to help with the accounting. Finally, I expect husband and wife to share responsibility for bringing up the children, especially on those occasions when Derrick is home, such as evenings and weekends.

We both agree to allow the other to pursue nonsexual friendships with either sex outside of the relationship. All of our friends need not be couple friends. The only limitation on this expectation is that these other friendships should not impose on our limited time together. Finally, when we are together, we should be companions to one another, and not simply engage in parallel play, e.g., watching T.V., writing letters.

Although Gary and Michelle conformed to a set of implicit rules in most areas of their marriage, they had great difficulties in the area of leisure time activities. Whereas household responsibilities, financial decision-making, child care, sex, and affection were all governed by a mutual, albeit unspecified, understanding of lines of authority and responsibility, power was always up for grabs on the question of how to spend leisure time activities. Anarchy reigned supreme in this area. Gary, who often preferred to remain at home alone with Michelle, frequently became angry at Michelle for making plans with friends without consulting him. Another problem which frequently arose involved two sets of weekend plans being made, where each spouse claimed to have received permission from the other to pursue their respective wishes. This perpetual conflict area between Gary and Michelle reflects a classic battle for control in an uncodified area of their relationship. Through the therapist's mediation, the following precedent was established:

> We, Gary and Michelle, must strike a balance between socializing with other couples and enjoying each other. On weekend nights, we will generally spend one night alone and one night with other people. If we are invited out for a particular night, and we both agree that it is something we would like to do, that will be all for the weekend socializing. Otherwise we will alternate weekends: On one weekend Gary will decide on the night and the company, and on the other next weekend, Michelle will decide. If one of us has already planned an evening, and then we get invited out for the other evening, we will say no!

* * *

Larry and Charlene spent the first three years of their marriage, which included the birth of two children, in a fairly conventional, traditional marriage. Over time Charlene became less comfortable with the arrangement, as the life of a housewife became less and less reinforcing. She joined a women's group, and grew to realize that she was not alone in her dissatisfaction with the role. Larry, on the one hand, was sympathetic to her expressions of discontent; yet he was reluctant to compromise on what to him had been a fulfilling, satisfying arrangement up until that time. As their arguments increased in frequency, Charlene decided to present Larry with an ultimatum: He either could enter therapy and begin to build a new relationship, or he could begin a new relationship with someone else. Their new marriage contract was a 20 page document, and will not be reproduced here. But the changes in it were quite sweeping and included a provision that each of them would would work part-time, that they would have no more children, and that many duties which had been the former province of one or the other would now be shared. Ultimately, the relationship was sufficiently important to Larry to justify the rather fundamental modifications in their relationship structure. Some couples, when faced with such a choice, would opt for separating since a sustained commitment involving the new terms would not justify the increased costs. Since men have been the primary beneficiaries of the traditional marriage, changes in the status of women, which result in increasing assertiveness on their part regarding benefits to be derived from marriage, have led to thousands of renegotiated marriage contracts at some short-term cost to husbands. Many relationships have terminated rather than accommodate to such sweeping demands for change. Larry and Charlene opted for radical alterations of their relationship, and thus have remained together.

In the above examples, the contractual terms tend to be relatively general and imprecise. The lack of specificity and elaboration in these agreements violates the spirit of negotiation training we advocate in the next two chapters. These contracts are not, therefore, finished products. Derrick and Pat, for example, formed the general contract that included a number of change agreements. They later negotiated each point individually for the purposes of clarification and specification. Nevertheless, the listing of expectations was valuable for both of them, and clarified the discrepancies in their views on what a marriage partnership was. When spouses are unaware of one another's wishes and expectations, the symbolic act of specifying them can be informative, cathartic, and progressive. Similarly, when changes in the marital context come about, the stimulus control deficit created by the lack of governing rules can be the primary problem. In contrast to when roles, responsibilities, and duties have been unclear and unexpressed, these contractual agreements can generate more predictable, more mutual, and therefore, more reinforcing behavior. At times they can adequately substitute for exceedingly inelegant, protracted intervention strategies.

SELECTING THE INTERVENTION

When implementing an increase in pleasing behaviors, the therapist needs to answer several questions about the couple she/he is treating to determine what type of intervention is most suitable. (1) Have the spouses' attempts to please one another slacked off? Interventions that are applied in this situation should produce a general upsurge in pleasing behaviors so that the partners have a greater sense of being cared for, attended to, and appreciated by one another: The giving of "love days" is one way to achieve these particular aims. (2) Are spouses not communicating their desires to one another in a manner that facilitates the other person's response? In this instance, the emphasis on fulfilling specific requests and writing exchange contracts is appropriate. (3) Is the lack of positive exchange related to a particular stimulus situation, such as a specific time, setting, or content issue? If such a relationship is discovered, it is best to work directly with the circumstances that trigger the depression in positive exchange by restructuring habitual lowspots or relationship rules. (4) Are the spouses ineffective at reinforcing one another such that positive behaviors are emitted but do not carry any reinforcing value? The goal in this case is to enhance the reinforcing potential of one or both partners by introducing more variability into the partners' range of pleasing behaviors or by instructing spouses to engage in shared activities that are inherently reinforcing. Occasionally it is also necessary to help one spouse become involved in a self-improvement program to make that person more attractive to his/her partner through weight loss, reduced smoking, fashionable attire, or the acquisition of a new skill.

ENGINEERING THE ACCELERATION OF PLEASING BEHAVIORS

In order to accomplish any of the described interventions, the therapist must maintain the directive stance we have discussed previously. The therapist bears the responsibility of introducing the intervention and supplies a good portion of the initial momentum. She/he must also structure the discussion so that the couple is prepared, by the end of each session, to work on a specific assignment at home.

The therapist can share with the couple his/her agenda for the session in the following manner:

"One of our goals for today is to look very closely at the information you have been collecting for several weeks on the types of pleasing behaviors that you provide for one another. I want to discuss what you see as the important aspects of your exchange that affect your partner's and your own satisfaction ratings. By the time you leave here today we should have a definite strategy to enhance the pleasing exchange between the two of you. Our plans will include activities that you can carry out during the next week at home."

By informing the couple of the structure of the meeting, the therapist enables them to work along with him to minimize sidetracking through irrelevant issues and keeps the session focused on the work that needs to be done.

The key to a well-received introduction lies in the way that the therapist relates the purpose of the intervention to the couple's stated concerns. The couple must be made to feel that the therapist is structuring the treatment as an answer to their unique concerns, in contrast to feeling that the therapist is blindly applying a random technique without attention to the unique facets of their own situation. It is thus helpful for the therapist to convey the reasoning that led to beginning therapy by accelerating positives and to indicate what type of effect this intervention might have for the couple. To do this, the therapist must integrate what the couple have verbalized and what their data reveal. Consider this example:

> As I recall from our very first session, Ellen, you mentioned that you would like to feel more appreciated by Jim. I think you said you wanted him to pay more attention to you. As I see it, this request relates very closely to the information you have given me on the SOC. Looking over the two weeks of data that you've collected, it is quite clear that the rates of consideration and affection pleases that you report for Jim are lower than many of the other areas. It looks as if Jim is doing a lot of things around the house but I guess those efforts are not as important to you as his showing appreciation. Likewise, Jim, you were concerned about the fact that the two of you rarely do things together. What is evident from your data is that the two of you actually spend a lot of time together but that you don't do many of the activities you would like. If you think in terms of your +1 to +3 ratings, you do many of those +1 activities, such as watching television or reading together, but not many of the +2 or +3 activities are happening. It is essential that you build up these two areas of appreciation and companionship and I recommend that we make the improvement of these areas our initial focus in therapy. That means that we must temporarily postpone working on sex and occupational issues, which you've identified as your major sources of trouble. I promise that we will get to these major areas but it will be easier once we've resolved some of the minor ones and established a basis of greater support and caring.

An important aspect of the above explanation is demonstrating how the therapist's conclusions are drawn directly from the client's data. The connection between one partner's behavior and the other partner's satisfaction rating is made even clearer through graphs that plot daily frequencies of pleasing behaviors and daily satisfaction ratings. Spouses can be instructed to plot aspects of their own data that have been defined as areas needing improvement. As shown in Figure 1, the wife was graphing separate frequencies of consideration and affectionate pleases as well as the occurrence/nonoccurrence of sexual intercourse and arguments. The husband was graphing companionship activities, his wife's positive statements regarding his work, and arguments. Sometimes graphing sheer frequencies of a particular type of behavior does not provide enough information, as in the case of companionship activities for this husband. Although the overall level of companionship pleases was satisfactory, a close examination of individual items revealed the low occurrence of highly desirable behaviors. The target for treatment in this instance was to increase a subsample of companionship events rather than the complete range of these activities.

Graphs like Figure 1 can be continued throughout therapy as a measure of the couple's progress. They provide feedback on the overall quality of the relationship and assess the effects of interventions for specific problems. The therapist should take note whenever an increase in a specific behavior or category is related to an increase in the partner's satisfaction. That association provides the motivation for continuing to emit those particular behaviors.

PROMOTING REINFORCEMENT BETWEEN SPOUSES

The procedures we have described for accelerating pleasing interactions are effective only if each spouse's efforts are acknowledged. If the partner ignores the new efforts or, worse yet, finds fault with them, they will rapidly dwindle. Sometimes a spouse's pleasure from the new efforts is obscured by his/her fear that the pleasing behaviors will stop as soon as the therapist no longer makes them an assignment. This concern is reflected in comments such as "How come you never did this before if it's so easy to do now?" or "You're only doing this now because you have to." The spouse who makes these types of comments must be convinced that his/her behavior determines whether or not the partner's efforts will continue. Adequate reinforcement will guarantee their continuance; questioning the giver's intentions or criticizing the giver's performance will guarantee their demise.

The therapist cannot assume that once the requested behaviors have occurred, the recipient will automatically express appreciation. On the contrary, a more likely assumption for distressed spouses is that they are relatively unskilled at reinforcing behaviors that they like. Yet, devising procedures so that spouses acknowledge one another's efforts can require the same degree of ingenuity as setting up the initial intervention. An explanation on the importance of reinforcement coupled with some minimal prompting may be enough to get some spouses acknowledging each other's pleasing behaviors. Other couples who are unaccustomed to positive feedback need more practice before positive feedback becomes a

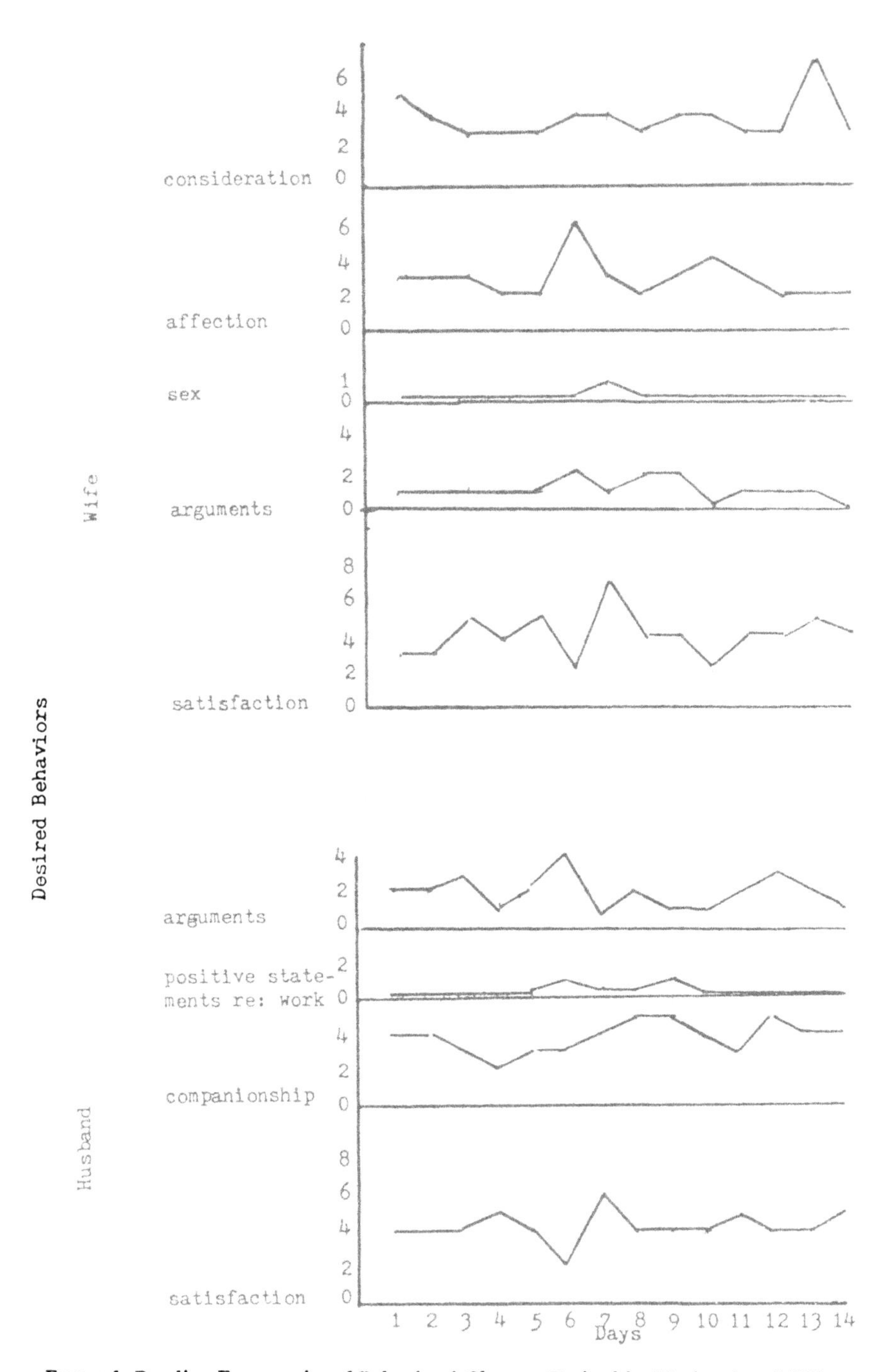

FIGURE 1. Baseline Frequencies of Behavioral Changes Desired by Husband and Wife.

natural component of interaction. One procedure to help spouses acknowledge each other's efforts is having the spouses read to one another the list of pleasing events they received that day. Here is a segment from a session with one couple who was to discuss the pleasing events each spouse had recorded. The wife had given her husband a gift and did not receive sufficient appreciation when he originally opened the package. Yet, when recounting the pleases the husband received that day, he included the gift.

T: What happened with the sharing of the pleases? I see that you did go through and check off pleasing events. Wednesday is the first night that you shared pleases. How did each of you feel?
W: I felt great!
H: Really great, because she asked me what I put down and I told her all the things. And I asked her the same thing.
W: And some of them really came as a shock.
T: Can you think of an example that really surprised you?
W: Yeah, buying a gift.
T: Is that something he told you was a please?
W: Yeah, buying him a gift. That was real surprising.
H: Well, you went out and bought me a shirt.
W: But then he told me the shirt was really weird. It was too small.
T: (*to husband*) So there were some problems with the shirt you got. Did you let Ellen know that you liked that she went out and bought you a gift?
H: I think I said it was a really nice shirt and I said "Thanks a lot, what's that for?" She said, "It's one of my pleases."
W: I signed the card "Mrs. Please."
H: At first, I couldn't understand the "Mrs. Please," but then it dawned on me, you know. I was really excited but got kinda discouraged myself when I saw it didn't fit me.
T: It's going to be hard to know what actually happened when you first discussed this but it's important that you let her know that you liked the card and the gift. (*To wife*) Did you have a sense that he liked it?
W: No, no.
T: You need more of that?
W: That he liked it? Yeah, I definitely do. I thought it was really nice of me.
T: Well, the way it's been discussed now, I get the sense your efforts were appreciated. But it's more important for you to get that feedback at the time.
W: Earlier it didn't come across like that to me. I bought something else, too. But then I know that he liked it. . . .
T: In that situation you knew he was pleased. What did he do to show that?
W: He said, "That was really nice of you. I'm not going to use it

until we get into the new house." (*To husband*) I mean you were really excited.

The situation presented by this couple is not uncommon. Perhaps the husband had not shown adequate recognition for his wife's attempt to please him by buying the shirt, even though he did not find the shirt altogether to his liking. Or, perhaps the wife responded too strongly to the husband's equivocal reaction to the shirt and did not hear the appreciation he did express. As this example illustrates, spouses can sometimes encounter difficulties with giving and receiving feedback that is appropriately positive yet candid.

Another couple was unfamiliar and uncomfortable with giving positive feedback and somewhat wary of this recommendation. The following statements summarize the wife's sentiments: "Why should I let him know that I appreciate something he is supposed to do? He should know I appreciate it if I asked for it!" The therapists decided to have this couple initially work on positive feedback before accelerating any other positive behaviors. In the first treatment session, the therapists asked each spouse to write an ending to the following sentence regarding the partner's behavior for the day: "I appreciated it when you. . . ." The therapists worked briefly with each partner to get a statement that was devoid of any hints of criticism. The appreciation notes read as follows: (*wife to husband*) "I appreciated it when you ate the sandwich I prepared for your lunch." (*husband to wife*) "I appreciated it when you handled the customer on the phone." The spouses commented upon seemingly mundane behaviors. Yet, upon exchanging notes, they broke into wide grins and the husband remarked, "I didn't even know that you had noticed." The spouses were instructed to leave one written note of appreciation for each other every day for the next week. Statements were to be written rather than verbalized to formalize the procedure and to keep the assignment distinct from the couple's other interactions. This assignment fulfilled the dual purpose of increasing the overall exchange of appreciation and giving feedback on specific behaviors that were well received.

The therapist cannot overemphasize the importance of positive feedback in trying to accelerate spouses' attempts to be more pleasing. It is a topic that needs to be dealt with in sessions with direct questions (e.g., How did you let your husband know that you appreciated his concern? How did she communicate her appreciation to you?) and with the rehearsal of such skills if they are lacking. In addition, the therapist can model how to give positive feedback by enthusiastically acknowledging spouses' efforts in the sessions and reinforcing their progress at home.

SUMMARY

This chapter describes a variety of procedures for increasing a couple's positive exchanges and enhancing partners' reinforcing value for one another. The spouses first learn to identify important relationship behaviors by monitoring their own behavior and its relationship to the partner's daily satisfaction. An increase in significant relationship behaviors is then engineered with the expectation that marital satisfaction will also increase. The overall strategy addresses both the erosion of relationship reinforcement and spouses' abdication of control over their relationship.

The couple's response at this stage is indicative of the degree of the flexibility that exists in the relationship. Some less distressed couples find they can resolve a wide variety of problems by employing only the strategies described in this chapter. It is best that we spare these couples our more advanced technology unless they absolutely need it. The more common situation is for couples to experience an initial boost from these procedures but be unable to move ahead until they learn specific skills to ameliorate their more difficult problems. There also are couples who have not obtained benefits after employing one or more of these interventions. Our first recommendation for these couples is renewed emphasis on developing a collaborative set, as described in the previous chapter. If there continue to be no gains, we recommend evaluating the spouses' reasons for being in therapy. When a couple makes no progress at this stage, one partner may be using therapy for a unilateral goal, such as convincing the mate that the marriage is over.

In addition to the inherent benefits of this type of intervention, it primes the couple for future change strategies. Spouses have been taught to take responsibility for requesting what they want from one another in nonthreatening, specific terms and for reinforcing the partner's efforts. Spouses have also demonstrated their willingness to risk greater relationship involvement which may also expose them to additional hurt. Participating in this initial treatment phase has the net effect of increasing spouses' investment in their relationship and the therapeutic process. In return, clients receive a demonstration of what therapy can offer. It should be clear that relationship improvement can be a pleasurable rather than painful experience and that at least some improvement is within their reach. These factors should encourage the couple to avail themselves of the potential benefits of upcoming therapeutic steps.

CHAPTER 7

Communication and Problem-solving Training

COMMUNICATION TRAINING is germane to any treatment program for relationship problems. Most theoretical perspectives on marital distress implicate communication deficits between marital partners as important areas on which to focus in therapy, either because such deficits are presumed to hold etiological significance, or because they are viewed as current manifestations of more primary interpersonal and intrapsychic conflicts.

Behavior therapy therefore has no monopoly on communication training. However, communication training from a behavioral perspective can be distinguished both by the *content* of skills which couples are taught, and by the *procedures* which characterize such training. Beginning with the latter, behavioral approaches to communication training can be distinguished by the systematic program of skill training involving provision of feedback, instructions, and behavior rehearsal. This method for skill training, briefly alluded to in Chapter 2, has been used in a variety of settings as a strategy for treating numerous interpersonal skill deficits. Its association with behavior therapy is by now familiar.

Although there is substantial overlap between the communication skills emphasized by behavioral marital therapists and those of other orientations, many of the skills taught in a behavioral program follow uniquely from a behavioral exchange model. This is particularly evident in *problem-solving* training, an important subcomponent of behavioral communication training. During problem-solving training, couples are taught behavior management skills in order to render them more effective in bringing about desirable behavior changes in the relationship through direct negotiation. Such a treatment emphasis is indicated whenever deficits in behavior change strategies are implicated as an important antecedent of relationship distress. Among other things, couples are taught to pinpoint target behaviors, to utilize behavior management strategies such as shaping, and to base their behavior change attempts on positive rather than aversive control principles.

Communication training has applicability far beyond the correction of deficits in problem-solving and behavior change skills. Distressed couples are often lacking in a variety of communication skills; since it is primarily through the medium of communication that couples provide benefits to one another, deficits in this area can often be instrumental in generating or maintaining an unsatisfying relationship.

Behavior therapists train couples in a variety of communication skills, using technologies which have generalized applicability across diverse content areas. The first section of this chapter will discuss procedures for training couples in communication skills, ignoring the content of the skills that are taught. Then, in a second section, we will discuss a variety of skills which can be taught to couples. Finally, in a third section, we will provide an extended discussion of problem-solving training, organized around a training manual which we have used with couples.

STRATEGIES FOR COMMUNICATION TRAINING

In this section we will elaborate on the clinical strategies which we use to train couples in a wide variety of communication and problem-solving skills. The skill training model that we emphasize is implemented sequentially, in a series involving three major training components: (1) *feedback,* where couples are provided with information about their current, presumably maladaptive, communication patterns; (2) *instructions,* where the therapist provides alternative, presumably more desirable, communication patterns for the couple; and (3) *behavior rehearsal,* where couples practice the communication patterns provided by the therapist. The three components form a circular relationship to one another, since couples continue to receive feedback during their practice attempts, and subsequently base further rehearsals on this feedback and further instructions (cf. Eisler & Hersen, 1973; Jacobson, 1977d; Jacobson & Martin, 1976; Margolin & Weiss, 1978b; O'Leary & Turkewitz, 1978).

Feedback

Let us define feedback as the provision of information to a couple regarding some aspect of their recently consummated behavior. In couples therapy feedback refers to the presentation of information about characteristics of their interaction, usually immediately or shortly after the interaction has been observed by a therapist. More specifically, in communication training feedback is based on a live communication exercise conducted by the couple. Feedback can be provided for either verbal or nonverbal aspects of performance. At times feedback occurs for specific behavioral units, for example, one statement uttered by the husband; in contrast to such molecular feedback, more commonly feedback is sequential, emphasizing an entire series of verbal exchanges between partners, and analyzing the relationship between these various exchanges. Other therapeutic approaches provide feedback to their clients; despite many similarities, behavioral feedback can be distinguished in at least two ways. First, behavioral feedback tends to be descriptive as opposed to interpretive. For example, a therapist might comment in the following way: "You praised her in your first statement. But then you criticized her for at least three things at the same time." In contrast, other approaches often treat behavior metaphorically or symbolically, and discuss its meaning, as perceived by the therapist or by the partner. For example, "You seemed to be saying, 'I'm going to praise you because the therapist told me to'; but your later remarks suggest that you were really trying to punish your wife for forcing you to be inauthentic earlier." Second, instead of focusing on the "message" conveyed by the behavior, behavior therapists emphasize the function of the behavior, in terms of its effect on other behaviors. The following therapist remark is illustrative. "The two of you were exchanging ideas pretty well until Judy made the remark about laziness; at that point things started to go downhill, and you began to criticize each other." Thus, feedback in a behavioral skills setting provides information about the nature of their interaction, the cues which seem to elicit particular responses, and the functional relationships between various aspects of the interaction sequence.

There are many dimensions along which feedback can vary. First, feedback can be *purely* descriptive or, at the other extreme, evaluative. "You interrupted him" exemplifies the former, whereas the latter is exemplified in the following statement: "Your interruption disrupted the communication." In problem-solving training, the therapist often labels particular behaviors as desirable or undesirable. Such judgments are based on rules identified for the couple, and are directed toward the goal of efficient, effective problem-solving. All critical remarks directed toward the couple are specific and limited to the context of the problem-solving situation. Since problem-solving is portrayed as a specialized kind of communication, even a technology, this kind of feedback is relatively easy for most couples to accept. It resembles instruction in other kinds of technical skills, such as learning to operate an automobile. Like any skill, critical feedback is often necessary before mastery can be expected; the therapist explains this to couples, and makes every effort to delimit his critical remarks in such a way as to reinforce the notion of participation in a technical, skill-building program.

Feedback can also vary according to its latency from the time in which the targeted response occurred. Some feedback is provided immediately following a response, whereas at other times it is delayed pending the completion of an entire interaction sequence. Delayed feedback is less disruptive of ongoing communication, and many couples report frustration following a high frequency of immediate feedback. Yet delayed feedback decreases the therapist's control over couples' communication, and allows couples to engage in a chain of disruptive behavior, which can be detrimental to the exercise and to treatment in general. Thus, immediate feedback not only allows the therapist to reinforce and punish partners soon after the occurrence of the behavior in question, but it disrupts aversive interaction early in the coercive chain, thereby preventing the usual negative outcome. *More often than not, the beginning stages of communication training should include a predominance of immediate feedback, since at this point, couples are minimally skillful and maximally primed for conflict.* As the relationship improves and couples develop skills, increasingly delayed feedback is both feasible and desirable, since it paves the way for termination and autonomy from the therapist.

Feedback can be either purely verbal, or augmented by the use of videotape. Since videotape feedback provides couples with added information, therapists often prefer it to simple verbal feedback. However, the few relevant studies are not supportive of its effectiveness. In an analog setting, Eisler, Hersen, and Agras (1973) found that instructions alone were as effective as instructions plus feedback in increasing eye contact among couples. Alkire and Brunse (1974), in a study plagued by methodological problems, reported an astoundingly high divorce rate among couples exposed to video feedback. These studies are not to be taken as definitive, and in fact probably bear little direct relevance to the use for which we are exploring video feedback. However, whatever benefits are to be derived by providing couples with such feedback have been difficult to document, and if anything we can conclude tentatively that videotape is a powerful tool, but that its effects are unpredictable. After all, it is not difficult to understand how such feedback could exert an adverse effect on a couple. Some partners are essentially unaware of their interactional style, and, assuming the role of victim, they view themselves as passive reactors to the other's malevolent behavior. Video feedback provides this kind of partner with a unique opportunity to view her/himself as an observer would view him/her; if the picture is less than flattering, and if the viewer had a considerably distorted view of her/himself in the interaction, the experience can be jarring.

This potential risk in using videotape is probably also the source of its greatest benefit, giving each partner an opportunity to view his/her own interaction from the vantage point of an observer. The *reciprocal* nature of the self-defeating interactions is often most obvious when one is not participating. We think that video feedback is, for this reason, worth the risk, as long as steps are taken to minimize the risks. Preparation should be routine, particularly before couples are accustomed to viewing themselves; advance warnings about the common shock of viewing oneself on tape should help mitigate the impact. Once the tape has been viewed, the therapist should accentuate all positive aspects of the interaction, and critique the performance as neutrally as possible.

This suggestion of combining positive and negative feedback leads directly to a fourth consideration in the use of feedback: providing feedback for positive as well as negative interactional behavior. Distressed couples provide so much negative interaction worthy of therapist comment that it is easy to forget the importance of reinforcing whatever desirable behavior couples exhibit when they enter therapy. Therapists are often understandably reluctant to add to the already extensive amount of feedback provided for negative behavior, since additional feedback increases the extent to which couples are disrupted in their communicative endeavors. Yet such feedback is vitally important; furthermore, disruptiveness can be minimized. Provision of positive feedback need not be as thorough and descriptive as negative feedback; one-word exclamations such as "fantastic" or "good," or nonverbal praise in the form of smiles or head nods often suffice. These types of stimuli are not disruptive. An additional strategy for providing positive feedback is to stop couples contingent upon disruptive behavior, and precede the criticisms with positive feedback for the behavior which occurred prior to the rule violations.

It will soon be apparent that, as the therapist provides feedback to a couple, she/he must utilize tactics reminiscent of the rules which couples are asked to follow while problem-solving with one another. We just mentioned the importance of presenting positive feedback prior to negative feedback, which is analogous to a guideline in the problem-solving manual that follows, where all complaints are prefaced with expressions of appreciation. Also, therapists should be critical only of behavior, not of clients: by confining feedback to behavioral descriptions and avoiding global attributions of motivation, the therapist increases the likelihood that the couple will be receptive to feedback. The intellectual challenge involved in instructional feedback should be minimized, so that clients are not straining to understand the therapist's point: the tendency to provide feedback in an overly intellectualized manner is a common mistake of novices. Finally, the therapist needs to constantly reassure couples that they are not "worthless" or "incompetent" as a result of their communication difficulties. They should be reminded that these deficits are common even among supposedly happily-married couples. The therapist must also communicate acceptance which is not contingent on couples' communication behavior; however difficult changing is for a particular couple, the therapist must communicate continued encouragement, confidence, and enthusiasm. These points are illustrated in the following excerpt:

W: When you say something, it almost always helps. You do a good job when you try to talk me out of it.
H: I don't always know when you're upset.
W: That's what I don't understand. How can you be so insensitive?
T: I liked the way you (*to wife*) gave him credit. Did you (*to husband*) notice that?
H: Not really.
T: She said you do a good job when you talk to her. If you had paraphrased what she said you would have caught it. Diane, your last remark sounded critical to me. How did you take it Rich?
H: I took it as criticism.
T: I think it was the word "insensitive" that did it. Also, you asked him an unanswerable question. Try it again—just tell him what you don't like and how it makes you feel.

The therapist's feedback is very specific, nonpunitive, and prefaced by praising the wife for her previous remark.

Coaching and Modeling

Once couples discover their mistakes, they need alternative responses; initially the therapist must provide them. The simplest way to do so is through verbal instructions, as in the following example: "This time, Amy, I want you to summarize what he says before responding." The line between verbal feedback and verbal instructions is not always clear; often the feedback implies what the alternative response should be. For example, noting that the wife neglected to express appreciation is tantamount to instructing her to include such an expression next time.

The therapist can also *model* alternative forms of problem-solving. Most commonly, the therapist will assume the role of one spouse, and engage in a dialogue with the partner; at other times, when co-therapists are working together, each assumes the role of one spouse and acts out the desired behavior. Modeling is an appealing alternative to simple instructions for a number of reasons. First, it is a very efficient way to provide information; instead of gradually approximating the therapist's instructions through trial and error, they can observe the desired behavior first hand.

Second, a therapist who has established her/his credibility can be a very effective model; as Eisler and Hersen (1973) have pointed out, the emulation of an esteemed model allows partners to change at minimal cost, i.e., without losing face. Third, modeling provides the therapist with a direct opportunity to demonstrate appropriate communication first-hand. With the therapist role-playing one of the spouses, the interaction sequence usually proceeds quite smoothly, and couples learn that it is possible to communicate effectively. Such demonstrations are even more effective when opposite-sexed co-therapists are role-playing together. Here is one situation where there seems to be a clear advantage in having two therapists present. Not only are demonstrations of desirable behavior more effectively modeled, but the danger of rivalry between spouses is minimized. With only one therapist modeling in a scene with one of the spouses, there is the danger that there will be an appearance of an alliance between the therapist and the spouse involved in the role-playing scene. The partner who is simply observing may resent her/his apparently lower status and become less susceptible to learning from the demonstration as a result. Conversely, the partner who is role-playing with the therapist may try to exploit the position of temporary superiority by becoming excessively critical of the partner and trying to behave as if she/he were a therapist. If only one therapist is involved, it is incumbent upon him/her to guard against this possibility by equalizing the amount of role-playing and observing engaged in by each partner.

The only major disadvantage of modeling is that couples may simply imitate the therapist(s), without actually apprehending the principles behind the modeled performance. In this case the couple will be unable to perform independently of the therapist, and generalization either to new situations arising in the clinical setting or to later home situations will be hampered. If modeling is used, the therapist must carefully structure the situation so that clients will be actively involved in the learning process. Discussions following the modeled performance can be very helpful in ensuring that this active involvement takes place. For example, a discussion can focus on those aspects of the model's behavior which lead to improved problem-solving. Or the discussion can pinpoint differences between the model's behavior and the prior behavior of the partner who is now observing the interaction. A brief excerpt from such a discussion is summarized below:

T: OK, now obviously that went very smoothly. Ed (*the observer*), what was different about how you did it and how I did it?
W: Well, you waited till I was . . .
T: (*interrupting wife*): Wait a minute, Lisa, let's hear what Ed has to say.
H: Well, you made sure that you understood what she was saying before you gave your two cents.
T: How did I do that?
H: Uh, by not interrupting, and then by summarizing what she said.
T: OK, so I let Lisa talk and then I summarized her remark. Good! What else?
H: You didn't bring up another problem the way I did.
T: What else did you bring in?
H: I got into the question of Michael watching television at night.
T: That's right. Your discussion got side-tracked onto whether or not Michael should be watching TV at night, even though that had nothing to do with the original topic, which was you and Michael discussing his math homework. Lisa, how do you think my behavior affected you in the interactions?
W: I felt as if you really cared about the problem and were willing to do something about it.
T: What did I do to make you feel that way?
W: You listened, and I knew you were listening carefully because you repeated back what I had said. And, uh, let's see, you didn't put it back on me. You didn't try to change the problem.
T: So, it seems like two very simple changes made all the difference in the world. One was my use of summary statements. The other was my avoidance of side-tracking. If the two of you could both remember to do both of these things, use summary statements, and stick to one problem at a time, 70% of the battle would be won. Try it again now, Ed. You can be you now, and I'll watch.

This excerpt illustrates a discussion following a modeling session where both partners are actively involved in the learning process, rather than passively watching and imitating the therapist. Notice that the therapist squelched the wife's initial attempts to play therapist, and insisted that the husband respond first to the question regarding the differences between his performance and the modeled performance. Notice also that the therapist insisted on specific, behavioral observations of these performance differences, rather than accepting such vague formulations as "you made me feel that . . ." Finally, the therapist was actively summarizing the observations of the partners, and repeated them a number of times, in order to maximize their impact. Discussions such as these, in between a modeling sequence and a segment of behavior rehearsal, will maximize the transfer of learning from the former to performance on the latter, and to subsequent performance in future communication.

Behavior Rehearsal

After couples have received feedback from the therapist, and alternative suggestions have been made, couples must practice the skills which have been suggested to them, either through verbal coaching or modeling. These practice sessions have traditionally been referred to as behavior rehearsal. Behavior rehearsal is probably the most important part of the triadic training sequence. For one thing, the process provides feedback to the therapist regarding the extent to which couples have understood the instructions, and the extent to which these instructions were translatable into behavior changes. More importantly, we believe that actual practice, with continued feedback and modeling by the therapist, is a necessary precursor to the mastery of new communication skills.

Behavior rehearsal can be thought of as a shaping process. One can expect an imperfect adoption of the therapist's initial instructions, whether these instructions are provided by coaching or modeling. Following an initial rehearsal segment, further feedback and instructions, including the reinforcement of whatever performance improvements have occurred, will lead to further performance increments in the next behavior rehearsal segment, and so on. Gradually, skills are refined and perfected. The actual rehearsal is instrumental in this shaping process. For example, in the excerpt below, the value of guided practice and feedback is illustrated:

T: Don't forget to indicate to her that you understand what she's saying. For example, Helen, tell me what you said you just told John.
W: I told him that . . .
T: No, say it to me, as if I were John, and I will answer as John.
W: I'm worried about what will happen when Don and Linda get back in town. We haven't seen them in seven years, and when we used to get together with them, the two of you ignored me and got very sarcastic.

T: You're worried that when Don and Linda get back in town, things will be like they were before. Is that right?
W: Yes.
T: OK John, go to it. Start again Helen.
W: (*repeats previous remark.*)
H: I can understand why you're upset, but . . .
T: No John, telling her you understand isn't the same as summarizing what she said. How does she know you understand? She has to take you on faith unless you tell her.
H: You're afraid that Don and I will get exclusive and ignore you and be sarcastic, but . . .
T: Check it out with her.
H: Is that what you said?
W: Um-hum.
T: Good.

Role Reversal

In closing this section on behavior rehearsal, we will mention one very effective role-playing technique called *role reversal.* Here partners switch roles, and try to discuss a particular problem as they believe their partner does. A couple can be asked to reverse roles and discuss a problem as it is usually discussed at home, as it was just discussed during the therapy session, or as it should ideally be discussed in the future. The benefits that can be derived from this technique are manifold. First, both the therapist and the partners can become more sensitive to each partner's misperceptions of the other's behavior. Since partners respond at least as much to their *perceptions* of the other's behavior as they do to the actual behavior, role reversals can clarify the nature of these misperceptions, and the therapist, as an objective third party, can then correct them. Second, assuming the role of the other partner broadens each person's perspective in much the same way as videotape feedback does. By focusing on the other rather than himself, the partner, often for the first time, empathically experiences the other person's position. As a result of this experience, the partner's perspective is often treated more sympathetically. Third, partners are often most articulate in informing the other about what behaviors they would like to see in the future during role reversal situations. Thus, couples can be instructed to imitate the behavior they would like to see in their partner while enacting the role of the partner.

Using Cues to Shape Positive Communication

In addition to the behavior rehearsal paradigm, positive communication can often be effectively shaped by using nonverbal stimuli to reinforce (and/or punish) specific communicative responses without interrupting the ongoing flow of interaction. For example, one of us (Margolin & Weiss, 1978a) has been experimenting with an electromechanical system for communication training, similar to the "SAM" system introduced by Edwin Thomas and his associates (e.g., Thomas, 1977). Although this system requires some technological sophistication, it is easily adapted to a clinical situation of more primitive technological capabilities. An example of such an adaptation is the "talk table" described by Gottman, Notarius, Gonso, and Markman (1976).

Basically, the system is one where "helpful" communication is defined spontaneously by the partners themselves. If the appropriate apparatus is available, couples simply press buttons identifying communication which they perceive as helpful. This can be done either concurrently, as they interact, or subsequent to their interaction, by viewing taped replays of the interaction. A pen recorder keeps track of each partner's sequential ratings of both his and his partner's communication. From these ratings information can be acquired regarding the "impact" of each one's communication on the other, as well as each person's perception of his own communicative responding (cf. Gottman et al., 1976). From these ongoing ratings, lists of helpful communications can be extrapolated retrospectively. Then, behavior rehearsal can be used, *along with continued feedback provided by spouses,* to shape helpful communication. Notice that the technology here, although helpful, is in no way essential to the identification process.

The system is also useful as a tool in the shaping and modification of desirable communication. For example, assume that buttons signifying helpful communications set off a pleasant tone, whereas a different button pressed following a disruptive communication signifies an aversive-sounding tone. Upon receiving a communicative response from the partner, the recipient presses one of these buttons (or, in the case of a "neutral" communication, refrains from button-pressing) depending on the valence of the communication perceived. The expressor thus receives immediate feedback on the impact of his/her communication in the form of a clear, unambiguous stimulus. The feedback is not disruptive to the ongoing communication process, and can be a very efficient procedure for shaping helpful communication. In the absence of a signalling apparatus, one can use signs ("helpful," "disruptive," "neutral"), which are held up by the receiver after the partner's response.

A more elaborate avoidance conditioning system was used by Margolin and Weiss (1978a). A pleasant tone would sound only when both partners agreed that a particular communicative response was "helpful."

If 1.75 minutes elapsed without the occurrence of a mutually agreed-upon helpful communication, an aversive buzzer would sound. The buzzer would continue until such a response occurred. By achieving a consenually recognized helpful communicative response at a rate exceeding 1/1.75 minutes, they could permanently avoid the buzzer. Notice that what is being shaped here is not only helpful communication but mutuality in understanding what a helpful communication is.

Margolin and Weiss found this exercise to be particularly difficult for couples, and in their illustrative case example, even after an intervention, there were still considerable discrepancies between the partners' identification of helpful communication. This suggests the major limitation of couples' defining their own helpful communication: a lack of reliability. Couples tend not to apply consistent criteria in their discriminations between helpful and unhelpful communication. The labelling process seems to depend on a number of uncontrolled factors, including immediate moods, situational context, level of fatigue, the quality of the preceding communicative sequence, and so on. With these *continuously* shifting preferences, the therapist must insert some stability and order to the shaping process. The extrapolation of general rules by the therapist is one way of eliminating "error variance." The following transcript illustrates how the therapist can create order and stability to this shaping process by establishing rules which represent commonalities in each partner's rating of communication as either "helpful" or "disruptive":

T: You seem to press the red button (disruptive) whenever Tim disagrees with you without telling you why. When he gives you a reason, you don't press the button.
W: That's true. I don't mind him disagreeing with me, as long as he explains it.
H: So Tim, perhaps you might try to remember the rule, "Always tell Ellen why you disagree with her when you do disagree with her."

It is important that these rules be based on a broad sample of interactions; otherwise an idiosyncratic response, based on a particular mood, time of day, or extenuating circumstance may lead to a rule which does not accurately reflect a spouse's general preferences. For example, on a day when Leslie was depressed, she labelled many of Dan's communications as "disruptive," whereas these same responses would have been called "helpful" on days when her mood was more favorable.

In summary, in this section we have summarized the prominent components of behavioral communication training. As we discuss particular aspects of communication training, more will be said of these strategies. In the following section, we will outline a variety of content areas which commonly serve as the focus for communication training. It should be remembered that the strategies described above are applicable to most targets for communication training. Behavior rehearsal is a vital cog in the machinery of interpersonal skills training. It is also, somewhat paradoxically, an efficient way to transform interaction from mechanical to natural. The process is an admittedly mechanical one at first; yet in order to disrupt extremely overlearned communication patterns and replace them with new patterns, the latter must be overlearned. As they become habitual, the mechanical underpinnings are eliminated.

VARIOUS TARGETS FOR COMMUNICATION TRAINING

In the paragraphs below we will list some examples of communication skills which can be mastered using a behavior rehearsal model. This list is not meant to be exhaustive, since communication deficits can be extremely diverse and idiosyncratic. However, it does provide a sense of the scope and breadth of deficits for which the behavior rehearsal model is applicable.

Empathy and Listening Skills

This heading covers a rather heterogeneous set of communication categories involving both listening to the partner more effectively and demonstrating to the partner that his remarks were "understood." The demonstration of understanding occurs through a paraphrase or a "reflection" of the other's previous remark. The key concept in the rationale for this kind of focus is the concept of "empathy," which helps elucidate the difference between a reflection and a paraphrase. Since empathy implies a direct apprehension of the other's experiences, especially the emotional component of the other's experience, reflecting, as a vehicle for the demonstration of empathy, includes an inference about the emotional state underlying the partner's remark. A reflection, in its pure form, is perforce inferential, since affect is not something that we directly observe, but rather something that we infer on the basis of both verbal and, particularly, nonverbal behavior.

In many ways, listening and empathy skills are more important and more *basic* than problem-solving skills. "Listening" and "demonstrations of understanding" are likely to be two of the most potent social reinforcers which a partner provides; they are prerequisites to intimacy and their absence, or low rate occurrence, is often lamented by the deprived partner. Another perspective from which to view these skills is as a strategy for teaching each partner to track the other's behavior more accurately. This is, of course, an important skill in and of itself, and deficits in this area may be important antecedents of relationship distress for some couples (cf. Weiss & Birchler, 1978).

Bernard Guerney (1977) and others (e.g., Rappaport, 1976) have developed an entire treatment strategy around the principles of training in empathy skills, an approach often called "conjugal relationship enhancement." By and large these skills have been applied to relatively nondistressed couples, and found to be effective ways of enhancing an already satisfying relationship. Our major caution in the use of empathy training with distressed couples is that one is essentially teaching mind-reading skills, since reflecting requires an inference about what is going on inside the partner. This is not necessarily a bad thing in and of itself; John Gottman's research (Gottman et al., 1977) has suggested that mind-reading can function in a variety of different ways in a relationship; in fact, distressed and nondistressed couples mind-read at equivalent rates. The difference lies in their use of mind-reading. In a satisfying relationship, mind-reading is used by partners to indicate attention and sensitivity to the other's behavior; mind-reading statements are likely to have the impact of an expression of concern or caring in such relationships. In a distressed relationship, mind-reading often serves a controlling, manipulative function. It is necessary to ensure that couples learn the appropriate discrimination here, and use reflecting only when it is appropriate. Consider the inappropriate use of reflections:

(1) *H*: Honey, I don't remember this bill. Have we received another copy of it?
W: Yeah, I guess I must have forgotten to show it to you.
H: Perhaps in the future you can put all the bills in one place so that I won't miss any of them.
W: YOU SOUND ANGRY.
H: No, I'm just trying to figure out a way to make sure that I see all bills when they first come in.
W: What I'm hearing is that you're angry at me, and are you possibly also blaming me for the debts we've accumulated?
H: If you keep reading my mind, I'm going to get angry.

(2) *W*: I'm sorry, John, I'm not in the mood tonight. I'm sort of fluish and achey, so let's go to sleep.
H: I can understand that you're upset. And I can be patient. I won't push.

W: No, John, that's not it. It's really just the cold.

In the first example, reflecting is used as a side-track. It is as if the wife is saying, "Let's not talk about my behavior; let's talk about your feelings." This almost inevitably happens when reflecting and problem-solving are engaged in simultaneously. An added subtlety of reflecting that is exemplified in the first example is that, if used in the wrong situations, it can have the opposite impact from what is usually intended. The object of the reflection can feel as if he is *not* being listened to, that he is *not* being understood, and he may become *more* frustrated and angry as a result.

In the second example, reflecting is being used to *contradict* the partner's causal explanation of her behavior. This is not "empathy." Both examples point out how infuriating it can be to be told what you are feeling when you are not looking for that kind of support, and especially when the other person is wrong and seems to be inferring your feeling to further his own interests.

Let us close this section with a pair of appropriate reflections. Their difference from the above examples is obvious:

A) *H*: Mr. Grant yelled at me today for something someone else did.
W: That must have been upsetting.
H: Yeah, it pissed me off! If that happens again, I'm going to say something to him.
W: Sounds like you're fed up. I don't blame you.

B) *W*: If this keeps happening, I'm going to begin to wonder. It seems like everytime I approach you, you pull away. There are only so many reasonable excuses that one can handle without beginning to see the handwriting on the wall.
H: Sounds like you're already beginning to wonder. You feel rejected by me, huh?
W: Yeah, would you?
H: Um, hum. I would.

Weiss (1978) has been most articulate in pointing out the importance of distinguishing between the "support-understanding" mode of couple interaction and the "problem-solving" mode. At times when a grievance is verbalized, the discontented partner wants simply to tell the other how she feels, without necessarily wanting to problem-solve at that moment. Couples should learn in therapy to distinguish between the two modes. All expressions of unhappiness need not be discriminative stimuli for problem-solving sessions. Couples need opportunities to talk about feelings, and on those occasions problem-solving is inappropriate.

Validating

Closely related to empathy skills is the concept of validation, discussed in detail by Gottman, Notarius, Gonso, and Markman (1976) in their self-help manual for couples. We find it useful to distinguish validation from both reflections and agreements. A partner's communication can be validated without agreement; in fact, ideally each and every remark in a transaction between intimately involved partners is validated, although disagreements may abound. To illustrate with a rather silly example, consider an outrageous idea by Mabel, expressed to her husband Steve:

> *W*: Steve, the baby-sitter of ours is really doing a lousy job. She keeps forgetting to change Karin's diaper, last night she fell asleep with the stove on, and two weeks ago she didn't even show up. I've been thinking about this, and I've decided what we should do. I think we should knock her off—kill her.

Steve has a number of choices in responding to this rather extreme solution. He can disagree with her in two basic ways:

> H_1: That is a ridiculous idea, and you are ridiculous for coming up with the idea.
>
> or
>
> H_2: I disagree with you this time honey, because killing her would be morally wrong, it would lead to our being sent to prison for life or executed, and there are less extreme solutions which would probably eliminate the problem for us.

The H_1 response might be considered a typical "pretest" response in a distressed relationship, whereas H_2 is more typical of a "posttest" response. The basis for the superiority of H_2 is obvious. However, neither of these responses is particularly "validating." Another possible response is a reflection:

> *H*: You are obviously very angry and upset at our baby-sitter.

Here we are getting closer to the notion of validation, since the response communicates empathy and understanding. Now, however, consider an authentic example of validation:

> *H*: I understand that you're upset at the baby-sitter and frustrated by our inability to change her. Your frustration is real and legitimate. I think, however, that your solution is not the best way to deal with the problem, and we should probably explore some alternatives.

The husband disagrees with his wife, yet he explicitly affirms not only the legitimacy of her feelings, but also her ultimate worth as a human being, despite strong disagreement with her specific suggestion. This is the essence of validation, to explicitly distinguish between a person and the person's behavior in such a way that whatever he says or does is deemed legitimate and understandable. Since the distinction between concepts like validation, reflection, paraphrase, and agreement can be subtle, extreme examples such as the one above are often the most powerful vehicles for illustrating the differences. If couples can learn that validation can be achieved regardless of the degree of absurdity manifested in the other person's behavior, the unique characteristics of the notion are likely to sink in. The above example also illustrates an ingredient of communication training which is of general relevance: the use of humor. Since the development of new communication skills can be both arduous and tedious, humor can be a useful mitigating component of the training program.

Validation is often an ideal response to a partner when she/he is emotionally upset, whether or not the partner's behavior has caused the feelings. For example, spouses are often at a loss in situations where their partner is depressed (Chapter 9). Typical responses to an expression of depression are either to try and persuade the depressed partner that there is no rational reason to be depressed, or to try and prescribe a solution to the current depression. Examples of each are presented below:

A) *H*: I was really hoping to get that promotion. I am so bummed out.
W: Oh honey, that's silly. I know you deserved that promotion more than Harry did. It's their problem if they don't recognize your competence.

B) *W*: It all seems so hopeless. Life is just an endless series of sunrises and sunsets; and all I see before me is an endless, interminable, boring existence.
H: What happened to the idea you had about taking up archery? I thought that was a good idea.

In both of these examples, the partner is playing therapist, by using cognitive restructuring in the first case, and by taking a more behavioral approach in the second case. Although, at certain times, both of these tactics might be helpful, on other occasions the depressed partner wants to know that he has permission to be depressed, that he is loved and cared for to the same degree when depressed as when feeling good.

Prescriptive responses do not serve this end. Validation, on the other hand, might be expressed as follows:

> I can understand how you feel. It must be awful to feel so sad and hopeless.

Caution: Depressive behavior may be viewed as operant behavior, reinforced by attention, concern, and solicitation. In those instances where depressed behavior is being maintained only by validating responses, validation is clearly inappropriate. The distinction is a difficult one, both for therapists and for couples: Is the partner depressed due to antecedent and/or consequent events which have little to do with the immediate consequences provided by the partner, or is the depressive behavior under the control of such validation? In the former case, validation is often the "treatment of choice"; in the latter case, validation is contraindicated, since it would be strengthening the depressed behavior.

Feeling Talk

Talking about personal feelings is not always necessary to a successful, satisfying marriage, except that in our psychologically-minded culture partners have attached great importance to feeling expression. A not infrequent refrain heard as a presenting complaint is "my husband (wife) doesn't open up to me; I seldom know how he (she) is feeling." Directed practice at talking about feelings can be a useful way for making feeling talk a part of the couple's repertoire.

The skill of talking about feelings is actually a four-stage process: first, spouses must be able to track their feelings and associate them with particular situations; second, they must be cued into talking to their partner in terms of these feelings; third, they must be able to recall feelings retrospectively; and fourth, they must be reinforced through validation, reflection, and generalized acceptance from the partner when they do talk about their feelings.

Many people are not accustomed to acknowledging feelings as events take place. By having them keep a diary where their task is to label events in terms of the feelings they evoke, such individuals can learn to track their feelings so that they become more noticeable. Checklists of various possible feelings (e.g., disgust, despair, amusement) can often help the person label particular feelings if she/he is not accustomed to doing so. Through tracking and recording relationships between events and feelings, another step in the process is facilitated, namely the subsequent recall of these feelings.

The insertion of cues into the persons' home environment can remind people to discuss feelings with their partners, especially when their habitual mode of conversation excludes feeling statements. A sign posted on the front dashboard of the car, thus forcing a partner to gaze at it as he returns home at night, is one example of such a cue. Although some might object to feelings that are expressed in response to such artificial cues for the unexpressive individual, spontaneity will result only subsequent to learning expressiveness skills. It requires dedication and practice to transform an individual from one who ignores his/her feelings to one who expresses them at a high rate. If a partner is dissatisfied with the amount of feeling talk in the relationship, she/he has to be willing to pay the price for change, namely a period of time where feeling expression is bound to be awkward and unnatural. Like any other relationship change, there is nothing magical about the process; it is simply a matter of effort and persistent practice.

Finally, the therapist must carefully focus on the interpersonal consequences which follow feeling expression in a formerly unexpressive individual. Often, past attempts at feeling expression were unwittingly squelched by a partner through punishing responses. Included among these are belittling the other person's feelings, accusing him/her of having inappropriate feelings, and simply ignoring them. At times, although one partner might be complaining about the partner's lack of feeling expression, she/he also enjoys the role of being the expressive spouse. When one partner begins to change, the other finds these changes difficult to accept. Thus, it is important that the therapist carefully structure the consequences that accrue to the person who is deficient, once change begins to occur.

Negative Feeling Expression

The pros and cons of encouraging direct expressions of anger in intimate relationships have been discussed in numerous contexts. Most marriage counselors encourage their distressed clients to express their angry feelings to their spouse in one way or another, assuming that the inhibition of these feelings, or their indirect and inappropriate expression, is either at the root of or at least helping to maintain marital distress. This belief reflects a pervasive conviction in our culture that catharsis eliminates or at least mitigates aggressiveness. It is assumed that anger, if not expressed, will fester and grow inside of a person, until at some point it will be released in uncontrolled, and presumably more destructive, ways. This belief persists despite a lack of supportive evidence as to its validity, and a great deal of indirect evidence suggesting that other models might be more viable. Research in social psychology (e.g., Schachter & Singer, 1962) has implications for this discussion: First, this research suggests that cognitions play an important role in our emotional experience; second, the evidence seems to suggest that a variety of allegedly distinct emotions are physiologically identical, and characterized by undifferentiated arousal of the sympathetic nervous system. If our emotional experience is largely a process of cognitive labeling, an alternative strategy for alleviating negative emotions is suggested, namely a cognitive restructuring process. If the physiological aspects of anger and aggression are similar to those of anxiety, anxiety reduction procedures might be generalizable to the elimination of anger (cf. Novaco, 1976).

At any rate, where does this leave us in regard to helping distressed couples handle their aggressive feelings? Recently, Gurman and Knudson (1978) criticized behavior therapists for their emphasis on positive control and structuring of positive exchange. The argument, familiar to us by now, is that behaviorists ignore the importance and inevitability of hostility in intimate relationships, and the necessity of allowing the expression of such feelings. They even intimate that putdowns, humiliations, and expressions of hatred are healthy in marriage since they are indicative of passion. It is clearly untrue that we deny the inevitability of hostility in intimate relationships. As one of us argued in a co-authored reply to Gurman and Knudson (Jacobson & Weiss, 1978), our task is not the clearly impossible one of eliminating conflict from relationships. Rather, *as a therapeutic strategy,* we temporarily focus on the enhancement of positive exchanges. Couples usually enter therapy with well-developed skills in partner-directed aggression, and need no help from us in "getting in touch with their anger."

However, it is often helpful to teach spouses different strategies for informing their partner that they are angry. When couples habitually maintain the privacy of their angry feelings, a great deal of potentially shared experience is lost. Opportunities for beneficial relationship changes are also lost when anger is not verbalized. Moreover, it is certainly true that it often "feels good" to tell a partner that one is angry. The problem is that distressed couples tend to express anger destructively, first, by augmenting their admission with threats, demands, and putdowns, and second, by speaking vaguely in regard to the antecedents of their anger. As a result of the style in which anger is typically expressed, the recipient does not attend to the other's expressed feeling, but rather focuses on his own victimization and responds by feeling wronged. Such a dialogue quickly degenerates.

Spouses can be trained to express their anger in simple "feeling-cause" statements (Kirwin, personal communication). The expression includes a statement of the feeling and the *behavioral* cause of the feeling. No threats, demands, or putdowns are included. First, here are some examples of "bad" anger expressions:

Expression	*Problem*
1. You fat slob! You ate all the steak.	1. A. Includes putdown.
2. I am furious; you better not let that happen again.	2. A. Excludes stated "cause" of feeling. B. Includes demand.
3. If that happens again, I am going to leave you.	3. A. Excludes "cause" of feeling. B. Includes threat.

Contrast the above examples with the "feeling-cause" statements which follow:

1. I am angry at you for not calling me to tell me you would be late.
2. Your just sitting there and watching TV while I move this heavy furniture pisses me off!
   (compared to: You asshole! Why don't you help me with the furniture?)
3. It made me upset to come home and find you drunk.

These latter "feeling-cause" statements include no extraneous material to distract the recipient. The reason for the anger is clear and delimited. The recipient has no wound of his own to attend to. He must accommodate to the other's feeling. Apologies follow feeling-cause statements with some regularity.

When people attempt to implement these new forms of anger expression, they frequently discover that the recipient has a profound investment in trying to induce threats, demands, and putdowns from the expressor, in order to avoid having to directly confront the other person's feelings. Thus, the following example is not atypical:

H: I'm mad at you for embarrassing me in front of Lois and Fred.
W: Are you saying that I'm a gossip?
H: I'm just telling you that I'm angry.
W: I was just kidding around.
H: OK, I just wanted you to know how I feel.
W: I suppose you want me to promise never to do it again.

Here the wife is trying to seduce the husband into putting her down, or, having failed at that, she attempts to transform his expression from a feeling-cause statement into a demand. The expressor must persistently adhere to the brief, direct format. The best way to ensure this is to encourage the expressor to terminate the discussion as soon as the feeling has been adequately expressed, by saying, for example, "We don't really need to talk about this anymore; I just wanted you to know how I feel."

Positive Expressions

One of the reasons for the immediate benefits so often reported when a behavioral program is implemented is the program's emphasis on producing interpersonal reinforcement. By refocusing couples' tracking behavior on positives and away from negatives, by asking couples to list the strengths of the marriage, by requests to increase positive behavior, the therapist is essentially saying, "The two of you have tremendous power over each other through your potential to administer positive reinforcement. When you use it, your partner will be happier. If your partner is happier, she/he will be nicer to you, and give more to you; therefore, you will be happier." Couples tend to underestimate the importance and the power of verbal reinforcements.

Affection and caring statements tend to recede with time in a marriage. Yet often in therapy at least one partner admits that she/he likes to hear remarks such as "I love you." Often, partners fail to express their affection not because they do not feel it, but because they assume that their partner is aware of their feelings. Whether or not they are right, it is still reinforcing to hear it firsthand from the partner. Another source of inhibition is the expressor's embarrassment at expressing love to his spouse, which in some cases is exacerbated by a dearth of ways to express love. This is where discussion in therapy, and perhaps some rehearsal might be useful. The receiver can make suggestions, say what she/he likes to hear, and embarrassment can be discussed and possibly alleviated.

Praise and compliments are also underemphasized by many couples. It is partly the discrepancy between not verbalizing positives and assiduously pinpointing negatives that creates the experience of "not being appreciated." *Expressing appreciation* frequently and, of course, being specific about the source of appreciation has an extremely powerful impact on a relationship previously devoid of such expressions. Again, initial progress may seem unnatural and awkward, since expressions of appreciation do not become immediately habitual. But couples' concerns about spontaneity can be assuaged by pointing out that they are not being asked to lie about their feelings, but rather simply to express feelings that already exist but up until now have gone unexpressed.

Assertiveness

Our experience has been that after one parcels out all the communication skills already discussed, very little remains in distressed couple's complaints which can be ascribed to a deficit in assertiveness. This certainly does not mean that partners seldom need to learn more effective ways of standing up for their rights. Rather, these skills are often best taught in situations other than that of conjoint relationship therapy. Individual therapy or, better yet, assertiveness groups seem more conducive to the production and perfection of assertiveness skills. For this reason, and because there is an abundance of sources describing assertiveness training elsewhere (Alberti & Emmons, 1970), we are not going to discuss assertiveness training any further.

We do wish to point out that it behooves the clinician who treats couples to avoid the assertiveness training bandwagon. Unless one defines assertiveness very broadly, to include feeling expressions, problem-solving skills, and the like, it is an issue which is of relatively minor importance as an antecedent of relationship distress. Couples in already satisfying relationships may present assertiveness as a major issue; but the kinds of couples who present themselves to mental health professionals lack much more basic skills. This is not to say that traditional husband-wife role divisions are not an important source of conflict in the contemporary relationship; and to the extent that the woman's lack of assertiveness is one way that the traditional relationship is manifested, it may serve as one therapeutic focus. However, *assertion deficits* per se are seldom prominent reasons for seeking therapy.

PROBLEM-SOLVING

As every chapter has mentioned in one way or another, one of the critical components in a behavior exchange formulation of relationship distress is that dissatisfied couples are often unskilled at generating changes in their relationship. They often seem to rely on aversive control tactics, especially punishment and negative reinforcement. In Chapter 2 we presented an illustration of aversive control in the example of conflict revolving around removal of garbage. Consider, as an additional example, the general use of verbal abuse as a tactic of behavior control. Threats, criticisms, and demands are used quite often in relationships, particularly in order to stop some behavior that is aversive to the abusive partner. These tactics are often quite effective at suppressing the aversive behavior to which they are applied. As the perpetrator of verbal abuse learns that these strategies "work," their use becomes more generalized. Thus, such strategies tend to multiply over time.

Not only does one spouse tend to increase his use of aversive control over time, but aversive control strategies tend to be reciprocated by the partner, as we saw in Chapter 1. Thus, a pattern of behavior change based on coercion, punishment, and negative reinforcement develops, and conflict is accelerated. However couples might respond to the influx of aversive interactions, unless the behavior change strategies themselves change, problems become exacerbated. If negative exchanges continue to predominate, the relationship is strained from two sources: the unsolved problems, which remain unsolved due to inadequate behavior change strategies; and the impact of the negative interchanges, which decrease the value of the relationship in various and sundry ways, mostly by increasing the costs of emitted behavior. If, on the other hand, problem-solving is effectively extinguished, negative feedback may be avoided, but problems remain unsolved.

This insidious pattern occurs despite the obvious negative impact of aversive control on the relationship. Couples are myopic in their perpetuation of this pattern: the negative impact is often subtle, insidious, and cumulative; in contrast, short-term changes are often successfully implemented, changes which are often immediate and dramatic. The immediate reinforcement provided by such short-term changes is considerably more powerful than the long-term negative consequences. In addition, many couples have no alternative to aversive control other than avoidance. To many citizens in our society, behavior change and aversive control are synonymous. At every level of our culture, including our criminal justice system as well as our child-rearing patterns, aversive control predominates. *Positive control* is seldom practiced, and when it is attempted, its implementation is sufficiently faulty so as to be unsuccessful.

Yet positive control strategies are required by distressed couples in order to emerge from the vicious cycle of aversive control and progressively increased discord. Systematic behavior management principles based on principles of reinforcement are extremely powerful skills in overcoming this undesirable pattern. Although there are a number of ways to teach behavior management principles to couples, we contend that the most expeditious area on which to focus is the *process* by which agreements are reached. Careful consideration of the adult dyad's uniqueness will reveal the logic of this focus. In dyadic interactions between parent and the young child, where the parent has almost total control (at least in potential) over the child's reinforcement contingencies, the parent can be taught behavior management skills and then be expected to implement them. In contrast, with adult couples reinforcement contingencies are seldom imposed, and verbal interchange is a necessary antecedent to behavior change. It is our belief that the characteristics of these antecedent conditions are among the most important predictors of successful behavior change. That is, how spouses discuss their problems is vitally important in determining whether or not change occurs, and also the exact nature of the change. Thus, the problem-solving interaction is a logical object of focus in teaching effective behavior change skills.

Focusing on problem-solving, or the process by which change agreements are reached, has many advantages. First, as we have just mentioned, it is an expeditious way of teaching behavior management. Second, given the expectation of learning an alternative way to discuss problems, couples can often cease their negative interchanges even prior to the acquisition of new skills, and experience some immediate relief. Another way of stating this is that problem-solving provides stimulus control over couples' conflict-related interactions, thus altering the quality as well as the connotations of such interactions. Third, in teaching problem-solving skills the therapist is also teaching couples how to communicate more effectively in a setting where effective communication is exceedingly difficult. The positive changes that occur in regard to problem-solving communication are likely to generalize to other areas of communication, and lead to increased satisfactions in areas only tangentially related to the actual training. Fourth, problem-solving training can serve a preventative function. Couples leave therapy with skills which they can apply in future conflict situations. In gradually acquiring self-management skills and thereby achieving autonomy, couples become their own therapists.

The remainder of this section is organized around a manual which we present to couples in conjunction with problem-solving training. The manual is reprinted in its entirety, with commentary provided for therapists who use it. The manual is not a therapy program in and of itself; we recommend its use *only* as part of a professionally-directed training program.

In the manual's introduction, we discuss both the *setting* and the proper *set* of problem-solving. The basic structure of problem-solving sessions and the conditions under which they are to occur, as well as the proper "attitude" with which to view problem-solving, are elaborated. This is consistent with our emphasis on establishing problem-solving as specialized, structured communication, dissimilar to other types of interaction. Couples must clearly discriminate problem-solving from their pretherapy communication; the more discrepant the settings, the more facile the discrimination process, and the less likely couples will be to apply their pretherapy social behavior to this novel situation. From the beginning, through such procedural instructions, the therapist assumes control over the couple's problem-solving interactions.

Thus, each spouse is instructed not to complain about aspects of the other person's behavior except during prearranged problem-solving sessions. These sessions are to have an *agenda,* and records are to be kept of the proceedings. Usually, we ask couples to tape all sessions conducted at home so that the therapist can bear witness to the interaction. Most importantly, the rules of problem-solving discussed in the manual serve the function of discriminative control, clearly demarcating the uniqueness of this activity.

Another noteworthy aspect of the manual is the emphasis on two distinct phases of a problem-solving session, a *definition* phase and a solution phase. During the definition phase, both partners develop a clear, specific definition of the problem. Until this definition has been specified, discussion should exclude proposals for behavior change. Then, once a problem has been defined, the interaction turns toward arriving at an acceptable *change agreement.* This aspect of the discussion is focused solely on resolution, and returning to definition interchanges is taboo.

Maintaining a distinction between these phases is extremely important. Distressed couples tend to perform impulsively while problem-solving, and are likely to argue about solution-related topics before the problem is well defined. Without a period of time devoted exclusively to definition, partners often entertain highly disparate conceptions of the problem, and unwittingly try to solve the problem, despite private discrepancies regarding what the problem is. Such a discussion is unlikely to prove fruitful. Equally counterproductive is a discussion of solutions to a problem contaminated by returns to definition and descriptive elaboration. Since change is difficult and often aversive, particularly to the object of a complaint, couples often revert to more benign interchanges, such as further discussion of the past. But problem-solving, subsequent to the definition stage, is future-oriented, and preoccupation with events of the past is extraneous, and also volatile, given couples' tendency to recall events of the past discrepantly. Hence, their efforts to confuse the past and the future must be thwarted.

What follows is the problem-solving manual, with corresponding commentary and guidelines. At the conclusion of the manual, we present a general discussion of clinical issues in problem-solving training.

PROBLEM-SOLVING MANUAL

All couples who live together over a long period of time face conflict now and then. Even in the most ideal marriage, periods of discord are inevitable. One of the hallmarks of a successful relationship is the ability to resolve these disputes smoothly and in a way that is satisfying to both parties.

Success at solving problems in your relationship means success at bringing about change. A relationship problem usually involves the desire for some kind of change on the part of at least one partner. The couple that can successfully make changes when they are called for is likely to maintain a flexible, satisfying relationship over a long period of time. A couple that is rigid and unresponsive to the inevitable need for change will eventually have significant problems. A long-term relationship is a struggle. It sometimes requires sacrifices, compromising, and even occasional restrictions on personal freedom. In order to continue to grow as a couple, the two people must collaborate. Collaboration and compromise are the key words in this program to improve your relationship. This manual is designed to teach you problem-solving skills so that you can better cope with the inevitable conflicts in a long-term relationship.

As you go through this program, keep in mind that problem-solving is a specialized activity; it is not like any other type of conversation. Therefore, it is not expected to be spontaneous, natural, relaxing, or enjoyable in the way that regular communication is. This is not to say that problem-solving cannot be fun; on the contrary once couples reap its benefits and become efficient at it, they report it as an enjoyable activity, an activity that brings them closer together and creates warm, loving feelings. However, at first problem-solving is difficult, complicated, and not rewarding in and of itself.

Let us define problem-solving as *structured interaction between two people designed to resolve a particular dispute between them.* Usually, but not always, the dispute is a complaint by one person concerning some aspect of the other person's behavior. Examples are one partner's desire that the other share more of the house cleaning chores, one partner's complaint that the other is inconsistent in his(her) methods of disciplining the kids, or one partner's complaint that the other drinks too much. Other types of disputes between couples involve mutual complaints where both partners object to the other's behavior in a particular situation. For example, when a couple gets together with their friends, the wife may complain that her husband withdraws from the conversation, while the husband might counter that his wife talks too much at these gatherings.

Problem-Solving Setting

Problem-solving is *structured* interaction. As such it should occur only in certain settings and not in others. The first thing you and your partner need to do to get ready for problem-solving is to set aside at time and a place in which discussions will be conducted. Usually couples like to hold problem-solving sessions at night, after children are either in bed or absorbed by an activity. This way they are less likely to be distracted by either the kids or the telephone. The two of you should be alone when problem-solving.

There should be an *agenda*. Ideally the agenda will be planned in advance. Husband and wife should alternate the responsibility for planning an agenda. While you are in therapy, these sessions are to be *the* time that problems are discussed. Don't attempt to resolve your disputes at the scene of the crime. Wait until the next problem-solving session. Trying to resolve a grievance *when* the grievance occurs is usually ill-advised. When we are emotionally aroused, as we are bound to be when our partner behaves undesirably, we are not at our best; we are unlikely to problem-solve in a rational manner. Discussing the issue at a neutral time, like during a prearranged problem-solving session, makes it more likely that it will be dealt with effectively. Tackling difficult relationship problems during structured problem-solving sessions brings new skills to bear on these issues. The guidelines discussed below, if followed, will make seemingly insoluble problems solvable. Later, when your problem-solving skills are well-developed, you can transfer them to the scene of the crime when minor, every day irritants come up. You should always save major problems for your scheduled problem-solving sessions.

Problem-solving sessions should be relatively short. If one problem is being discussed, thirty minutes should be the maximum. You should allow no more than an hour for two problems. Never attempt the resolution of more than two problems in a single session. Problem-solving is difficult; don't exhaust yourselves.

Buy yourselves a notebook, and record the important elements of each problem-solving session. At the top of the page, write the date. Underneath, record the problem discussed, along with the agreement reached.

Problem-Solving Attitude

The purpose of each and every problem-solving session you have is to improve your relationship. Each time a relationship problem is solved, the relationship improves, and each partner becomes that much happier. It is in the interest of both partners to *collaborate* during these sessions. Every problem discussed, whether it be a gripe on the part of woman or man, is a *mutual* problem. These two notions, that problem-solving is *collaborative* and each problem discussed is a *mutual* problem, are absolutely critical. Typically, when distressed couples deal with conflict, the event takes the form of a power struggle. If the wife has a gripe about the husband, he adopts a rigid posture and regards her gripe as a threat. If he agrees to change, he becomes less powerful in the relationship, he loses face. He waits for his partner to change *first*. It is easy to see how couples reach stalemates with this view.

The rigid posture adopted by distressed couples makes some sense. After all, in the short run a partner who agrees to make a change in his or her behavior is sacrificing something. Such changes are costly, particularly if they are not reciprocated by changes on the part of the partner. However, this view is extremely short-sighted. In the long run, the refusal to change is self-defeating for one's own personal happiness. As long as the relationship remains distressed, he will be unhappy. By changing in a way which the partner suggests, any short-term cost will be more than outweighed by the advantages of an improved relationship. His partner will respond more positively to him because she is happier, and in the process will provide him with reinforcement which is often more important than anything that he got out of the old behavior.

To take a simple example, consider the wife who asked her husband to take over the responsibility of playing with their three-year-old son between 5:30-6:30 every evening. This was the period of time when the husband first came home from work, and he looked forward to this as time to relax, read the paper, drink a beer, and unwind. The thought of having to spend this time interacting with his rambunctious son was aversive to him. In the short run, it is clear that he would have been giving up an important period of leisure time by assuming this responsibility. Thus, it is not surprising that he was reluctant to agree to her request. Now add to this the dynamics of this couple's power struggle.

They were in the middle of a period in their relationship filled with conflict and discord. He figured that most of the problems were her fault. Why should he agree to her request when it will make his already miserable existence a bit more miserable without her prior commitment to changing in ways which he would find desirable?

The answer is that any positive change, whoever initiates it, will be beneficial to both parties. If the husband agrees to his wife's request, she will experience some relief from the rigors of child management. Not only will she be more relaxed as a consequence, she will be grateful to him. This restructuring of the couple's child responsibilities is bound to have repercussions for the rest of the relationship. Her increased relaxation is likely to make her a more pleasant person to be around. Her gratitude will lead to her doing nice things for her husband. Finally, she will likely reciprocate by making some changes in her own behavior to accommodate his wishes. All in all, it adds up to a more pleasant existence for the husband as well as for the wife, despite the short-term costs.

Again, since all potential marital problems have implications for both partners, every problem is a mutual problem. Collaboration is in the interest of both parties; therefore, each change agreed to by a partner will make his(her) life more pleasant in the long run. Collaboration pays off and for this reason it is the essence of problem-solving.

Our plea for collaboration does not mean that you must *always* agree to behave in a way that is satisfying to your partner. Some requests for change are unreasonable; at times the problem may be in the mind of the person who registers the complaint more than in the behavior of the person who acts as the object of the complaint. The plea is simply that each partner remain open to the possibility of behavior change in response to the other's wishes. A readiness to consider changing to make one's partner happier must be viewed in terms of its long-term benefits to the relationship, rather than simply in terms of its immediate costs to the person who is changing.

Problem Definition versus Problem Solution

A problem-solving session should have two distinct, non-overlapping phases: a problem definition phase and a problem solution phase. During the problem definition phase, a clear, specific statement of the problem is produced, a definition which is understood by both parties. No attempt is made to solve the problem during this phase. During the solution phase, discussion is focused on the elaboration of an agreement designed to rectify the problem; one or both parties agree to change their behavior in some way so that the problem will be eliminated.

This means that initially no solutions will be proposed. Until both partners have defined the problem the task is confined to problem definition. Then, once the next phase has begun, returning to the definition phase should be avoided. First, couples should avoid analyzing the problem's causes during the solution phase. Second, couples should avoid further examples of the problem's occurrence during the solution phase.

The distinction between phases is important because couple's problem-solving communication tends to be chaotic and ambiguous. Focused discussion tends to be more efficient. More importantly perhaps, discussing solutions is positive and forward-looking, whereas problem definition is more apt to be negative and backward-looking. The spirit of collaboration and compromise is unnecessarily dampened by excessive focus on past misdeeds. While an element of this latter focus may be necessary during the definition stage, it should not protrude into the elaboration of solutions.

DEFINING A PROBLEM

Guideline 1: In Stating a Problem, Always Begin With Something Positive

The way a problem is first stated sets the tone for the entire discussion. If you are about to say something which your partner might interpret as critical, you want to make sure that you say it in such a way that you don't make him/her angry. You want to maintain your partner's co-operation and collaborative spirit. Since it is difficult for all of us to accept criticism, since most of us immediately want to defend ourselves when we are criticized, and since we are likely to argue and counter-attack when we are defensive, you must make every effort to minimize your partner's discomfort.

One very effective way of doing this is by beginning the statement of the problem with a positive remark, such as an expression of appreciation. Mention something about the other person that you like before mentioning the problem that is currently upsetting. To illustrate what we mean, below are lists of initial problem statements with and without positive beginnings (+):

With +	*Without +*
1. I like it when you hold me while we watch TV. But I feel rejected when you aren't affectionate in other situations.	1. I feel rejected by you because you are seldom affectionate.

2. I often look forward to coming home because I can unload all of my tensions on you by telling you what a rough day I had. It always has made me feel close to you. You have always been such a good listener. But lately you haven't expressed much interest in hearing about my day.

2. Lately you haven't expressed much interest in hearing about my day.

3. I appreciate the way you've been helping me around the house lately. Don't think I haven't noticed. My only remaining gripe is that you don't help me clean up after dinner.

3. You don't help me clean up after dinner.

4. You and Sheila get along so well. And you are very good with her. I think she really misses you when you spend so little time with her on week nights.

4. It concerns me that you spend so little time with Sheila on week nights.

5. I love you, even though sometimes you make me so mad. The thing that I'm angry about now is the way you've been coming home late and not letting me know.

5. It makes me mad that you've been coming home late and not letting me know.

The differences between the above statements with and without expressions of appreciation are readily apparent. People tend to take the positive qualities of their partners for granted. They assume that their partners don't need to hear about them. Nothing could be further from the truth! Human beings need praise; we all need to know that people recognize and appreciate our positive attributes. This recognition is particularly important when we are being criticized without such recognition; your partner is likely to feel attacked. The positive remark reminds the partner that you care about and appreciate him(her), although you find certain behaviors distressing and unacceptable. This kind of specific criticism is much easier to accept than criticism which does not include a positive component. If your partner is able to accept your criticism, she/he will remain in a collaborative spirit; otherwise, a countercriticism or statement of self-defense is likely to follow. In this case, the problem-solving session can quickly deteriorate.

Ideally, the behavior which is being praised will be directly related to the behavior being criticized. In the first four examples, the expression of appreciation deals with the same behavior about which the partner is dissatisfied. However, it is not always possible to praise someone for something *related to* the problem. Rather than be phony and invent a compliment, we recommend that you express appreciation in a more general way in such instances by reminding the other person that you care about him, that your criticism of his behavior does not signal your rejection of him as a person. Example five illustrates such an expression of appreciation.

The manual does not recommend phony praise. Most couples do not need to invent expressions of appreciation. You probably appreciate many things about your partner, although you may seldom feel the need to express it. We are merely suggesting that a problem-solving session is an opportune time to express this appreciation. Actually, telling your partner what you like about him is a good thing to do frequently. If expressions of appreciation occur with some frequency in a relationship and not just during problem-solving sessions, they are more likely to be accepted at face value when they occur at the beginning of a problem definition.

Commentary

Couples often question the apparent deception and the manipulative quality of this rule. In regard to the deception, it should be emphasized that we are not suggesting that expressions of appreciation be invented; rather, only those aspects of the partner that actually are viewed positively should be verbalized. The suggestion merely involves transforming covert appreciation to overt appreciation. To the extent that these expressions are viewed primarily as strategies for attenuating criticism, they may be interpreted as manipulative; but if they are viewed as simply an elaboration of relevant positive qualities, which place the subsequent critical remarks in a more realistic perspective, they are less likely to be viewed as such. Without some form of affirmation of the other's positive qualities, problem formulations are likely to be interpreted as being more comprehensive than they were intended to be, and reactions such as "everything I do is wrong," "you think I'm worthless," or "you've forgotten how hard I've been trying" are commonplace. Collaborative behavior is unlikely to follow from such reactions, since cooperation would imply a tacit endorsement of these sweeping attacks.

Guideline 2: Be Specific

When defining a problem, make sure that you describe the *behavior* of your partner that is bothering you. If you try hard enough you can almost always state your needs and your gripes in terms of specific words and actions. What is it exactly that your partner does or says which disturbs you or upsets you? Or what would you like your partner to do in order to make you happier? The problem should be described in such a way that its presence or absence can be clearly determined by an observer. In other words, one should be able to either see it or hear it. Notice the contrast below between specific and vague problem definitions.

Specific	*Vague*
1. You seldom ask me questions about how my day was.	1. I get the feeling you aren't interested in what I do.
2. Most of the time I initiate sex.	2. You don't want to sleep with me anymore.
3. We talk about day-to-day happenings, but rarely do we talk about how we feel.	3. We don't seem to make contact anymore.
4. You talk to me while I'm cooking and I can't do two things at once.	4. You don't know me very well.

Notice that in each of the vague examples, it is unclear what the problem is. The partner who is being criticized can not be certain what it is that leads the other to the conclusion that she/he is uninterested, not desirous of sex, out of contact, or unknowing. It is very difficult to get anywhere when the problem is defined in terms of the other's internal state. When you can be specific, on the other hand, the other person will know exactly what you are referring to and communication is much clearer. Let us be clear about one thing: the impressions you and your partner form of one another are based on what he or she says and does. They don't come from "vibrations" or "out of the blue." The key to understanding the feelings and reactions you have to your partner includes identifying the specific words and actions which bring out these feelings. Learning to pinpoint the correspondence between behavior and feelings is an important skill in understanding your relationship.

There are many pitfalls in defining a relationship problem, many ways to be vague and imprecise, and thereby to confuse the communication. Two of the more common examples are discussed in the paragraphs below:

Derogatory adjectives and nouns. One way to be vague in a problem formulation is to use derogatory labels as substitutes for descriptions of the behavior which bothers you. Consider the following examples:

1) You are inconsiderate.
2) You are lazy.
3) You are cold.
4) You are dogmatic and intolerant.

In none of these examples do we know what the accused partner has done to warrant these labels. The labels themselves are not only vague, they are provocative. If your purpose is to make your partner angry and alienate him(her) from the task of problem-solving, there is no better way to do it than to substitute a derogatory label for a behavioral description. Since such name calling leads to a feeling of being attacked, the response is usually a counterattack (for example, "So I'm lazy, eh? Well at least I'm not insensitive and cold the way you are"), or a self-defense (for example, "I'm not lazy!"). In either case, the problem-solving session has become, at best, a debate, and, at worst, an argument.

If, on the other hand, your purpose is to maintain the other person's cooperation and keep communication clear and unambiguous, simply describe the behavior which displeases you, and forget the labels. Consider the advantages of redefining the four examples listed above in terms of *behavior*.

1) When you fix yourself something to eat at night, you often neglect to ask me if I want something.
2) Today you didn't make the bed, you left your dirty clothes on the floor, and you left used dishes in the living room.
3) In the past month, you have seldom touched me except during sex.
4) I've noticed that lately, when we discuss important decisions, you often interrupt me and insist upon your point of view.

If you find it impossible to give up these derogatory adjectives, you'd better reexamine your purpose in bringing up the problem. The chances are that you were more concerned with expressing anger or getting back at your partner than with solving the problem.

One final word about the use of labels rather than behavioral descriptions in defining a problem. Our culture teaches us to try and view people as having personality traits which explain their behavior. Thus, when our partners act in ways that upset us, we are likely to call them "repressed," "hysterical," "overprotective," "sadistic," "introverted," and so on. Often, there is a tendency to define relationship problems as either or both partners' possessing an undesirable personality trait. These labels have all the drawbacks of derogatory adjectives and nouns. In addition, their use creates pessimism about being able to change, because personality traits are often thought of as permanent or fixed. Don't forget that we infer the existence of personality traits on the basis of behavior. The important question is not "What personality trait does this person have?", but rather, "What is it about your partner's behavior that displeases you?" The behavior often leads to the inference. Why not stick to the behavior? *Behavior can be changed!*

Overgeneralizations. Couples often exaggerate the scope of their complaints. Words like "always" and "never" are typical ways that such exaggeration is accomplished. For example, "You *never* clean up the messes you make"; or "you're *always* late." Not only are these overgeneralizations imprecise from the standpoint of communication, but they are seldom accepted by the object of such a criticism. In response to an overgeneralized complaint, the receiver is likely to dispute the overgeneralization, rather than discuss the problem *per se*. Whether the problem occurs *"all"* of the time or *some* of the time, it is a problem. Debates about frequency are usually not to the point. Avoid overgeneralizations.

Guideline 3: Express Your Feelings

> "I feel rejected and unloved when you don't include me in your Friday night plans."
>
> "It's very frustrating to me when I want sex but have to wait for you to initiate it."
>
> "I get angry when you leave your clothes on the floor."
>
> "I get upset when I think the time is right but you don't show me affection—like after we go to see a romantic movie."

Almost always, when you find some aspect of your partner's behavior objectionable, it is because the behavior (or lack of it) leads you to become emotionally upset. If the behavior didn't displease you, it would not be the subject of a problem-solving session. It is important to make these feelings known, in addition to pinpointing the behavior which leads to the feelings. When aware of your discomfort, your partner is likely to be more sympathetic. Don't assume that the feelings are obvious; if you state them directly, your partner can avoid the hazardous, and often not very reliable, task of trying to guess what your feelings are. Good problem-solving communication means sharing your feelings as well as openly admitting to the behavior that upsets you.

Guideline 4: Admit to Your Role in the Problem

This is the first of our rules which applies to the receiver of the problem definition as well as the one who has stated the problem. In the competitive disputes which all too commonly substitute for problem-solving, each partner tries to deny the validity of the other's point of view. In a real problem-solving session, where couples are collaborating to solve a *common* problem for the mutual gains that follow from an improved relationship, both partners adopt the stance of accepting responsibility rather than casting blame. The difference in problem-solving styles, depending on whether or not couples accept mutual responsibility, is striking, as the following contrasting examples illustrate:

Example 1: *W*: I would like to see you spend more time playing with Linda.
H: I already play with Linda more than you do. Besides, whenever I try to play with Linda, you interfere.
W: That's not true.

Example 2: *W*: I know that I can make it hard for you to play with Linda because I sometimes step in and interfere. It would be nice if we could do something about this problem, because I would like to see you spend more time playing with her.
H: You're right, I don't spend a whole lot of time with her these days.

In example one, each partner competes to point the finger at the other. They are struggling rather than collaborating. In contrast, both partners in the second example are being self-critical and recognizing their own role in creating the problem. Again, we are not suggesting that you must accept responsibility for a problem when you feel such acceptance is unjustified. Nevertheless, when couples are truly collaborating, it is almost always the case that some responsibility can be legitimately shared for any given problem.

Commentary

The word "responsibility" has many connotations in our culture, and in problem-solving training some educated spouses object to the notion that one spouse accepts responsibility for behavior which bothers the partner. The argument is that if partner A is upset by partner B's behavior, it is partner A's problem, and partner A's responsibility to cope with it. This argument, though elicited by Guideline #4, transcends this particular rule and challenges the very foundations of a treatment program which places value on behavior change.

The philosophy that partners can not justifiably request change from one another is diametrically opposed to our belief that such requests must be forthcoming if a relationship is to remain satisfying and viable. This ideology must be conveyed to couples when such objections are raised, without simultaneously imparting the inaccurate notion that one has complete license to request any change he wishes from the partner. Accepting responsibility for engaging in a particular behavior which is upsetting to the partner does not NECESSARILY imply changing that behavior. As the manual suggests in the sections on problem solution, couples have many options once a problem has been defined, ranging anywhere from complete behavior change to acceptance of the status quo on the part of the partner who initiated the complaint. The important point is that problem-solving must occur, and both partners must be committed to the principle that behavior change is at times a responsibility of each, and that behavior change is in the interest of their satisfaction as individuals and as a couple.

Guideline 5: Be Brief When Defining Problems

In general, problem-solving is oriented toward the future. The question which pervades most problem-solving sessions is the following one: "Something is troubling one of us; what can we do in the future to prevent a recurrence of this discomfort?" The only exception to this focus on the future is at the very beginning of the problem-solving session, when the problem is defined. Since problem definitions describe behavior that upsets one or both partners, they must make reference to things that have occurred in the past. But the object is for this phase of problem-solving, the problem definition phase, to be as brief as possible, so that the focus can quickly shift toward the future and a resolution of the current conflict. The problem must be defined clearly; both partners must understand what the problem is. Beyond this, the focus should immediately turn to "what do we do about it?"

Couples often become bogged down in this definition phase. They spend an excessive amount of time engaged in an unproductive focus on the past. This makes the probability of an argument higher. It also lengthens problem-solving sessions unnecessarily, thereby making them less enjoyable and more tedious. Finally, these discussions often contribute *nothing* toward the ultimate solution. "Talking about" the problem may be interesting; but it is not problem-solving. Don't confuse the two. Here are common ways that couples devote excessive time to *describing* rather than *solving* a problem:

1) Couples mention as many examples as they can remember of the problem's occurrence, and then argue over the details of the particular examples;
2) Couples analyze their problem and try to come up with the *cause* of the problem;
3) Couples ask "why" questions: "Why are you so stubborn?", "Why can't you just remember to be on time?", "Why do you hold your feelings in?", etc.

There is no need to list example after example of the problem's occurrence in the past. There is no constructive purpose served by this process, and it lends itself to irrelevant disputes about the details of the examples. Nor is it relevant to uncover the past cause of the problem. Usually there is no one cause to a particular problem, and the attempt to find one is a fruitless task. For example, "I get upset when you stay out until 1:00 a.m. because my parents used to leave me with babysitters a lot, and it made me feel insecure." This connection between a childhood event and current behavior may or may not be accurate; in either case it makes little difference in terms of coming to agreement on what to do about the problem. Many couples enjoy discussing the possible cause of their behavior; we do not mean to imply that these discussions are inappropriate or uninteresting, simply that they are irrelevant in a problem-solving situation.

There is another type of "cause" which *is* relevant to a probable definition, and should not be included in our general caution about irrelevant digressions. These are "immediate" causes, or events which occur along with the defined problem which seem to have some relationship to the defined problem. Below are some examples:

"I don't intentionally hide my feelings from you; it's just that it seldom occurs to me to share them with you."

"I have trouble thinking of things to do with the kids. That is one of the reason that I spend so little time with them."

"I am afraid to initiate sex because I always think you will reject me if I do."

In other words, mentioning the apparent reason for the occurrence or nonoccurrence of some behavior often adds to an understanding of the problem from the perspective of the person whose behavior is being focused upon. Although these factors should be mentioned, make sure that the discussion does not shift to them. The focus should remain on the defined problem, although the eventual solution may take these immediate causes into account. The danger is that one partner will *blame* his/her behavior on the immediate cause, and thereby deny reponsibility for doing anything about it. Immediate causes are factors to be taken into account, not reasons for avoiding a direct focus on the problem.

"Why" questions are specific invitations to focus on the alleged cause of the problem rather than ways to solve it. In addition, "why" questions are usually experienced as critical. The recipient of a "why" question is likely to feel threatened and "set up." Stifle such questions, and expend your energy changing the situation so that the behavior ceases to be a problem.

Commentary

The various ways to violate Guideline #5 often fall under the heading of "verbal masturbation"; although such conversations often seem gratifying to both interactants, they contribute little toward either defining or solving the problem. The therapist should beware of couples who insist upon "insight" or understanding as a prerequisite to behavior change. First, such couples may be exemplifying the well-known aphorism "a little bit of knowledge can be a dangerous thing." Well-educated couples, familiar with pop psychology, and likely to be labeled as "psychologically minded" by mental health professionals, believe that understanding the historical origins of their relationship problems must precede behavior change. Such couples have been greatly influenced by the psychodynamic thinking which is so pervasive in our culture. We try to gently disabuse couples of the notion that such historical insight is either necessary or a relatively efficient way to solve relationship problems. There is an obvious parallel here between the specific goal of changing couples' problem-solving focus from discussions of historical etiology to focusing on present and future behavior change and the general distinction between insight oriented psychotherapy and behavior therapy. Surely, if the couple has bought into the general paradigm, this rule will be accepted with relative ease.

Second, couples may be focusing on the past as a way of avoiding change, because the anticipation of the latter is anxiety-inducing or aversive in some other sense. A couple in this situation is acting in a way similar to many men who have erectile difficulties: such men often prefer masturbation to sexual encounters, despite knowledge that if they could become sexually functional the ultimate gratification would be greater. The anxiety connected with the sexual situation perpetuates the avoidance. Despite awareness that they would be much happier with their problems solved, there is often tremendous anxiety associated with behavior change.

The distinction between historical and immediate causes is difficult for many couples to grasp. The therapist wants to ensure that couples not parcel out relevant information about the problem in their quest for brevity and in their zeal to avoid descriptive elaboration. Factors associated with the problem's occurrence, such as situational events, feeling states, and even the other person's behavior, should be included in the formulation of a problem. However, it is important to ensure that couples not become side-tracked onto these related but tangential factors, so that these additional factors never become the primary focus of a problem-solving session. An example below illustrates such an attempt on the part of a couple, and the therapist's attempt to counter it:

H: It is very important that you be sensitive to those things. When you don't act excited or show appreciation, I feel as if you don't care about me.
W: But when you let me know what you want from me, you always get it, don't you? Like when you ask me directly I always come through.
H: Yes, that's true.
W: Well, why can't you state your needs directly more often?
T: Hold it, Cathy. You are about to change the problem.

It is one thing to identify an S^D or S^Δ for a targeted behavior. It is quite another to then redefine the problem in terms of the S^D or S^Δ. The former is in the service of specific and precise problem-solving. The latter is an avoidance of responsibility.

Conclusions: A Well-Defined Problem

A well-defined problem includes a description of the undesirable behavior, a specification of the situations in which the problem occurs, and the consequences of the problem for the partner who is distressed by it. A list of well-defined problems follows:

1) On Sundays when neither of us work, you seldom help me plan daily activities. I end up feeling like the responsibility for our leisure time is all on my shoulders, and I resent it.
2) The problem is that, although we have been talking a lot more

lately, we have not been communicating about things that are really important to me. You still don't talk to me about your feelings, and I still get little appreciation from you. I tend to turn off to you when I don't get this, and I feel closest to you when I do get it.

3) When you get up in the morning, you don't say anything to me, like "hello" or "good morning" or "would you like some coffee?" I feel very distant from you at that time of the day.
4) We have a limited amount of time together now, and I don't think we have been spending enough time talking. When you come home at 10:30 p.m. and watch television, I get upset.
5) There is not enough physical affection in our relationship.
6) I get pissed off when I notice that the checkbook is not balanced, particularly when you have let it go for more than two weeks.
7) I get criticized by you a lot for the housework I do, particularly the dishwashing. It really irks me when you do that, since I do 90% of the housework, and you give me very litle credit for doing a good job.
8) When you let a week go by without initiating sex I feel rejected.
9) You seldom ask me questions about my day, even though I listen and show interest when you talk about your day. I often feel cheated after we have supposedly caught up on each other's activities.

In the first example, one partner names the other's unwillingness to plan activities as the problem. The situation in which the problem occurs is Sundays when both of them are free from work. The consequences of the problem are that she feels resentful. As an exercise, go back through the remaining examples and identify 1) the problem; 2) the situations in which the problem occurs; and 3) the consequences of the problem. In each of the examples, the problems are clearly defined, and the couple is ready to move on to the solution phase of the problem-solving session.

Summary: Commentary on Defining Problems

The primary rationale for designating a problem definition phase is to allow a circumscribed period of pinpointing behavioral excesses or deficits. The period serves as a springboard for behavior change negotiations, and the latter should occupy the couple for the major portion of their problem-solving effort. Thus, problems should be defined as quickly and expeditiously as possible, in a way which fosters collaboration during the negotiations which follow. In maintaining couples' cooperation during this phase, the most difficult obstacle lies in their concern about being stifled. For example, the partner who serves as the object of the complaint may not have the opportunity to express his opposition to the other's complaint. Or he may not be allowed to elaborate to his satisfaction on his EXPLANATION for the behavior. Similarly, the complainer may lament the lack of input from the partner and constraints imposed on such exchanges by the rules in the manual.

In counteracting these concerns, the therapist must emphasize that these types of comments fall outside the task of problem definition. The problem definition phase exists simply for the delineation and clarification of the problem. The person whose behavior is being pinpointed is attempting SIMPLY to understand what behaviors on his part are of concern to the partner. The fact that the other is distressed is sufficient to legitimize the problem as an area to be negotiated further. By agreeing to negotiate, the partner is not necessarily agreeing to change his behavior; he is simply acknowledging that he knows what the problem is and is willing to problem-solve about it, simply because the other is distressed. In "accepting responsibility," the partner is simply admitting to complicity in the pinpointed behavior; he is not necessarily admitting his "guilt" nor promising to change his behavior. The spirit of collaboration requires that each partner commit himself to NEGOTIATING; but this is the only commitment required in coming to an agreement on the existence of a problem. Therefore remarks such as "I don't see why you're upset about this" or "I don't think that my changing would accomplish anything" are inappropriate. The point is that the other person is upset because of something he is doing or not doing, and a solution must be found. If the partner whose behavior is being focused on is uncomfortable, the following remarks might be appropriate: "I feel uncomfortable about this thing that you've brought up, but I'm willing to negotiate with you BECAUSE it's upsetting you."

The logical question then becomes HOW and WHEN does one deal with this partner's discomfort. The answer is, during the solution phase of the problem-solving session. Within the context of discussing possible ways to alleviate the problem, concerns on the part of either partner can be raised. Put within the context of discussing the specific pros and cons of proposed solutions, such discomfort can be handled in a more productive way, in a way which will likely serve the goal of an improved relationship more satisfactorily. This subject will be taken up again in the commentary on Guideline 11.

GENERAL GUIDELINES

Before specifying the optimal strategies for generating good solutions to relationship problems, we will identify some general rules which should be observed during all phases of a problem-solving session, whether the immediate task is one of problem definition or problem solution. These rules are equally applicable to both phases.

Commentary

All of these rules could have been included in the section of the manual on defining problems, since, if not followed, problem definition phases can be significantly impaired. However, since they are equally necessary during the solution phase, we decided to list them in a separate section. Therapists should introduce these rules in conjunction with defining problems, and continue to emphasize them during the discussion of forming solutions to problems.

Guideline 6: Discuss Only One Problem at a Time

In a given problem-solving session, only one problem should be discussed. When an additional problem is brought in, it is referred to as *side-tracking.* Couples are frequently guilty of *side-tracking,* to the point where it often occurs without either party being aware of it. It takes many forms, as the following examples suggest:

1) *W*: The problem is that I would like you to be nicer to my mother.
   H: Since when are you nice to *my* mother? *(Side-track).*

2) *W*: I wish we had more interesting conversations.
   H: What can we do about that?
   W: Maybe if you had more outside interests. That's another thing I've been meaning to talk to you about. (*Side-track*).

3) *H*: We have to try to show each other affection.
   W: I think you're right. It would be hard at first . . .
   H: It would be good for Michael as well as for ourselves to see us being more affectionate.
   W: That sort of disturbs me. Because I feel that Mike and I are very close, but that you and he have no relationship. I wish you could somehow get to know him a little bit. (*Side-track*).
   H: I know, you're right. It is difficult for me to get to know Mike.

4) *W*: I think we should panel the walls, and then buy furniture.
   H: I think we should buy the furniture first, and then panel the walls to match.
   W: Don't forget this house was your idea in the first place. (*Side-track*).
   H: Well, it was either moving or having to put up with your brother living right across the street.
   W: You have never really given him a chance.

In each of these examples, the couple has drifted from the original topic to a new topic. In the first example, a discussion of the relationship between the husband and his mother-in-law is refocused on the wife and her mother-in-law. In the second case, the couple is discussing how to have more interesting conversations and is side-tracked to whether or not the husband should expand his leisure time activities outside the home. In the third instance, the topic moves from affection to the husband's relationship with his son. Finally, in a "double side-track," the couple begins by discussing the interior design of their home, turns to the question of whose decision it was to buy the house in the first place, and terminates on the topic of the wife's brother.

The reason for restricting discussion to one problem at a time is simple. Solving two problems simultaneously is twice as difficult as solving one problem in isolation. One of the reasons couples find problem-solving so difficult is that they cannot talk about a problem without bringing in every problem in their relationship. Such a task is overwhelming. It is amazing how simple and straightforward problem-solving can be if discussion is limited to one problem at a time. When you recognize that either you or your partner has drifted off the track, bring it back to the problem by saying "We're supposed to be discussing. . . ."

At times it is difficult to draw the line separating a side-track from a statement which merely pinpoints a related problem. For example, consider a situation where the husband defines the problem as the wife's nagging him about household tasks. The wife responds by pointing out that she only nags him after he has procrastinated for a day or more. Is this side-track? Clearly, she is bringing in a new problem, which is our definition of a side-track. Yet, she is also doing something which we have previously labeled as good practice when defining a problem, namely she is identifying the situations in which nagging occurs. Whether or not this is to be viewed as a side-track depends on two factors: first, how it is brought into the situation, and second, how the problem-solving session proceeds from that point on. If the wife were to have said, "You're right, I do nag you, and I know I shouldn't do that," she is indicating an acceptance of responsibility for her role in the problem. If she follows this remark by adding, "I think it would be helpful if you recognized that my nagging only occurs after you've delayed a task for at least a day," it is fairly clear that she is not trying to change the subject or *blame* her nagging on the husband, but simply providing information which may help them reach a workable solution. However, if her response had been "You deserve to be nagged because it takes you so long to complete tasks," she would be side-tracking, because here she is redefining the problem in a way which implicates her husband as the one who is misbehaving.

The discussion should continue to focus on the nagging rather than the procrastination. Switching to a discussion focusing on the procrastination would indeed be a side-track. However, given this new information provided by the wife, if the couple can return to a discussion of the nagging and stick to it, they have successfully avoided a side-tracked discussion. Later, the procrastination problem may be taken into account in their solution to the problem.

Thus, the key to staying on task is to not let yourselves become diverted onto related but distinct problems. If another problem is mentioned because it relates to the problem under discussion, it should not become a new focus for problem-solving. Below is a list of both legitimate and illegitimate ways to temporarily bring in a new problem in order to clarify the problem under discussion. You will notice that the primary difference between the two is that side-tracking remarks seem to blame the problem on some *new* factor and imply that this new factor should become the focus of discussion.

Legitimate	*Side-track*
1. I know that I am often late for dinner. Sometimes I guess wrong about when dinner is going to be ready, and so I turn out to be late. I don't mean to blame it on you, I'm really just trying to get you to understand what's going through my mind on those days when I'm late.	1. If you could have dinner ready at the same time every night, then I would know when I have to be home. If you get your act together, I would get mine.
2. You're right, I do let the kids get away with things, and I don't enforce rules consistently. Usually, when I get lax, it's when I don't agree with one of your rules. But that's not a good way to show my disagreement with you.	2. I don't enforce rules because I don't agree with them. They're usually your rules. I think you are too strict with the kids. So this is really *your* problem.
3. I apologize for putting you down in front of our friends. When I'm angry at you for being withdrawn, I could probably wait until we get home to tell you how I feel.	3. If you would talk more in those social situations then I wouldn't be mad at you, and I wouldn't put you down.

Commentary

The focused, discriminative, goal-oriented nature of problem-solving requires that couples avoid this pervasive tendency to bring additional problems into their discussions. Since couples are seldom accustomed to discussing their problems in this selective fashion, they find such restrictions uncomfortable and unnatural at first. Yet it is virtually impossible to resolve disputes when the focus shifts from problem to problem. Also, a ban on side-tracking places a prohibition on cross-complaining, the phenomenon where a spouse counters a critical remark by criticizing the initiator about some other matter. Cross-complaining is simply one type of side-track.

A therapist must be somewhat flexible with this rule. The manual includes a qualification to the effect that, under certain conditions, it is advantageous to acknowledge relationships between problems. These conditions can be thought of as instances where another problem reliably covaries with the problem under discussion. Examples are presented: Practically any relationship problem is under environmental control, and when one spouse's undesirable behavior occurs under the stimulus control of a particular aspect of the partner's behavior, or when the undesirable behavior is being maintained by a particular spouse behavior, these behaviors must be pinpointed along with the targeted problem, in order to define the problem completely. The acknowledgment of such functional relationships in no way sanctions a refocusing of the discussion on these antecedent and consequent spouse behaviors. The manual explicitly contrasts legitimate and prohibitive use of these additional behaviors in a problem-solving session.

Side-tracking is an important and subtle problem in communication training, because it coincides with partners' tendency to view their dysfunctional behavior as being a function of the other's dysfunctional behavior. Each mate views him/herself as a victim, a passive reactor to the other person's tendency to provide discriminative stimuli and reinforcing control for "bad behavior." This set induces spouses to view their own changing as possible only after the partner has removed his(her) own inhibitory stimuli, i.e., by changing first. Thus, when wife accuses husband of "seldom taking the kids off my hands," and the husband points out that "whenever I do take the kids you interfere anyway," he may be quite accurate in pointing out a correlational relationship. However, he must be discouraged from either 1) insisting that her interference CAUSES his inactivity with the kids, or 2) suggesting that she stop her interference PRIOR TO his increase in activity with the kids. Instead, he should agree to spend more time with the kids, AND (independently) she should agree to divert herself from interfering when he is in charge. Since they began the discussion with the wife's AGENDA, which was his "inactivity," this is the agreement that should first be formed. Notice that an alternative would be to form a "quid pro quo" contract, where each change was cross-linked to the other (see Chapter 8). Moreover, she could offer to "help you change" by ceasing her interference. But the essential point is that his arbitrary definition of causality must be squelched.

Here is where the strategic use of cognitive restructuring, discussed in Chapter 5, becomes important. The therapist must persistently and consistently confront spouses with the notion of RECIPROCITY, and its implications for problem-solving dilemmas such as this one. It is certainly demanding, and possibly even a bit utopian, for the therapist to expect spouses to adopt this new correlational view of their behavior vis à vis the partner. However, one thing is certain: without tenacity in "calling the couple" on their inappropriate views, the therapists will be perceived as inconsistent, she/he will lose credibility, and such cognitive changes definitely will not occur!

Guideline 7: Paraphrase

We are about to suggest a rule which may seem silly to you, and a bit mechanical. First, from the beginning until the end of the problem-solving session, every remark which your partner makes should be summarized by you before you respond. Second, after your summary statement, check its accuracy with your partner. If it was accurate, fine. Go ahead and give your response. If your partner does not think your summary statement was accurate, she/he should repeat the original remark, and you should try it again, until you both feel that the summary and the original are one and the same. Below are examples.

1) *W*: I feel very close to you when you express interest and support in my activities outside. Lately, I've been feeling rejected by you when I try to talk to you about work; you haven't been asking questions or making supportive remarks.

   H: You like it when I show interest and support for your job experiences. And lately you feel that I haven't shown much interest. Is that what you said?

   W: Yes.

   H: I wasn't aware of that. I can understand how that would be upsetting to you.

2) *H*: You're very physically responsive to me at times. That is very important to me. But I've been noticing lately that when I initiate affection you don't respond. That hurts me alot, and I feel unloved.

W: You're saying that you've had some doubts lately about whether or not I love you.
H: No, I know that you love me. But you are not affectionate to me unless you are the one that initiates it.
W: Oh, so you're upset about my not returning affection when you initiate.
H: That's it.

Summary statements are powerful ways of clarifying and improving communication. First, knowing that you will have to summarize forces you to listen carefully. Second, the summary statement ensures that you will understand what the other person has said; if you don't, the misunderstanding will be immediately corrected. Third, summary statements minimize the likelihood of interrupting the other person's speech. Fourth, summary statements help you see things from the other person's perspective. You should paraphrase *all* of your partner's remarks, not just the initial formulation of the problem.

Commentary

Paraphrasing is a valuable problem-solving tool both because of its reinforcing function and because it helps clarify communication. Most spouses like to be heard; it is punishing to be engaged in an interaction with another person and receive incontrovertible indications that the person is not listening carefully to your remarks. Conversely, for most couples, confirmation that the partner has been LISTENING, and, better yet, that she/he UNDERSTANDS, enhances collaboration. At the very least, summary statements demonstrate attention. The paraphrasing directive increases the likelihood of listening, and also requires a demonstration of listening.

Paraphrasing clarifies communication primarily by serving a pacing function. Distressed spouses often respond impulsively to the partner's remarks; their responses are often based on only a portion of the partner's statement. Instead of listening carefully, they are covertly formulating their reply, and important elements of the message elude them. Paraphrasing minimizes the likelihood of this common deterrent to effective communication.

Notice that there is an important distinction between a "paraphrase" and a Rogerian "reflection" (Guerney, 1977; Rappaport, 1976). A reflection is an attempt to include in a summary statement the affect apparently underlying the remark. This type of response serves a different function than a paraphrase, a function which limits its use in problem-solving negotiations. Reflections are inferences; because they are inter-

pretive, they are generally to be avoided in a problem-solving situation, for reasons enumerated below.

Guideline 8: Don't Make Inferences—Talk Only About What You Can Observe

> "I don't think you're mad at me because I criticized your driving. I think it had more to do with my refusing to have sex with you last night."
>
> "There's a lot of anger inside you waiting to come out."
>
> "You're trying to get me to do things that you *know* I shouldn't have to do for you."
>
> "As soon as I become more independent, you're going to leave me. That's why you're coming to therapy."

All of the above examples constitute attempts on the part of one spouse to speculate about what the partner is thinking or feeling. We refer to this practice as *mind-reading*. Problem-solving is hindered by mind-reading since the entire process is built on being specific, and relying on what you can observe. Also, people often don't like to have their minds read. Mind-reading may be perfectly appropriate in some situations; all we are saying is that it is inappropriate in a problem-solving situation.

A particular form of mind-reading which is both common and dangerous to problem-solving is the attempt to infer the partner's intentions from his/her behavior. Consider the following example:

> *W*: When you made fun of me in front of Rick and Barbara, it really pissed me off. I don't like it when you crack jokes at my expense in front of other people. *You were trying to humiliate me.*
> *H*: I was not trying to humiliate you.

The wife is not only describing to her husband the behavior that was upsetting, but she is accusing him of *bad intentions*. She has no way of knowing what his intentions were, and by insisting that he intended, by his remarks, to humiliate her, she is focusing on the wrong issue. The husband is now obliged to defend his benevolent intentions, and the conversation has been diverted into an unproductive area. Disputes about what people are thinking or feeling cannot be resolved; only one partner has direct access to such an inner state. The real issue is his behavior, which was upsetting to her regardless of his intentions. Whenever one partner's behavior is upsetting to the other, it is legitimate to focus on it; but it is not legitimate to leave the behavior aside and instead focus on the person's motivation. Stick to behavior; this is the simplest and most effective way to problem-solve.

The confusion of *intentions* with *behavior* can interfere with problem-solving in still another way, as illustrated in the following example:

H: I don't like it when you criticize my housework.
W: But I'm just trying to be helpful.
H: But I don't like it.
W: But don't you see? I really don't mean any harm.

Here the wife is justifying her behavior on the basis of her good intentions. She is claiming that, given her good intentions, she does not have to change her behavior. But the husband is really asking her to stop certain behaviors, regardless of whether or not her intentions were to be critical. Although her *intentions* were constructive, her *behavior* is destructive. If her behavior is upsetting to her husband, it is a legitimate problem regardless of her intentions.

Commentary

"You know her intentions only through her behavior. Only behavior can upset you. Therefore, your problems are solved if behavior changes, so don't worry about intentions." We have uttered this refrain in one form or another so often that we could be accused of overkill. Yet, spouses need to be reminded repeatedly that their interest must necessarily be in their partner's behavior, since that is the only way they have access to his intentions. Mistakes occur on both sides. One partner may define a problem as "She's trying to humiliate me," that is, inferring his wife's "underlying motivation," instead of simply verbalizing the observation that led him to the motivational inference. Then, the wife will likely dispute his interpretation, and they are wasting energy on an unresolvable, counterproductive issue. Often, these discussions are brought to their logical extreme when, to stay with this example, the husband insists that behavior change would not help, because "she would still WANT to humiliate me." Here the meaning that he has attached to his wife's behavior has become autonomous from the behavior itself. Since this inference resulted from her behavior, the therapist can assume that if the process is reversed, that is, if the behavior changes in a desirable way, the husband will gradually change the inference in correspondence with his wife's behavior. Thus, the only attitude change that must precede this behavior change is a suspension of judgment, a willingness to enter-

tain the therapist's hypothesis and allow the behavior change to occur. We have found, and the evidence seems to support our intuitions, that if the behavior change persists, most spouses do change their inferences.

The other side of this issue involves the use of "good intentions" as a defense against behavior change assumed by the accused. One example in the manual illustrates this ploy. The husband's "jokes" upset his wife, despite their alleged humorous intent. Her discomfort, regardless of his intentions, justifies her request that he change his behavior. This is generally true in problem-solving despite the existence of an alternative option, namely the wife altering her reaction to this well intentioned behavior. In theory, therapy could focus on the latter, by using cognitive restructuring techniques to have the wife change her reaction by helping her relabel the behavior as "humorous." However, this would be quite difficult, and other than pointing out the possibility of such an alternative way of labeling the behavior, or having the wife rehearse such novel reactions, it is not immediately clear how one would efficiently bring about such cognitive changes. The perpetrator of the instrumental behavior, in this case the husband, has much more control over his behavior than the wife has over her largely involuntary reaction. Therefore, the path of least resistance is to focus on behavior change.

Be cautious, however, lest one spouse use this rule of thumb as a ploy. If partners are given blanket permission to request change of any behavior that they claim causes them discomfort, some spouses may "cry wolf" by incessantly pleading discomfort as a way to manipulate their partner into changing during therapy. Or, if one partner's reality testing is poor, he/she may interpret almost any behavior as malevolent. In these instances, the therapist must temporarily become a "reality tester" for the afflicted or manipulative spouse, and point out that in his/her objective, expert opinion, the spouse's inferences are inaccurate and her/his discomfort should be modified through direct focus on the appraisal of the partner's behavior.

Many of our previous examples involve specific manifestations of spouses' tendency to guess what their partner is thinking or feeling. In addition to the frequent controlling, manipulative function of mind-reading, it is not consistent with effective problem-solving. At best, mind-reading is a digression from the task at hand, which is to pinpoint and then solve relationship problems. At worst, mind-reading is a tactic for avoiding change. There certainly is a place for mind-reading in intimate relationships, particularly in the context of supportive, empathic explorations of feelings. But problem-solving is not the time to delve inside the head of the partner.

Guideline 9: Be Neutral Rather Than Negative

When couples are fighting rather than collaborating, their interaction is frequently punctuated by attempts to put down, humiliate, or intimidate the partner. Such power struggles constitute the antithesis of problem-solving. As such, their presence serves as a clear indication that at least one partner is really more interested in winning a battle than in problem-solving. Verbal abuse can take an infinite number of forms, many more than we could possibly enumerate in this manual. The most prominent forms of verbal abuse that occur during arguments are put-downs, threats, and demands. All three categories share the function of removing the receiver of such a remark from a collaborative stance. People respond to insults, threats, or commands with counterinsults, counterthreats, or counterdemands. It is unlikely that agreements will be reached under these circumstances, and even if they are, they are unlikely to be successfully implemented; agreements reached after a great deal of bickering and arguing are unlikely to be enacted by either party. Instead of using threats or demands, simply describe the behavior that is upsetting you and the changes you would like to see.

SOLVING PROBLEMS AND FORMING CHANGE AGREEMENTS

Guideline 10: Focus on Solutions

Once a couple has agreed on a definition to a problem, the focus should henceforth be on *solving* it. The discussion should be future-oriented, and should answer the question, "What can we do to eliminate this problem and keep it from coming back?" Returns to problem definition should not occur, and in fact, there should be no further discussion of the past.

The most effective way to maintain a focus on solutions and on the future is by *brainstorming*. This means couples go back and forth, generating as many possible solutions to the problem as they can think of, *without regard to the quality of the solutions!* In fact, some of the proposed solutions should be absurd. The important point is that you use your imagination and say anything that comes into your mind, without censoring anything, no matter how silly or unworkable it may seem. Each proposed solution should be written down.

The next step is to go through the list and eliminate the proposals that are ridiculous or absurd. What remains is a list of reasonable solutions which can now be discussed at greater length.

The reasons brainstorming is so effective are twofold. First, it keeps couples focused on the task of arriving at a solution to the problem.

Second, if the rules are obeyed, couples are less inhibited in suggesting things. People often hold back from suggesting solutions because a given proposal may seem inadequate when it is considered privately; yet, when it is verbalized and later considered publicly, it often contains at least some merit.

As an example, consider the couple who had difficulty in social situations with another couple because the husband of the first couple did not like the wife of the second couple. Even though the wives were close friends, almost every time the four of them got together the first husband would either withdraw or make nasty remarks toward the second wife. After brainstorming, the couple came up with the following list of solutions (John and Helen are the couple in therapy, whereas Sam and Connie are the second couple):

1) We will not socialize with Sam and Connie anymore.
2) We will socialize with Sam and Connie only when other couples are present.
3) John will have an affair with Connie.
4) John will make a flattering remark to Connie at the beginning of an evening to set the mood.
5) The foursome will engage in activities which don't require entire evenings of conversation (e.g., movies, theatre).
6) Sam and Connie will enter therapy with Dr. Jacobson.
7) The foursome will hold a joint problem-solving session.
8) John and Helen will relate positively to one another, and not split up enough to allow opposite-sexed pairings between couples.
9) The couples will stay close to one another physically and sit so that John and Connie are not close together.

From this original list, proposals #3, 6, and 7 were eliminated as absurd, and #1 and 2 were eliminated since both John and Helen agreed that the foursome was worth preserving. This left them with #4, 5, 8, and 9. The eventual agreement was as follows:

"In future evenings with Sam and Connie, we will make sure that we function as a couple and not allow Sam and Helen or John and Connie to pair off. Physically, we will sit next to each other and put Helen in between John and Connie. We will suggest activities which provide us with breaks from an entire evening of conversation (e.g., movies). John will start the evening off by complimenting or flattering Connie."

Consider, as another example, Tim and Elaine, who had been plagued with a problem for years: Tim had a tendency to engage in extramarital affairs. A brainstorming session uncovered two factors which had never been brought out into the open before: First, the sexual aspects of Tim's affairs were really unimportant compared to Tim's wanting to maintain a diversified social life with people of both sexes; second, Elaine's concerns were not so much the relationships themselves, but the understandable feeling she had that she was being rejected for these other women. Here were the specific proposals generated during the brainstorming session:

1) Tim will sleep with any woman whom he is attracted to.
2) Elaine will start to sleep with men she is attracted to.
3) Tim will tell Elaine when he is attracted to another woman, and they will discuss it.
4) Tim will not form any kind of relationship with other women.
5) Tim will have platonic relationships with other women, but will not sleep with them.
6) Tim and Elaine will both have sex with the women whom Tim is attracted to.
7) Tim will discuss his daily social interactions with Elaine at night.
8) Tim will get together with other women only during the day.
9) Tim will see other women only in public places or at his home, when Elaine is there.

From this list of solutions, the following agreement was formed: "Tim agrees to forever stop sleeping with other women. He has the right to pursue friendships with women, under the following conditions: 1) He will get together with them only during the day; 2) he will get together with them only in public places or at his home, when Elaine is present; 3) he will discuss his activities upon coming home, on days when he gets together with a woman. In return Elaine will refrain from making suspicious or mistrustful remarks regarding Tim's activities."

Commentary

Brainstorming is particularly useful for those problem-solving sessions in which the couple is simply "stuck" at the solution stage, although the session has been relatively smooth and devoid of acrimony. The problem in such cases is often a reluctance to verbalize suggestions that, when considered privately, seem to contain little validity. Or the inhibition may be due to fear of the partner's reaction. In the above example involving the husband with a history of extramarital affairs, his initial silence resulted from a fear that his wife would not accept his suggestion, namely a proposed compromise whereby he would maintain platonic relationships with other women. Brainstorming instructions are often liberating, and elicit proposals which at times appear more reason-

able after being subjected to a discussion. The therapist usually encourages at least a few patently absurd or silly solutions, both for a touch of levity and as a point of contrast, so that couples will learn to discriminate between an actual absurd suggestion and one which is imperfect but worth considering further. To instigate both humorous and realistic proposals, the therapist will often suggest examples of either variety to be included in the list.

Brainstorming has never been systematically evaluated, and it remains somewhat controversial. At times, as a close friend and colleague put it, "Brainstorming just gives you a longer list of bad solutions." Such objections notwithstanding, we have found it to be a useful technique. At the very least, it is a structured technique for inducing the fundamental problem-solving behaviors, namely the discussion of proposals for behavior change.

Guideline 11: Behavior Change Should Include Mutuality and Compromise

In the spirit of collaboration and cooperation, whenever possible problem solutions should involve change on the part of both partners. This is even true in situations where the problem is clearly pointing to change on the part of one person. One reason for this is your partner is more likely to be willing to change if he/she isn't doing it alone. Another reason is that a partner can often help the other person change by providing feedback or teaching the partner some skill. In this sense, providing feedback or teaching a skill is the change to which the second partner is agreeing. Finally, at times some behavior on your part may be serving as a reward for the behavior of your partner which you find undesirable or you may be able to do something following the change which you are asking for which will serve as a reward for that change.

As an example of the first reason mentioned, consider the husband who was upset because his wife left clothes on the floor. After battling over this problem for years, the husband finally asked, "How can *I* help you change?" They quickly reached an agreement which permanently settled the issue. Each night prior to bed the husband and wife walked through the house together, hand in hand, picking up clothes. It became a game which they both enjoyed.

The second reason for offering your services in your partner's change efforts is that you can provide valuable feedback and instructions which may help the process of change along. Consider the husband who, as far as the wife was concerned, spent an insufficient amount of time playing with their three-year-old daughter. One factor which emerged from their problem-solving discussion was that the husband felt incompetent as a father, and had difficulty thinking of things to do with the daughter. The wife offered to help her husband by planning activities for the husband and his daughter to engage in. With her help he found it much easier to interact with his daughter, and quickly became independent of his partner's instructions.

The third reason for changing at the same time as your partner changes, even when the problem is defined in terms of the other person's behavior, is that your behavior may be related to your partner's behavior in such a way that your change would make it more likely that he(she) would change. For example, another couple was in conflict over who should do *what* with the kids. The wife wanted her husband to put the kids to bed at night. In the service of her own request, she granted him complete control over this task; she would leave him alone while he put the kids to bed. This was a big help, since in the past she often interfered with his efforts out of fear that he would do something wrong. When she agreed to leave him alone, he unburdened her of this responsibility.

As a rule of thumb, whenever you are discussing a problem involving some aspect of your partner's behavior which upsets you, begin the solution phase with an offer to change some aspect of your own behavior. Like the above examples, this offer can take one of two forms; either you can offer to help your partner change, or you can change some aspect of your behavior to make it more likely that your partner will behave in a way which is satisfying to you. Thus, if you are brainstorming, your first reasonable proposal should involve an offer to change some aspect of your own behavior, prior to requesting a change from your partner.

You should also remember that you must be willing to compromise if you expect your partner to change. It is difficult to change. The more complete the change that we request, the harder it will be for the person who is supposedly changing. Yet spouse's often act as if they have to have it all immediately, or otherwise they don't want it. The wife who felt that she carried the full child-rearing load suggested, for example, that her husband take on 50%. Helen suggested that Jerry change from a quiet partner to a man who talked about his feelings on a daily basis. Pam expected Al to change from a procrastinator to someone who fulfilled all of his responsibilities on time without being reminded. Jackie asked Mark to give up drinking beer completely, even though beer was his favorite drink. Distressed spouses frequently demand sweeping changes from their partners, changes which seem so overwhelming that the partner simply refuses.

Consider another strategy. How about starting with less than what you would ideally want, but something which seems possible to your partner? She/he may be more willing to agree to such a request. Later, you may want to ask for more, but by that time your partner will have already moved in the direction you want, and the request will not seem as overwhelming. Or you may even find that you are perfectly content with the original reduced request.

Whenever you want to see a change in your partner, formulate the problem in two ways:

1) What do I ideally want?
2) What am I willing to settle for?

The answer to question #2 should always be somewhat different from the answer to question #1. Otherwise, you haven't obeyed this principle.

Mark and Pennie only had Sundays together. Pennie virtually always planned their Sundays for the family, and wanted Mark to play a role.

1) Ideally, she wanted to trade Sundays, so that every other Sunday it was Mark's responsibility to plan their time together.
2) As a compromise, she suggested that Mark plan one Sunday per month. He agreed, and she turned out to be satisfied with this solution.

Tim complained about Ann's high frequency of verbal criticism. He defined her nagging as "Reminding me to do things or commenting on the fact that I haven't done what I said I would do."

1) Ideally, he wanted her to drop such verbal comments from her repertoire entirely. She found this extremely difficult.
2) He was willing to settle for a change in the "content" of her verbal comments. They agreed to set a deadline on particular tasks, and she agreed to comment only on the fact that the deadline had been reached, when, in fact, the task was not completed within the alotted period. The agreement worked, but it was never necessary to really test it out, since the setting of specific deadlines eliminated the problem of Tim's not completing tasks.

Mark had a tendency to drink a lot of beer on weekends. On a Friday night, he might consume a six pack of beer, for example. This would result in his becoming tired early, which in turn would lead to an unwillingness on his part to engage in sexual activity. He would also become verbally abusive on occasion.

1) Ideally, Pam wanted Mark to stop drinking beer entirely. This wish was based on her belief that he could not control his beer drinking once it started. Since Mark really liked the taste of beer, he refused to give it up.
2) She was willing to settle for his limiting his consumption to two beers during the course of an evening. Mark agreed to this and was able to stop with two.

In all of these examples, the complaining spouse was willing to settle for less than what she/he would have insisted on in the past. The partner was able to honor the new requests without cramping his style to any great degree, whereas the original, sweeping changes which were suggested were more than the partner was willing to make. More often than not, the complaining spouse is so happy with the changes that the original request is no longer deemed necessary.

An exercise that is often valuable during a problem-solving session is to explicitly tell your partner what you would ideally want, in the best of all possible worlds. Then your partner can respond by telling you how close he is willing to come to granting you your ideal wish.

Commentary

One should not underestimate the reinforcing power of offering to aid the other person in the change process. This offer of reciprocity is often sound contingency management. In the example where the wife offers to help her husband construct activities for father-daughter interaction, she is providing him with a skill which, up until now, he did not possess. Skill deficits often account for less than adequate behavioral rates. When this is the case in a relationship dispute, as it often is in cases where there is about to be a shifting of roles and responsibilities, the skillful partner's participation is imperative. Also, when the targeted behavior of partner A covaries with some behavior on the part of partner B, it is obvious that certain changes in partner B will facilitate desirable change in partner A. For example, if the wife frequently rejects her husband's sexual initiations, changing her rate of acceptance will obviously facilitate his increase in rate of initiations. Or if nagging is one of the setting events for alcohol abuse, the nagger's cooperation will remove an important discriminative stimulus for drinking.

An astute reader might recognize the operant notion of shaping in our discussion of the discrepancy between what spouses WANT and what they are willing to SETTLE for. Shaping conveys the flavor of setting preliminary goals which are then gradually changed to progressively approximate the desired, terminal behavior. A major deterrent to effective problem-solving is the tendency to view the partner's behavior in all-or-none terms. He either drinks or doesn't drink. The partner either shares child-rearing responsibilities or does not. This is a residue of the tendency to view behavior as being a manifestation of a personality trait. The exercise where spouses state their ideal wishes for their partner's behavior, and then set preliminary goals which involve less extreme changes on the partner's part is a valuable one. Change is more likely to occur under such circumstances largely because the partner is more likely to agree to change. Immediately, she/he will anticipate lower costs incurred from changing than if the ideal change had been requested; thus the changer is less anxious about the prospect of change. Also, at the level of implementation, shaped goals are EASIER for the changer to meet; this renders the agreement more viable. Later, if the degree of change is deemed insufficient, further negotiations can occur.

Guideline 12: Reaching Agreement

Once brainstorming and related exercises have generated a series of possible solutions, the task becomes one of combining those solutions in such a way that change agreements are reached. Ultimately, the ability to agree on and implement behavior change is the acid test of effective problem-solving. Discuss the advantages and disadvantages of each proposed solution on your brainstormed list, including the consequences of each proposal for each of you and for the relationship. Then combine the proposals into a final agreement. Keep in mind the following points:

A) *Final change agreements should be very specific. They should be spelled out in clear, descriptive behavioral terms.*

The agreement should clearly state what each spouse is going to do differently. Too often couples agree to vague changes, and subsequently it is unclear exactly what the agreement was. Each person walks away with a different interpretation of the agreement, and future clashes over what was meant by the terms of the agreement frequently occur. Along the same lines, disagreements can arise in the future over whether the agreement was complied with.

Change agreements should not be open to interpretation. From the terms of the agreement the behaviors that are required for compliance should be absolutely clear. The terms should include a description of the exact changes to be made, along with *when* these changes are expected to occur, and if possible, the frequency with which the new behaviors are to occur.

Here are some examples of bad agreements and the modifications that would be necessary in order to make them conform to this rule:

1) *Bad*—Jerry agrees to come home on time from now on.
Good—On Monday through Friday, Jerry will be home by 6:30 p.m. If for some reason this is impossible on a particular night, he will let Marlene know by 4:30 p.m., and at that time will tell her when he will be home.

2) *Bad*—Mike will show more interest in Holly's day.
Good—Each day when Holly and Mike get home, before dinner Holly will speak with Mike about the events of her day. Mike will ask at least five questions of Holly regarding her day. He will also avoid the use of put-downs and other derogatory remarks, which to Holly imply disinterest.

3) *Bad*—John will make an effort to talk more about his feelings to Helen.
Good—On Tuesday and Thursday nights, John and Helen will engage in "feeling talk" sessions. Helen will model feeling talk by going through the days since the last session and describing feelings she had in the various situations she was in. Then John will do the same things with his past few days.

4) *Bad*—Dana will try to do more of her part around the house.
Good—Dana will be responsible for washing the dishes (to be completed within an hour of dinner), walking the dog (twice per day, 7:30-8:00 a.m. and 9:30-10:00 p.m.), and sweeping the floor (every other evening before bed).

5) *Bad*—Patty will not be as apprehensive about the future, and will have more confidence in Don.
Good—Patty will respond positively to Don when he initiates conversation about his job. During these conversations she will not make pessimistic remarks about his future with the company.

6) *Bad*—Don will be more understanding when Laura is depressed.
Good—Don will actively listen and "reflect" Laura's verbalizations of her depression. He will not offer suggestions unless she asks for them. Nor will he express annoyance or frustration.

You will note that these agreements are quite structured. Often couples have a difficult time accepting such structure in their agreements. It seems mechanical and artificial. Well, it is true that to some extent these kinds of agreements are mechanical and artificial. However, don't forget that you are in many cases trying to change very long-standing habits. Such habits are very difficult to change, and *the changes do not come naturally*. If the changes are to occur, a good deal of structure is necessary *at first*. Later, after the changes have been in occurrence for a while, they will become more natural and the need for such explicit structure is reduced. But don't let the structure scare you away. The chances are that clarity and structure were frequently missing from your previous attempts to deal with your problems, and you know how much success you've had in the past.

B) *Final change agreements should include cues reminding each of you of the changes that you have agreed to make.*

In many instances, the problem is not that an individual is unwilling to comply with his/her partner's request, but when the time comes he/she simply forgets. This is particularly true with long-standing habits involving behavior which is incompatible with that which the partner wants to see. In such cases, the agreement should include some way of reminding the other person of the behavior to which he/she has agreed. Sometimes the agreement itself, written down and posted at a location where it is likely to be seen, is sufficient. At other times the agreement can include reminders from the spouse. One of the more inventive uses of an external cue involved a husband's placing a sign on the dashboard of his car which read "EXTJ"; translated this meant, "express feelings to Judy." This cue served as a reminder for Henry to talk about his feeling to Judy.

C) *Final change agreements should be recorded in writing.*

This has been mentioned before, and it is very important. First, writing down agreements avoids the necessity of relying on our memories. Our memories tend to distort in directions which are most beneficial to our interests. Second, when you write down your agreements, you will be more precise; ambiguities in communication will become more obvious and be more easily ironed out. Third, the written agreement, conveniently posted somewhere in the house, will remind you of what you have agreed to.

Let problem-solving become a part of your routine. Even after you have solved your major problems in therapy, you should have time put aside for problem-solving sessions at least one night per week. This should be the time that you deal with any conflict that has arisen since your last problem-solving session. Also, you should use this time to go over prior agreements and discuss how they are working. If an agreement is not working well, it should be renegotiated.

* * *

CONSIDERATIONS IN PROBLEM-SOLVING TRAINING

Collaborative Set

Most couples, when they first enter therapy, are not ready for the cooperative, intensive effort necessary for successful problem-solving training. The implicit assumption in the discussions thus far in this chapter are that the clients are two individuals recognizing a common deficit for which they are equally responsible, and that it is in the interests of both partners to change their behavior in ways required to correct the deficit. Unfortunately, seldom do couples enter therapy entertaining these assumptions. One of the nearly inevitable concomitants of a distressed relationship is the gradual derivation of two separate, mutually exclusive world views regarding the relationship. Each spouse views her/himself as a victim of the other's destructive behavior; if they admit to transgressions of their own, they are usually seen as a reaction to the other's misbehavior. Since the other is the *cause* of the current relationship distress it is usually the *other* from whom change is expected. If the "victim" expresses any willingness to change, it is usually only after the other person has changed. With each partner adopting this position, the therapist is clearly at a disadvantage in implementing a treatment program which assumes cooperation and collaboration.

Thus, the discussion of the *collaborative set* in Chapter 5 is particularly relevant to problem-solving training. At the very least, a suspension of judgment is required on the part of each partner: that is, even if they cannot be convinced that they are each viewing the relationship from a biased perspective, and that in reality the problems are consistent with the assumptions behind a problem-solving training program, the couple must be convinced to at least suspend those behaviors that follow from *their* assumptions, and act *as if* the therapist is right. The problem-solving situation has to be established from the onset as an arena within which interaction will occur only under a set of rules, no matter how couples feel about the other person at the time of the problem-solving session. Otherwise, problem-solving will simply become another forum for their pretherapy behavior, including accusations, denials of responsibility, and nonnegotiable demands for unilateral change.

This minimal collaborative set will not emerge magically; it must be induced by the therapist. At times, if sufficient expectancies are generated by the assessment period and the therapist's analysis of the relationship—including his/her emphasis on its strengths—the couple's initial commitment will result in a collaborative spirit. Usually, however, it will also be necessary for the therapist to establish stimulus control over couples' problem-solving behavior, to ensure maximum discrimination between problem-solving behavior and other areas of interaction. If problem-solving occurs only under special, well specified conditions, couples are more likely to adopt the requisite collaborative behavior. As the manual suggests, couples should attempt to talk about marital problems at home only during prearranged problem-solving sessions. These sessions should be time-limited, and should occur at a time and place where couples will not be distracted. Highlights of each session should be recorded in writing, and initial sessions should be taped for the therapist. At no other time should relationship conflicts be discussed.

A fringe benefit of the stimulus control instructions described above is that couples will not be discussing their problems during periods of peak emotional arousal. Particularly during the initial stages of training, the least desirable time to attempt problem-solving is "at the scene of the crime." At the point where an event occurs which angers one or both partners, the emotional arousal is likely to preclude effective problem-solving at that time. Postponing such discussions until a prearranged problem-solving session results in a discussion at a time when both are less aroused, more rational, and thereby better able to resolve the difficulty.

The therapist cannot overstructure these problem-solving sessions for a couple at the beginning of therapy. The more rules that exist to govern the problem-solving behavior for the couple, the easier it is to discriminate between problem-solving behavior and other types of interaction; and the easier the discrimination, the more likely that problem-solving decorum will be adhered to. With rules and tight structure, the therapist's control is extended beyond the therapy hour into the couple's attempts to use problem-solving techniques at home. If couples complain about the highly formal, mechanical nature of these problem-solving rules, the therapist can remind them that the procedures are temporary, and will disappear as the couple acquires problem-solving skills. Indeed, the fading of this structure as couples become skillful is not only feasible but desirable, since the dissipation of structure probably facilitates maintenance of problem-solving once therapy has terminated.

As another strategy for increasing the likelihood of collaborative problem-solving behavior, the therapist should encourage couples to begin by working on minor problems, which are less likely to elicit the prepotent, unproductive verbal exchanges characterizing their interaction prior to therapy. For some couples, even minor problems will prove to be excessively volatile at the beginning of therapy; in such cases, the couple may begin practicing their skills on hypothetical marital problems rather than on those problems characterizing their relationship.

Another alternative to these strategies already discussed is to delay problem-solving training until positive changes in the relationship have already occurred following other therapeutic interventions. These initial positive changes usually result in greater collaboration and commitment during the problem-solving phase of therapy. For example, some of the general strategies for increasing positive behavior discussed in Chapters 5 and 6, along with other more basic types of communication training (discussed earlier in the chapter), could be emphasized at the beginning of therapy.

The therapist must use his/her clinical judgment as to whether problem-solving training can or should be delayed. One major advantage of problem-solving is that, although it is a generalized set of skills, in the process of acquiring these skills salient areas of discord are also addressed. Generalized procedures for increasing positive relationship behavior often do not sufficiently address particularly prominent presenting complaints. By not attending to these circumscribed complaints from the beginning, couples may become discouraged and terminate prematurely. When fairly circumscribed content issues are presented which are viewed as *the* issues by couples, they should usually be addressed immediately through either problem-solving training or some other direct procedure. However, more often than not the complaints are more generalized and diffuse, and are adequately addressed by the procedures discussed in the previous chapter.

Therapist as Teacher

In problem-solving training the therapist is teaching skills to couples. The *sine qua non* of a successful problem-solving training is the couples' ability to use the skills independently of the therapist. To the extent that couples' improved problem-solving does not generalize beyond the presence of the therapist the job has not been completed. This limited form of improvement is possible in the type of treatment program outlined above; by providing couples with constant cues, prompts, and reinforcers, problem-solving behavior might change in the therapy setting, yet couples may not learn to function effectively without the stimuli emanating from the therapist. At times, this limitation may be difficult to ascertain, since couples show progressive improvements in problem-solving behavior during the course of therapy, and solve most of the problems relating to their presenting complaints; it is only subsequent to therapy termination that such couples distinguish themselves, since they have not learned to function independently of the therapist. These couples will revert to old strategies when new problems arise, and as a result will gradually deteriorate. This is true despite the obvious reinforcement they derived from successfully solving old problems while in therapy. And it is understandable, since often the long-term reinforcement is more than outweighed by the short-term costs of problem-solving, a difficult undertaking requiring continuous effort. The only way to overcome the powerful prepotence of pretherapy behavior is to systematically program generalization into the treatment program, and insure that the couples have learned the skills to the degree necessary for them to maintain themselves independently of a therapist.

What is most critical in setting the stage for generalization is to make sure that couples have learned generalized skills, as opposed to the more limited ability to simply anticipate the therapist's suggestions with decreasingly explicit prompts. The couple must abstract a set of strategies for their own use in order to monitor their own problems once therapy has terminated. Let us examine some methods for maximizing the likelihood that such strategies will be learned and adopted.

First, the couple should be responsible, from the beginning of therapy, for providing the content of their own behavior change agreements.

This point highlights an important aspect of behavior rehearsal, its contribution to the provision of mastery experiences in therapy. Through the gradual shaping and prompting provided by the therapist, the couple eventually *solves* a relationship problem during the therapy session. The experience of mastery during the therapy session probably contributes to couples' perception of self-efficacy regarding their problem-solving abilities (cf. Bandura, 1977). Ultimately, the success or failure of this training approach will hinge on couples' willingness to utilize it in response to real-world conflict. That is, at its best, problem-solving is a preventative coping skill which couples will apply to future conflict situations. Mastery experiences during therapy sessions can play an important role in creating expectancies of generalized mastery regarding these skills. Since the therapist has almost total control over the couple's problem-solving behavior during the therapy session, and since this degree of control is lacking when the couple practices at home, the therapy session is really the only opportunity that the therapist has to provide such mastery experiences. Their importance is paramount.

It is primarily because of the importance of providing couples with such mastery experiences that the therapist must not solve the couple's problems for them. There is a great temptation for a therapist to impose solutions on a couple, and in the short run therapist-provided solutions can greatly benefit a relationship besieged by conflict. But it is important to recognize that when the solution to a marital problem is generated by the therapist, the nature of the treatment has been qualitatively altered. Now the treatment approach is essentially that of crisis intervention, where the therapist has expeditiously intervened to ease current tensions, but has not in any way prepared the couple to handle future problems independently of a therapist. Behavior rehearsal—along with modeling and feedback—is a *process* approach; couples learn skills to solve their own problems. This allows them to be their own therapists if and when problems arise in the future. In order for this goal to be realized in therapy, couples must arrive at their own problem solutions in therapy. This does not mean that the therapist can not and should not veto inadequate solutions when they present themselves. On the contrary, veto power is part of the shaping process. But learning, and subsequent generalization to the real world, will be maximized only if the couple learns *from their own mistakes,* not if the therapist, by imposing solutions on the couple, prevents them from making mistakes.

Second, therapy sessions should be faded, both in terms of the interval between sessions and the degree of therapist directiveness. Rather than ending the sessions abruptly following weekly meetings, the sessions should be faded from existence so that they are biweekly and then monthly just prior to ultimate termination. In fact, with some couples periodic booster sessions might be advisable. Also, as problem-solving training progresses, the therapist should become less *active* and less *directive.* This allows the couple to gradually assume control of their own problem-solving behavior and make the transition from therapist mediation to situations where they must function on their own.

Third, in a number of ways, through the process of training, the therapist must ensure couples' active involvement in the learning process. Active involvement means more than nodding affirmatively or in other ways reinforcing a therapist's instructions. It also means more than performing in response to therapist-provided discriminative stimuli. Remember that the goal is to teach *principles,* and that the behavior will generalize to and be maintained in the home only if such principles are mastered. Active involvement on the part of clients begins at the point where problem-solving deficits are pinpointed: During the orientation session, the time when the therapist first outlines problem-solving as an area of focus, couples should be asked to produce examples of ways in which they are deficient in problem-solving abilities, and situations where such deficiencies have plagued them in the past. During problem-solving training sessions, each practice session should conclude with both partners' elaborating on everything they have learned about problem-solving during the practice session. This exercise helps couples transfer successful interaction from a concrete practice session to future problems, since they are required to derive principles from the concrete instructions from the therapist. An exercise which serves a similar purpose involves the therapist role-playing some aspect of problem-solving, with the couple assigned the task of critiquing the performance. Finally, periodically the therapist should ask clients to explain the rationale behind a given set of instructions. All of these suggestions involve ways of actively involving couples in the learning process, and serve to complement the performance aspects of a training program. Their effectiveness will be felt particularly after therapy is over, as couples become their own therapists in an attempt to maintain the gains realized in therapy.

We often encourage couples to hold their own weekly therapy sessions at home, after treatment has ended. These sessions, prearranged and held at the same time each week, are essentially maintenance meetings, where couples assess the status of the relationship, and deal with any new problems that have emerged, hopefully, by using the problem-solving skills discussed in this chapter. Additionally, past problems and change agreements are noted, and discussed if these agreements are not working. These sessions can serve a variety of other functions—such as a forum for emphasizing positive spouse behaviors—but we mention them here as a convenient vehicle for generalization, which the therapist can begin to encourage as he begins fading the treatment sessions.

Overview of Problem-Solving Training

Problem-solving training has been, in our experience, a very powerful treatment strategy for a wide variety of distressed couples. Systematic research into the efficacy of behavioral marital therapy seems to support our intuition (see Chapter 10). Its power seems to stem from two primary sources. First, it focuses simultaneously on *process* and *content*. Couples solve presenting problems as they acquire problem-solving skills, and at the same time they acquire skills which lead to more reinforcing interaction and allow them to solve their own problems more effectively in the future.

Second, problem-solving training epitomizes the reinforcing power of collaboration. In the process of mastering the art of solving relationship problems, couples learn that they will be much happier working together on their relationship than dealing with their conflicts as adversaries. The key to successful training lies in inducing spouses to behave as a team so that the advantages of collaboration have an opportunity to present themselves. Every guideline in the manual is designed to circumvent the typical subversive strategies which couples use when they approach conflict resolution as adversaries. Reluctance to adopt specific guidelines defines the refusal to collaborate; any spouse who knowingly adopts the former stance must accept responsibility for the latter.

The therapist should notice that the rules and guidelines are interdependent, such that the adoption of one facilitates performance on another. For example, when couples obey the directive to refrain from problem-solving at the time some undesirable behavior occurs, the conflict often disappears. Couples report that if they postpone the discussion to the next scheduled problem-solving session, by the time the session occurs the problem seems trivial. The conflicts created by unproductive verbal exchanges can be considerably more destructive than the persistence of the problem which served as the impetus for the discussion. Thus, deferring the discussion to a prearranged problem-solving session diffuses it and often eliminates the need for the discussion; at the very least, it transfers the discussion from a situation likely to produce a negative outcome to one where the potential for a favorable settlement is much greater.

Perhaps the most difficult response class to modify in a problem-solving session is the tendency of spouses to defend themselves and their transgressions. The most common instance is the accused spouse attempting to either deny the legitimacy of the other's complaint, deny responsibility for the action or inaction on which he is being called to task, or enumerate circumstances which render the behavior beyond his control. The guidelines for problem definitions attempt to circumvent this tactic by designating the function of this phase as one of simply pinpointing the target behavior. The legitimacy is *assumed,* since one partner is upset, and there is no need for evaluation. The spirit of collaboration obviates an evaluative focus. This does not mean that the receiver of a complaint agrees with the problem nor does acceptance of a problem definition obligate one to change. The solution phase will determine what is to be done about the problem. The point is that the destructive debate centering around the justifiability of the proposed problem is deflected. This is likely to frustrate couples, but their opportunity to evaluate the problem will occur during the solution phase, where the couple considers the pros and cons of various strategies for solving the problem, which may include maintaining the status quo. The advantage of deferring this type of discussion until the solution phase is that by this time, if all the guidelines have been followed, the response of the receiver of the complaint is likely to be mellowed. She/he has not been attacked, the complaint has been confined to a specific pinpointed set of behaviors, and the mutuality of problem-solving has remained intact.

Another fringe benefit of problem-solving training is that it forces couples to confront their *real* goal in discussing relationship problems. If they cannot, will not, or do not observe the guidelines, they are tacitly endorsing the combative, adversary type of interaction. These discussions occur in all relationships, and perhaps they are functional; but they do not lead to changes, and relationships are seldom enhanced in the long run. The important discrimination couples must master is the difference between fighting and problem-solving. It is not incumbent upon them to stop fighting, but simply to separate fighting from problem-solving. If a couple is fighting rather than problem-solving, they should be taught to acknowledge what they are doing, relabel the session as an argument, and reschedule the problem-solving session. During therapy sessions, we have couples move to another part of the room if they insist upon arguing rather than problem-solving, to emphasize the discrimination. We also encourage them to use two distinct locations at home for problem-solving and arguing; they are instructed to move to the arguing locale if they cannot persist in a problem-solving endeavor.

Finally, problem-solving training follows smoothly from the less intensive focus on increasing positive behavior which occurs earlier in therapy. Often, our treatment program begins with general instructions to identify and increase pleasing behavior, followed by a more specific focus on exchanging specific behaviors, and concluding with problem-solving to deal with major problems. Couples' success in prior, less demanding stages fosters greater collaboration in subsequent phases. Occasionally, the major presenting problems can be resolved without problem-solving training. In these instances, the therapist can terminate, or, given an ambitious couple, problem-solving skills can be taught for preventative purposes.

COMMUNICATION TRAINING IN GROUPS

It is not uncommon for communication skills to be taught in a group format; this approach has been endorsed by many as a useful format for treating couples (Guerney, 1977; Miller, Nunnally, & Wackman, 1976).

Generally, the advocates of group training have reported findings for relatively nondistressed couples. There is very little information on the efficacy of group therapy for distressed couples. Behavior therapists have not contributed much to the literature on group marital therapy. This may reflect a certain reticence about treating distressed couples in groups, perhaps because the empirical evidence for the efficacy of behavioral marital therapy is less compelling for couples treated in a group format (cf. Jacobson, 1978b; see also Chapter 10). Despite the obvious cost effectiveness of group therapy, it is difficult to duplicate the intensive nature of behavioral marital therapy in a group setting, with the therapist's time necessarily divided among the various participating couples. It is also difficult to reconcile the idiographic emphasis of a behavioral analysis with the standardization requirements inherent in a group format.

Let us examine the potential advantages of a structured group for a therapeutic endeavor such as problem-solving training or communication training. First, there is the cost effectiveness factor, a point which needs no elaboration. Second, there is the potentiality of multiple models. Despite overlap between couples in the communication skill deficits, there are usually substantial differences in the strengths and weaknesses of particular couples, and therefore each couple can learn from the others' communication strengths as well as from their weaknesses. An additional related factor is the potential for exposure to a greater variety of both positive and negative aspects of problem-solving, which can foster generalization. Couples spend more time observing in this format, and even more importantly, they observe at a greater distances since they watch others rather than themselves. Since they can maintain a relatively objective stance in their observations of other couples, the learning of problem-solving principles can be facilitated. The opportunity to comment on and provide feedback to other couples can further enhance the learning process. All of these factors may, in many instances, compensate for the less intensive focus on each individual couple and, in the long run, increase the likelihood that the skills learned in therapy will be practiced outside the meeting room once therapy has terminated.

The other potential advantages of group problem-solving training are more closely related to the nonspecific considerations discussed in Chapter 5. First, anxiety connected with the hopelessness partners may feel in regard to solving their problems in therapy can be mitigated by the presence of other couples who are struggling with their own significant problems. Second, the group can become a very supportive environment for behavior change, and can create its own norms and expectations which will support a collective collaborative set. A subversive or resistant spouse now must contend with an entire group, and noncompliance with assignments, to take one example, often becomes more difficult. Moreover, counterproductive or noncollaborative behavior during therapy sessions is often less likely, since such displays become public in a group format. Group pressure can maximize the likelihood of initial collaborative behavior, which will often be self-perpetuating once it is initiated.

Groups should be as homogenous as possible, in order to minimize the danger that a focus on one couple will be irrelevant to another couple. Compromises which provide the best of both idiographic and nomothetic worlds might be considered. For example, couples might be treated alone during the initial stages of therapy until the point where collaboration has begun and some positive changes have been achieved. Then, if problem-solving training is indicated, the couple could be referred to a group.

One possible group format which utilizes our manual is an eight week format where three sets of skills are taught: problem definition, problem-solving, and change agreement skills. Session one involves an introduction to the program without any specific training. During this session couples discuss the strategies they have used for dealing with conflict in the past, as well as a variety of other topics designed to build cohesiveness and allow couples to become acquainted. Sessions two and three are devoted to mastering the skills of problem definition, along with the general guidelines such as "paraphrasing." We have worked with videotapes which couples made prior to the first group meeting, replaying the videotapes for the purposes of feedback, and then instructing the couples to practice the new skills during the therapy sessions, with continued feedback provided both by therapists and by other group members. We have begun with less threatening role-playing of "hypothetical" relationship problems in Session 2, and have utilized couples' actual problems in Session 3. Homework assignments reflect the activities which occurred during the previous group meeting. For example, between Sessions 3 and 4, couples practice defining various relationship problems; but they are instructed to stop after the problem is defined without moving onto the solution phase. Sessions 4 and 5 are devoted to the practice of brainstorming, with the first of these two meetings again utilizing hypothetical problems and the second using problems from the couples' own relationships. Sessions 6 and 7 are devoted to the negotiation of behavior change agreements; but this time the sessions are confined to "real," as opposed to "hypothetical," problems. We have allowed a two-to-three week break between sessions 6 and 7 to allow couples some time to consolidate and practice the skills, applying them to various relationship problems. The final session is a review session, with an opportunity to discuss relevant issues not covered by problem-solving training. It is also a session which concerns itself with generalization. Couples are urged to continue the practice of weekly problem-solving sessions, which contain an agenda including a monitoring of previous change agreements, a renegotiation of agreements which are not working, and an attempt to resolve new problems.

We think that the group format is an extremely promising one for teaching problem-solving skills to couples. However, it is a relatively recent development in the practice of behavioral marital therapy, and is still very much in its experimental stage. In the coming years, we expect to find a proliferating literature on group training, along with data suggesting the optimal strategies for helping couples improve their relationship in a group setting.

SUMMARY

In this chapter, communication training with couples has been discussed in detail. The standard skill training triad of feedback, coaching, and behavior rehearsal was discussed, along with a more recent development in shaping positive communication using unambiguous cues provided by the couples themselves. Then, various applications of communication training were enumerated. A specific application, problem-solving training, was discussed in detail, with the discussion centered around a manual for couples, reprinted with commentary in the chapter. Nonspecific clinical considerations, including formation of a collaborative set and the importance of teaching generalized skills, was discussed next. The chapter concluded with a brief outline of communication training in groups.

CHAPTER 8

Contingency Contracting

THE BEHAVIOR CHANGE contract has become a symbol for the behavioral approaches to treating relationships. Historically, its roots lie in the application of operant conditioning procedures to clinical problems, and its first published application to marital problems was Stuart's (1969) classic paper. However, the idea of couples' forming contracts and negotiating for terms of the relationship began as a metaphor used by communication theorists (cf. Lederer & Jackson, 1968); in fact, the widely-used contractual label "quid pro quo" began with Lederer and Jackson. The communication theorists viewed marital relationships as based on contingent agreements between partners which were often not verbalized. Marital quid pro quos were seen as beneficial to both parties, and sufficiently stable that any attempt by either party to alter its terms would meet staunch resistance. The marriage contract has also been used as a metaphor by psychoanalytically-oriented theorists, for example, Sager (1976), to describe an unconscious agreement by each partner to fulfill the other's needs, both rational and neurotic. Traditionally, the term "collusion" has been invoked by psychoanalytic theorists (cf., Gurman, 1978; Meissner, 1978) to describe an unconscious agreement between marital partners whereby each helps the other maintain his/her own self-image and defensive structure.

Thus, there is a well-established precedent in theories of marital interaction to view the relationship as being under the control of contingencies or agreements, although views differ as to the level at which the agreements are formed. It is also true that all major theoretical orientations toward marriage recognize the importance of renegotiation as one component of improving a distressed relationship (cf. Lederer & Jackson,

1968; Sager, 1976). Behavior therapy has carried this tradition perhaps to its most extreme, literal form, in its advocacy of written change agreements as a primary method for bringing about change in a distressed relationship.

This section will begin with a definition of a contingency contract, and a rationale for its use. Then two major forms of contingency contracting will be discussed, parallel contracting and quid pro quo contracting. The advantages and disadvantages of each form will be enumerated, along with some a priori rules for optimal use of contracting procedures. A third section will offer a critique of contingency contracting procedures, based on both conceptual and clinical considerations.

WHAT IS A CONTINGENCY CONTRACT, AND WHY BOTHER WITH IT?

A contingency contract is a particular type of agreement between spouses. First, it is an agreement in writing. Second, it is an agreement which specifies a change in the relationship, usually a behavioral change by one or both partners. Third, and of greatest theoretical import, it is an agreement in which contingencies for compliance with the contract (and sometimes for noncompliance) are explicitly written into the written agreement.

The agreement need not be a *change* agreement although in practice contracts are used in therapy to formalize and specify the resolution of problems which the couple brings into therapy. Explicit contingency contracts are not needed in those problem-free areas of the relationship, although implicit agreements of a similar variety may be largely responsible for successful functioning in those areas. In therapy, contracting often represents the last phase of problem-solving, the formalization of an agreement which results from a successful problem-solving session. The use of contracting in therapy presupposes skill in problem-solving. To introduce contracting prior to training in problem-solving skills, assuming that problem-solving deficits exist, works against the spirit of a behavioral approach, which is essentially oriented toward step-by-step training in self-management skills. If couples are unable to effectively and reciprocally produce solutions to their problems, from where will the solutions to be contracted for emerge? They must perforce come from the therapist, and if this be the case, the approach has become one of crisis intervention. On the other hand, for a couple who can problem-solve successfully but is deficient in the ability to form viable agreements, contracting skills may be taught without a prior focus on problem-solving.

More than anything else, contracting is used to enhance the likelihood of behavior change. Distressed couples who are fortunate enough to reach agreement on solutions to marital problems seldom form viable agreements. Furthermore, even on those rare occasions when viable agreements are reached, they are seldom implemented successfully. Contracting skills are aimed both at facilitating the formation of viable agreements, and increasing the likelihood that the agreement will be successfully implemented.

Recording an agreement in writing serves both of the above goals, as described in Chapter 6.

The use of explicit contingencies specified in a written contract follows directly from a behavior exchange model of marital distress. It is believed that the behavior of both members in a relationship is controlled to a large extent by consequences provided by the partner. Current undesirable behavior in a distressed relationship is therefore thought to be maintained by reinforcers provided both by the spouse and by factors outside the relationship. An example already mentioned in different contexts is the use of aversive control. Verbal abuse provided by one spouse is often an effective means of controlling the other's behavior in the short run. Thus, such behavior is immediately reinforced by the partner's compliance. More importantly for the purposes of an approach to therapy based on increasing positive behavior, many of those spouse behaviors pinpointed as positive by the partner fail to occur with sufficient regularity or frequency because they are not reinforced by the partner. Dick complained, for example, that he wanted Pam to initiate sexual activity more often; yet upon careful inspection of their sexual rituals, it was revealed that he was responsive to her only on those occasions when he was the one who initiated sexual activity. At other times the partner may inadvertently reinforce behavior which is incompatible with the behavior which she/he claims to want. Sally was affectionate to her husband Rob only when he behaved in a cold and aloof manner toward her, despite her expressed wish that he behave more affectionately. Finally, partners may actually punish those behaviors which they desire to increase. Donna complained that Phil did not help her with the children enough; yet on those rare occasions when he did take over the primary management responsibilities, she interfered by constantly advising and directing his paternal behavior.

Given the lack of suitable contingencies for bringing behavior in accord with spouses' expressed wishes, it is naive to expect simple directives from the therapist to lead to behavior change. Unless environmental contingencies are restructured so that only desirable behavior is reinforced, there is little reason to expect relationship behavior to conform to each spouse's desires. The question facing the therapist is how best to elicit suitable changes in reinforcement contingencies. One way is to explicitly reprogram these contingencies as spouses agree to change their behavior. By setting explicit consequences for change in a written contract, it is ensured that spouses receive some immediate return on their investment in change. Although it is hoped and expected that over the long run the new behavior will be maintained by the natural contingencies inherent in a greatly improved relationship, in the short run some immediate payoff seems to be necessary. The relationship does not improve overnight, and the replacement of old well-established, habitual behavior patterns with new, costly positive behaviors will not endure during the often protracted transition from a distressed to a nondistressed state without short-term reinforcers.

Thus, the rationale for contingency contracting is that spouses will not change simply to please one another or the therapist. The consequences of initial change efforts will be critical for the upholding and maintenance of these efforts. Contracting is seen as a *temporary* way of structuring the environment so as to support each partner's new, therapy-induced behavior.

THE QUID PRO QUO CONTRACT

Historically, the oldest form of contingency contracting has been what Weiss, Birchler, and Vincent (1974) called the "quid pro quo" contract. Early publications in the area advocated this contracting form (e.g., Knox, 1971; Rappaport & Harrell, 1972; Stuart, 1969). The quid pro quo (QPQ) contract involves the direct, simultaneous exchange of behaviors. In the exchange each partner alters some aspect of his/her behavior in accordance with the other's wishes. Reinforcement control is derived from the contingent nature of the exchange. For example, Jim and Holly formed a QPQ contract designed to accommodate two areas of expressed dissatisfaction in the relationship. Holly complained that Jim seldom expressed interest in her day at work. Jim complained that Holly was seldom willing to play games which he enjoyed at night. Their contract took the following form:

a) Jim agrees to spend between 10-15 minutes each week night, between 5:00-6:00 p.m., discussing Holly's day at work. During this period, he will ask her at least five questions about her day, based on what she says. He will not make derogatory remarks during this period (e.g., "big deal"). Holly will be the judge of whether or not a remark is derogatory, based on the impact of the remark on her.

b) Holly agrees to play a board game of Jim's choice on Tuesday and Thursday evenings between 9:00-11:00 p.m.

If Jim complies with his end of the contract on Friday, Monday, and Tuesday, Holly must agree to her end of the contract on that Tuesday evening.

If Jim complies with his agreement on Wednesday and Thursday, Holly must agree to her end on that Thursday evening.

If Holly fails to participate in the game suggested by Jim on days when he has earned it, the work conversation is automatically suspended until the next scheduled game, at which time the work conversation will resume, as long as Holly participates in the game which Jim chooses for that evening.

What qualifies this contract as a QPQ are the following:

1) Each partner is agreeing to change some aspect of his/her behavior desired by the other;
2) Each partner's behavior change is to be reinforced by the other's behavior change.

In the paragraphs below we will discuss various aspects of QPQ agreements.

Explicit Behavior Change Agreements

As we indicated in the problem-solving manual, change agreements must be specific. This certainly holds true for the agreements comprising a QPQ contract. The agreement must specify exactly what the changed behavior is, when the new behavior should occur, how frequently it must occur, or for what duration it should persist. Consider the following QPQ agreement:

a) Bob agrees to spend more time with the children.
b) Carol agrees to be nicer to Bob's parents.

Clearly this agreement is ambiguous. How much time spent with the children will satisfy Carol? Does "spending time" consist simply of being in the same room with the children, or does it necessitate direct activity with them? How will Carol's "niceness" toward Bob's parents manifest itself? Who is to determine whether Carol has been sufficiently "nice"? Since the agreement is so nebulous, it is quite conceivable that Bob and Carol will enter into a dispute over whether or not either or both of them have delivered on their promises. Each, either in good faith or for manipulative purposes, can define the terms in a self-serving manner. Now consider a revision of the above agreement:

a) Bob will play with the children each day from the time he arrives home from work until dinner time.
b) Carol will speak to both of Bob's parents when they call on the telephone, and will ask each of them how they are and also ask "What's new?"

Now, in the revision, it is much clearer what each partner's requirements are. Although it is far from a perfect agreement (e.g., "play with" the children is still a bit vague), the specifications of the behavior expected of each are much more precise. While such precision lends the appearance of greater rigidity to the agreement, it also renders the agreement much more likely to be fulfilled. *Remember that such specified agreements are always viewed as temporary expedients, adopted for their strategic value.* It is assumed that once behavior change is well under way in a variety of areas, the contracts will become less necessary as the natural reinforcers associated with an improved relationship take over.

The therapist can and should be flexible in determining the necessary degree of specificity. In general, the more distressed the couple is, the more specificity is required in the contract. At times it is acceptable to tolerate a less specific agreement in less distressed couples, provided that the couple can agree on the criteria for compliance and noncompliance. For example, for mildly distressed couples, or couples in the latter stages of a successful therapy program, "being nicer to Bob's parents" may be sufficient for the above contracts, as long as each partner can answer questions such as "What does this mean?" or "Are you likely to disagree on when this has occurred?" to the therapist's satisfaction.

Contingent Relationship between Behaviors

The QPQ is distinguished by virtue of the contingent relationship between behavior changes undertaken by each spouse. Thus, each behavior change is assumed to be reinforced by the other's change. This cross-linking of target behaviors provides automatic contingency control, as Weiss et al. (1974) have pointed out.

It is important that the nature of the contingency be spelled out in the contract. Consider the following change agreement:

a) Don agrees to plan all weekend activities.
b) Jean will assume responsibility for finding a babysitter for all weekend activities.

It is not clear from the above agreement exactly how the two behaviors are to be related to one another. If they are to be used as reinforcers for one another, details of how and when each behavior change will be provided and withheld are essential. Under what circumstances should Jean reinforce Don by finding a babysitter? How much "finding" must Jean engage in before Don agrees to plan a weekend activity? This is clarified in the provision enumerated below:

> Once Don has presented his plan for a weekend activity to Jean, and she has agreed to it, she will then find a babysitter. If the activity must be cancelled because Jean has not found a babysitter, she must take responsibility for weekend activities until the next time she finds a babysitter.

A statement of the exact contingency is necessary in order that these behavior changes really do have the opportunity to act as reinforcers for one another. The therapist, along with the couple, must decide on the direction of behavior change, that is, who is to change first? This should not be left to chance since, as Weiss et al. (1974) have aptly pointed out, in a distressed relationship, mistrust abounds. Neither partner is willing to unilaterally engage in costly behavior change efforts, and they both seek evidence that the other is going to change *first.* Since it is impossible for both to change at exactly the same time in a truly contingent agreement, the therapist must help structure the contingency. The therapist can take steps to minimize the "who goes first" problem by equalizing the order of change across contracts; if the husband was the first one to change in contract one, then the wife should be the one to change first in the next contract. Also, contingencies can be arranged so that there is a circular, reciprocal connection between the two behaviors. Although one person must start, the relationship is not, in this instance, simply one where spouse A changes in order to be reinforced by spouse B. In the reciprocal contingency, not only does spouse B reinforce spouse A, but spouse A then reinforces spouse B. In the Jim and Holly example, although Jim is first agreeing to talk with Holly about her work, he only continues to do so if Holly complies with her end of the contract. Thus, although Jim must start, once the sequence begins the relationship is reciprocal, and each person's continued behavior change depends on reinforcement from the other.

Considerations in the Use of QPQ Contracts

The therapist must make sure that the behaviors engaged in by each spouse in a QPQ contract are of approximately equal cost, and that they are equally valued by the other. If partner A's change is exceedingly difficult and aversive, and/or partner B's behavior change is of minor importance to partner A, the reinforcement provided by B's minor change will clearly not compensate for the cost of making the major change. For example, Jack and Marion worked on an arrangement where Marion agreed to take over all household responsibilities, and in return Jack took responsibility for keeping the checkbook balanced. The agreement quickly broke down, perhaps because Jack's change was not a particularly powerful reinforcer for Marion, and the change that she was undertaking was particularly aversive and costly to her. Major high-cost changes should be reinforced by reciprocated major high-cost changes.

The most efficient kind of QPQ contract involves a situation where the behaviors being changed by each spouse are complementary. For example, husband agrees to spend more time with the children and the wife agrees to yield total child control to the husband on those occasions when he is spending time with them. This agreement, which involves a problem area of mutual concern, is likely to be successful because it mirrors a real-world quid pro quo. That is, rather than creating artificial arrangements between husband's behavior and wife's behavior, the above arrangement involves behaviors which are functionally related to one another in the real world. Unfortunately, it is not always possible to arrange for such exchanges. But, as a first step, it is always a good idea to look for exchanges which simply improve on those already existing in the life of the couple.

Certain behaviors in a marriage are not always conducive to contractual exchanges. In particular, contracts involving an increase in sexual activity can be problematic. Sexual behavior is consummatory and thereby produces its own reinforcing and/or punishing consequences independent of additional specified contingencies. Thus, whether or not an increase in sexual activity is reinforcing will depend on the consequences of that increase for the enjoyment of the sex act itself. Couples who engage in a low frequency of sex usually find higher rates punishing, for whatever reason. It is clinically unwise to attempt to change the frequency of these behaviors by altering their consequences; rather, in order to improve sexual and affectional aspects of a relationship, it is usually necessary to focus on the behaviors themselves, and attempt to bring about a change in each spouse's ability to enjoy them (see Chapter 9 for a complete discussion of this problem).

In any form of contracting, including the QPQ, the focus is on increasing positive behavior rather than decreasing negative behavior. Behavior therapy with couples focuses on teaching positive control strategies; positive control strategies are most appropriate for increasing positive behavior. In order to bring about decreases in negative behavior, aversive control strategies are necessary. Since distressed couples rely excessively on aversive control to begin with, it is usually not clinically advantageous to program additional aversive control into the relationships. When high frequency negative behaviors need to decrease, the most desirable strategy involves reinforcing the occurrence of behavior which is incompatible with the high frequency behavior. For example, one wife wanted her husband to stop spending money playing pool after work. Instead of contracting for a decrease in pool-playing, which would have necessitated the use of punishment or extinction, the husband was rewarded for contributing a certain amount of money each week to a common family fund, an amount which could be produced only by severely curtailing pool expenses. The specific terms of the contract were as follows:

> *Husband* agrees to place five dollars into the family safe deposit box every Thursday.
>
> *Wife* agrees to spend ten hours per week doing non-essential household tasks which are pleasing to husband.
>
> When the $5.00 check is not deposited on a given Thursday, a week's abstinence from non-essential tasks will follow, and will resume only upon deposit of the next $5.00. If wife does not complete tasks by a given Thursday, the next deposit is delayed until the tasks have been completed.

Another couple contracted for a reduction in the wife's nagging and the assumption by the husband of certain household duties. But instead of attempting to punish or extinguish nagging, the husband reinforced non-nagging remarks by engaging in the very household tasks about which she had formerly nagged. Note that this contract exemplifies a complementary quid pro quo:

> *Wife* agrees to praise her husband for all tasks completed around the house during the past 24 hours. The praise will occur at the end of each evening (between 9:00-10:00 p.m.).
>
> *Husband* agrees to complete the following tasks: walking dog (morning and evening), wash dishes immediately after dinner (before moving to the living room) and do one additional daily task of his choice from the list of daily tasks.
>
> Praise occurs only if all tasks are completed. If praise does not occur by bedtime, husband does not complete any of the tasks on the following day.

The preference for increasing positives and avoiding change agreements which decrease negative behavior is not absolute. In fact, arguments can be mustered which support regular inclusion of the latter. Wills, Weiss, and Patterson (1974) and Jacobson and Waldron (1978) found that pleasing and displeasing behaviors were relatively independent, that increases in pleasing behavior would not automatically lead to a decrease in displeasing behavior, and vice versa. Moreover, displeasing behavior accounts for an inordinately large proportion of the variance in marital satisfaction, according to data from these studies. These data would imply that ultimate improvement in marital therapy depends on the success of attempts to change negative behavior, either directly or by prompting increases in specific positive behaviors which are incompatible with the targeted negative behavior. However, Margolin and Weiss (1978b) found that a variety of treatment approaches successfully brought about decreases in displeasing behavior without direct attempts to decrease such behavior, whereas only behavioral approaches increased positive behavior. Behavioral treatments resulted in the greatest overall relationship improvements. Thus, a decrease in displeasing behavior seems to be a natural consequence of many forms of couples' therapy, even without directly focusing on such changes. Increases in positive behavior, on the other hand, must be systematically programmed into treatment. They do not automatically follow from decreases in negative behavior, and although a marriage can be greatly enhanced simply by the removal of aversive behavior, the data seem to suggest that increasing positive but low frequency behaviors adds a great deal to a treatment program.

What about very prominent presenting problems involving behaviors which are extremely aversive to one spouse and threaten, by themselves, to destroy the relationship? Behaviors such as alcohol abuse, physical beatings, and extramarital affairs fall into this category. These behaviors often create such an aversive impact that, even if they could be gradually eliminated by a persistent focus on increasing positive behavior, there is such desperation associated with them that something must be done immediately. An additional difficulty in dealing with these behaviors is that it is difficult or impossible to use them in exchange contracts, simply because there are no comparable behaviors to exchange for them. Often, these behaviors must receive early and immediate focus, and the rule of focusing on increasing desirable behavior must be temporarily suspended. More will be said about modifying these types of behaviors in Chapter 9.

To summarize, quid pro quo contracts involve the direct exchange of behaviors pinpointed by each partner as relationship problems. Each change serves as a reinforcer for the partner's change. Usually, although the contract specifies that one partner must start, once change has been generated, the relationship between each partner's behavior change is a circular one, such that each partner's changes reinforce the other's changes. Failure of one partner to comply with his(her) end of the change agreement sanctions the other to abdicate his(her) own contractual responsibility. The discussion now moves to parallel behavior change agreements, the so-called "good faith" contract (Weiss et al., 1974).

PARALLEL CONTRACTS

The parallel or "good faith" (GF) contract was recommended by Weiss et al. (1974) as an alternative to the quid pro quo. As the term "parallel" implies, couples each form independent change agreements, agreements where partners' behavior changes are not made contingent upon one another. The parallel contracts are said to be independent rather than functionally related.

Although parallel contracts do not involve explicit exchanges of target behaviors between spouses, parallel contracts are contingency contracts, since explicit rewards are specified for compliance with the contractual terms. Below are illustrations of change agreements and their respective contingencies in QPQ and GF contracts:

COUPLE #1

QPQ

Husband agrees to clean the bathroom every Saturday. *Wife* agrees to do laundry every Sunday. Wife does laundry on Sunday only when husband has cleaned bathroom on Saturday. Husband cleans bathroom only if wife did laundry on previous Sunday.

GF

Contract A
Husband agrees to clean bathroom every Saturday. On those Saturdays when he does, he chooses the activity for the evening, and the wife assumes responsibility for reservations and a babysitter.

Contract B
Wife agrees to do laundry every Sunday. When and only when she does, husband will assume all responsibility for children on Sunday nights, including baths, undressing, and putting to bed.

For this couple, the husband's complaint that the wife did not do laundry with sufficient frequency, and the wife's desire that the husband clean the bathroom regularly, were both behaviors targeted for change. In contrast, the two rewards used in the GF contracts were not target behaviors, but rather favors that each spouse suggested as appropriate reinforcers for increases in the respective target behavior.

COUPLE #2

Target Behaviors

a) Husband should be home for dinner by 6:00 p.m., or have called to say he will be late.
b) Husband wants wife to pick up clothes from floor before going to bed.

QPQ Contract

a) Husband agrees to be home for dinner by 6:00 p.m. every evening, unless he has phoned her by 5:00 p.m. to tell her that he will be late.
b) Wife agrees to have all clothes off the floor by bedtime.

If the husband either arrives home by 6:00 p.m. on a particular evening, or phones by 5:00 telling his wife that he will be late, she will pick up her clothes by bedtime. Whenever he fails to either arrive home on time or call in advance, she does not pick up her clothes. On nights when she is obliged to pick up her clothes, if she fails to do so her husband is relieved of his obligations for at least a day, and until all the clothes have been removed from the floor.

GF Contract

Contract A
Husband agrees to be home for dinner by 6:00 p.m. every evening unless he has phoned her by 5:00 to tell her that he will be late.
Reward: On those evenings when the husband complies, the wife will fix him a drink when he arrives.
Punishment: Husband must wash dishes on those evenings he is late and fails to call in advance.

Contract B
Wife agrees to have all clothes off the floor by bedtime.
Reward: Back rub on nights when clothes have been removed from the floor.
Punishment: Wife cannot shower on mornings after she has failed to comply.

COUPLE #3

Target Behaviors

a) Wife spending time with husband.
b) Husband's willingness to go out on week nights.

QPQ

a) Wife agrees to stay home on as many week nights as possible.
b) Husband agrees to go out more with wife on week nights, at her request.

On those nights when wife is home, husband will go out with her for at least an hour whenever she suggests that they go out.

GF

Contract A
Wife agrees to stay home on as many week nights as possible.
Reward: Husband will wash dishes and give baths to the children on all nights when wife is home.
Contract B
Husband agrees to go out with wife on at least two week nights, although he can choose which nights.
Reward: Sex games of his choice, one for each week night he accompanies her.

The reinforcers used in parallel contracts are not restricted to spouse-provided stimuli. In fact, the reinforcers are virtually unrestricted except that they should not consist of target behavior changes on the part of the spouse. And this is the major distinction between GF and QPQ contracts. Since spouses are not exchanging pledges to alter their behavior, at least theoretically the "who goes first" problem is eliminated. An additional supposed benefit of a GF contract is that the breakdown of one agreement is less likely to initiate further breakdowns. Since each agreement is independently negotiated, the failure of one agreement implies no disruption in any other agreement. In contrast the QPQ contract actually obliges spouse B to desist from her/his change efforts if spouse A fails to meet his/her contractual obligations.

As the examples suggest, when the spouse is providing reinforcement in a GF contract, the distinction between the two forms can become nebulous. In fact, there is nothing in the topography of the reinforcing stimuli which differentiates GF contracts from QPQ contracts in these instances. Rather, the distinction is based on the expressed *meaning* of a particular behavior to the recipient. If the reinforcer consists of behavior provided by the spouse which would alleviate a presenting complaint on the part of the recipient, the contract is a QPQ contract. If, on the other hand, the reinforcer simply involves spouse-provided behavior which, for whatever reason, is believed to be appealing enough to the recipient to strengthen a desired target behavior, the contract is a GF contract. The same behavior, when used as a reinforcer, will constitute a QPQ contract for one couple and a GF contract for another.

For example, consider the agreement where one spouse reinforces another by assuming responsibility for the children. Since some people enter therapy complaining that their partner is insufficiently involved with the children, this reinforcer would automatically render a contract a QPQ if used with such couples. On the other hand, for couples who do not complain about unequal distributions of child-rearing responsibility, but who would be reinforced by some extra "time off" from the children, a contract including such a reinforcer would be considered a GF contract.

Such distinctions do not always hold up under careful scrutiny. It would seem that any effective spouse-provided reinforcer in a GF contract would be behavior which the recipient desires, whether or not the absence of that behavior was mentioned as a presenting complaint. When viewed in this light, GF contracts seem quite similar to QPQ contracts. Perhaps rather than attempting to make categorical or qualitative distinctions between QPQ and GF reinforcers, it might be better to think of the distinction quantitatively or relativistically. Given a low frequency spouse behavior whose absence is relatively *salient* to the recipient of the behavior, the couple is agreeing to a QPQ contract when such a behavior is used as a reinforcer. When less salient, but nevertheless desirable, spouse behaviors are used as reinforcers, the contract is a GF contract.

In forming parallel contracts, most of the considerations mentioned in the previous section are relevant. Behavior changes should be explicit and specific. The contingent relationship between the behavior change and reinforcement should be clearly spelled out. Like the QPQ, it is generally desirable to emphasize positive control by reinforcing increases in desirable behavior rather than punishing decreases or extinguishing undesirable behavior. Despite all of these similarities, some special consideration must be given to the GF model by virtue of its reliance on sources of reinforcement which are outside of the target behavior exchange in the QPQ model. The next section discusses issues connected with the quest for effective reinforcers in GF contracts.

Considerations in the Specification of Reinforcers for GF Contracts

Reinforcement describes a process whereby the presentation of some stimulus following a behavior leads to a strengthening of that behavior. In an experimental laboratory, where the investigator completely controls the environment of the subject, including all potential reinforcers, this process can be identified empirically. Strictly speaking, before we can designate a given stimulus as a reinforcer, we need to demonstrate that there is, *in fact,* a functional relationship between a given response and that stimulus such that the response will be reliably strengthened when the stimulus is contingently available, and weakened when the stimulus is unavailable.

In a marital therapy setting, where the therapist controls neither the environment nor the couple's sources of reinforcement, such prospective, empirical demonstrations are impossible. The therapist, in collaboration with the couple, is reduced to guessing as to what stimuli will function as effective reinforcers for behavior change. Therefore, in a GF contract, it is a misnomer to designate the consequences specified in a contingency contract as *reinforcers* or *punishers*. Rather, they are simply *hypothesized* reinforcers and punishers. Once a contract is implemented, one might argue, its effectiveness or lack thereof will verify the effectiveness of the chosen consequences. Unfortunately, even changes in behavior subsequent to contract implementation cannot be attributed to the chosen consequences. Other factors cannot be ruled out as causal elements in behavior changes, such as characteristics of the problem-solving session itself, or other reinforcers inadvertently delivered by the spouse.

Thus, in a very real sense, therapists function in the dark as they help couples form good faith contracts. While it is quite easy to induce couples to report what they enjoy or what feels good, it is extremely difficult to uncover the effective reinforcers in a marital relationship. The *real* reinforcers in most adult intimate relationships are terrifically complex and subtle, and thus very difficult to specify discretely and on demand. The typical reinforcers described in studies using GF contracts, such as back rubs, reduced therapist fees, and relief from household tasks are unlikely to be important reinforcers in most marriages.

In other words, it is one thing to describe a particular stimulus as "pleasant" or "desirable," and quite another for that stimulus to function as an effective reinforcer, that is, as a stimulus for which couples will make costly behavior changes. People in adult relationships seldom emit behavior because of *discrete* pleasant stimuli; rather they respond to cumulative totals of such stimuli, or ratios of such stimuli to aversive stimuli, and so on. It is our guess, based on both our clinical experience and our understanding of operant psychology, that creating a reinforcement "menu," by asking spouses "what they like," generates long lists of stimuli which spouses find pleasant, but yields few effective reinforcers. Probably the only stimuli of this nature which are powerful enough to strengthen behavior are those unusually salient "pleasures" which are labeled as targets for change in therapy, i.e., those used in QPQ contracts.

What then is the function, if any, of those stimuli which are commonly specified as reinforcers in GF contracts? Again, we must speculate, as there are no data to bring to bear on this question. The back rubs and the other pleasures received by couples in exchange for behavior change possess cue functions; they are discriminative stimuli which bridge the gap between behavior change and reinforcement contingencies. For example, a spouse who receives a drink for coming home on time may be more likely to arrive home on time in the future, but the drink is best viewed as a cue rather than *a reinforcer.* A variety of stimuli act in concert to maintain this behavior change, including any behavior changes on the wife's part which accompany the presentation of the drink, or which follow his behavior change. The drink cues both spouses to the fact that changes have been made, and signals the likelihood of other reinforcers from both parties.

Again, we admit to the speculation in which we are indulging, for there is little evidence for our view of the function of spouse-provided pleasant stimuli in good faith contracts. Furthermore, even if these stimuli were not actually functioning as reinforcers, their value as cues or discriminative stimuli would be sufficient to recommend their use. However, here the therapist must ask himself exactly what the desired goal of the contract is. If the clinician believes that it is necessary to build in a *reinforcer,* spouse provided-pleasant stimuli may not be the best bet. On the other hand, if the therapist concludes that the reinforcers are likely to occur outside of the formal contractual boundaries, she/he may still opt to include a specified consequence for its discriminative value.

Assuming that, for whatever reason, the therapist has decided to use spouse behaviors as specified consequences in a GF contract, she/he should follow some common guidelines. First, the reward should not be costly or aversive to the spouse who is providing it. To the extent that the provider experiences the provision of the reward as burdensome, she/he enters into a conflict of interest. The benefits derived from having one's spouse change his/her behavior may be outweighed by the costs of providing the reward. If this is the case, the agreement will either dissipate, or be upheld with the paradoxical result of decreased satisfaction for the spouse who provides consequences, For example, Lisa and Peter attempted to contract for a change in Lisa's tendency to be late for engagements. She would agree to be on time for a number of specified appointments, and Peter would reward her with physical affection. However, Peter found affectionate interaction with Lisa displeasing at the time the contract was first implemented, and as a result he began to subtly encourage Lisa to be late, thus undermining the agreement. Another example involved Greg's rewarding Pam by taking over certain household duties which were normally hers. He found the duties so odious that the agreement, although successful, rendered him even less satisfied with the relationship. Thus, it is important that, when the consequences of a GF contract are provided by the partner, the provision of the reward is not punishing to the partner. The difficulty of uncovering spouse-provided rewards which are both powerful and of low cost to the provider may limit the viability of this contracting form for some couples.

Another important consideration in the formation of GF contracts is whether or not to include consequences for noncompliance along with the rewards for compliance. Some of the examples presented above include "punishment" for failure to comply with the terms of the contract. Common punishers in GF contracts include assignment of odious household tasks or loss of certain pleasant privileges, such as a night out with the girls (or boys). At times the inclusion of aversive consequences for noncompliance will strengthen a change agreement. The danger of using aversive contingencies is that they may be more powerful than the positive contingencies. In this case, even though the agreement has been strengthened, the behavior change is being maintained primarily by the specified punishment for noncompliance; this amounts to programmed aversive control, a state of affairs to be avoided in marital therapy for reasons already mentioned. Punishment for noncompliance should be included only in those instances where the therapist is reasonably certain that his contingencies for compliance are at least as compelling as those for noncompliance.

So far in this section, we have suggested that spouse-provided pleasant stimuli may not function as reinforcers in the literal sense of the term. This certainly should not preclude their use in GF contracts, since they may be of symbolic or discriminative value even if they do not in themselves strengthen the behavior which they follow. However, if the therapist is convinced that he needs actual *reinforcers* for a particular contract, she/he might consider alternatives to spouse-provided pleasant stimuli. These alternatives fall into two general classes: reinforcers coming from sources other than the spouse, and high frequency behaviors.

There is no reason for insisting that positive consequences for compliance in GF contracts stem from stimuli provided by one's partner. Indeed, the distinction between GF and QPQ contracts is clearest when GF contracts rely on stimuli provided by sources other than the spouse. One alternative mentioned by Weiss et al. (1974) is to use therapist-provided reinforcers, such as reduced fees contingent on compliance. Such reinforcers circumvent many of the difficulties discussed in previous paragraphs, such as concerns about the cost to the spouse who provides the reward. It remains an empirical question, to be determined individually for each couple, whether or not these financial incentives would be effective as reinforcers for behavior change. An additional limitation of therapist-provided incentives is their inherent transience; such reinforcers are not available once therapy has terminated, and their widespread use during therapy may retard generalization. Privileges which do not directly involve the spouse may be effective as reinforcers in GF contracts. Spending one night out of the house per week with same-sexed friends would be one example; another would be financial rewards, taken from the family's earnings, which could be used in either a specified way or at the discretion of the spouse who has earned it. The broader one's perspective regarding the scope of potential contractual rewards, the more likely that effective reinforcers will be uncovered. This is the main rationale for considering money and outside privileges. It should be pointed out, however, that these reinforcers have some of the same potential problems as spouse-provided reinforcers. They can be costly to the partner, regardless of whether or not they actually emanate from the partner. Consider the husband whose presenting complaints include the wife's excessive time spent outside the home. For him, a reinforcer allowing her further outside privileges would be aversive, and turn the behavior change which earned this reward into a mixed blessing.

Now let us consider the use of high probability behaviors as reinforcers. Premack (1965) demonstrated that high frequency behaviors can be used to reinforce lower frequency behaviors if somehow the opportunity to engage in a particular high probability behavior is made contingent on the emission of the targeted low probability behavior. The *Premack Principle* has sweeping implications for operant psychology since it sharpens our conception of reinforcement as a relative process, and properly alters our focus from the intrinsic properties of particular stimuli to the relationship between various responses and the environment. Earlier applications of learning principles to marital therapy were guilty of the former trend, that is, looking for effective reinforcers in the intrinsic properties of stimuli which are designated as pleasant on an *a priori* basis (e.g., Weiss et al., 1973). The Premack Principle, along with other research on complex reinforcement schedules (e.g., Morse & Kelleher, 1970), cautions against the inherent attribution of reinforcing properties to specific stimuli without taking into account the complexities of learning history and particular behavior-environment relationships.

The Premack Principle has been applied to a variety of clinical problems (cf. Danaher, 1974). Most commonly, individuals are instructed to engage in various high probability behaviors (e.g., drinking coffee, smoking cigaretes, urinating) only after emitting the behavior which the client is desirous of increasing. Todd (1972), for example, instructed a depressed cigarette smoker to precede all smoking with a positive self-statement (e.g., I am a worthwhile person). The rationale was that positive self-statements, which were believed to be incompatible with depression, would occur at a higher rate if a high frequency behavior (smoking) was made contingent on their occurrence. The effectiveness of this type of clinical procedure has not been demonstrated. Yet it does suggest a possible strategy for uncovering effective reinforcers which might be used in GF contracts.

A day in the life of a couple includes a number of behaviors which are important to each spouse, but which are not typically thought of as inherently rewarding or punishing. A few examples of such behaviors include going to work, taking showers, opening mail, the after-work cocktail, after dinner coffee, reading the newspaper, etc. These behaviors occur at high frequencies and would be missed, were their occurrence prohibited. Many of them are potentially effective reinforcers for behavior change. Consider the following examples:

1) Frank can leave for work in the morning *contingent* on kissing Colleen goodbye and telling her what time he will be home.
2) Terry has the privilege of showering in the morning *provided that* he has removed all of his clothes from the floor.
3) Marian can open her mail *only if* she arrives home at the time she has announced.
4) Amy can drink coffee after dinner *once* the dishes are washed.

In each of these examples, high frequency behaviors which were formerly rights are now considered to be privileges, to be allotted on the basis of performing certain desirable behaviors. The obvious appeal of the Premackian strategy is based on two factors: First, the privileges will often be effective reinforcers, if the therapist can ensure their occurrence only on the basis of performing the requisite behaviors; second, such reinforcers are plentiful, and thus can provide the icing on many a contractual cake. The critical issue in deciding on their use is whether, for any given couple, the ends justify the means. For in order to utilize these daily events as reinforcers, the therapist will have to produce an extraordinary commitment from a couple; essentially she/he must persuade them to cede control of normally noncontingent events in their lives. It is a skillful therapist indeed who can induce a couple to undergo this kind of voluntary deprivation in the service of therapy, and the initial cost of this procedure makes it risky.

In contrast to the already discussed paradigm, where at least in theory the spouse receives an added benefit in exchange for compliance, now he is emitting costly new behavior, with no new benefits to compensate for those costs. These contracts are likely to break down, since a failure to comply may not prevent the spouse from indulging him/herself in the customary privilege anyway. The wife who is late in arriving home from work may simply read her mail anyway. Or, the contract may be upheld, but with the undesirable consequence of strong resentment on the part of the person who is working for favors which used to be free. The couple who is highly committed to therapy may tolerate these restraints on a temporary basis, but these contracts, if used, should be faded out as soon as behavior change has begun to occur, and replaced with rewards comprising something new. We would also suggest that in one's initial treatment contract with a couple, any perceived potential for use of Premackian principles should be mentioned and agreed to by the couple in advance. Once they have committed themselves to the use of Premackian reinforcers, the contracts are less likely to be problematic.

To summarize this section, we have tried to elucidate the theoretical and practical difficulties associated with GF contracts, especially the difficulty of uncovering reinforcers. We have asserted that many of the pleasant spouse-provided stimuli used to consequate compliance are not really reinforcers at all, but may still have some role in maintaining behavior change through their cuing functions. Stimuli that can be chosen for this task are limited since they must not be costly or aversive to the spouse who provides them, yet must still be powerful incentives for the spouse who is making behavior changes. Contracts can often be strengthened by adding aversive consequences for noncompliance, although there is some danger that these aversive consequences will fundamentally alter the character of the agreement, such that the couple may be inadvertently programming additional aversive control into the relationship. Two alternatives to spouse-provided reinforcers were considered, privileges stemming from other sources, and high probability behaviors formerly available on a noncontingent basis. In the next section we will summarize the relative advantages of each of the two major contracting forms.

ADVANTAGES AND DISADVANTAGES OF GF AND QPQ CONTRACTS

The QPQ contract is a simple exchange by the two partners, each complying with a request for change on the part of the other. The contracts are often efficiently constructed, since the reinforcers have already been pinpointed, and the only remaining task is to specify exactly how the pair of behavior changes are to be related. In addition, there is usually little question as to the potency of the reinforcers, since they constitute the very behaviors which propelled the couple into therapy. In contrast, the construction of GF contracts is cumbersome, since specifying the behavior to be changed is only the first step in an often protracted, trial and error process of uncovering effective reinforcers. The inefficiency is exacerbated by the need to form two GF contracts for every QPQ contract, since the latter specifies changes in at least two problem behaviors. Finally, it is often very difficult to find powerful reinforcers to specify in GF contracts.

Given these clear advantages of the QPQ contract, it has to be considered the contracting form of choice unless there is reason to believe that GF contracts are more effective under certain circumstances. Weiss et al. (1974) have argued that for severely distressed couples, the "who goes first" dilemma precludes the effective use of QPQ contracts, and they favor the use of GF contracts in such instances. However, we believe that this is a pseudo-issue. As we have already indicated, the "who goes first" problem can be minimized by the therapist's making that decision. Once one partner begins to initiate change, the contingent relationship becomes reciprocal. Then, by alternating the order from contract to contract, it is possible to equalize the amount of change initiation engaged in by each partner. It might also be pointed out that a "who goes first" problem also exists with GF contracts—unless contracts for each of the spouses are established at the same time. The other major drawback of QPQ contracts is not so easily mollified: each time one agreement breaks down, at least two target behaviors are affected, since each person's compliance is required only as long as the other complies. This problem can be dealt with in the specification of the contingency, by minimizing the disruptiveness sanctioned by one partner's failure to comply. For example in the QPQ by Jim and Holly at the beginning of the section on QPQ contracts, Jim's noncompliance legislates Holly's noncompliance only on one occasion; the contractual relationship could remain unbroken, and Jim could reinstate the contingency by, for example, complying on the next two days. In the specification of the contingency, complete breakdowns are prevented by including rules for reinstating the contingency following noncompliance. Also, it should be noted that in practice any two GF contracts are probably somewhat dependent on one another despite the lack of an explicit relationship. If one contract breaks down, the other is often affected.

In order to justify a preference for GF contracts, in light of all the above-stated reasons for choosing the QPQ, the former's greater clinical effectiveness must be demonstrated. In the only study comparing the relative effectiveness of the two forms, Jacobson (1978a), treating moderately distressed couples, found no differences between them. Although it is still possible that the GF form may be more effective with severely distressed couples, there is no evidence to suggest this at present.

The GF form still has a place in certain specified situations. At times, as we have indicated, it is impossible to generate an equitable QPQ exchange. Certain behaviors play such a prominent role in a distressed relationship, such as excessive drinking or physical abuse, that no corresponding change by the partner would be equitable. If exchanges involving approximately equal costs are not possible, GF contracts may be preferable. Also, some couples may simply find the GF format more acceptable, given the "tit for tat" nature of QPQ contracts. The GF format is an acceptable substitute for such couples. Finally, some couples present unequal numbers of complaints. If 75% of the presenting complaints are voiced by one partner, only a minority of the problems can be negotiated with QPQ change agreements. GF contracts may figure more prominently with such couples.

GENERAL CRITIQUE OF CONTINGENCY CONTRACTING

In deciding whether contingency contracting is clinically indicated, two issues need to be addressed: First, does contracting add anything to the therapy regimen; second, are there clinical hazards associated with contracting which contraindicate its use in lieu of other strategies capable of achieving the same treatment goals?

The primary rationale for contingency contracting is that it restructures the relationship environment to create a milieu supportive of behavior change. There is no doubt that relationship environments need to be altered in order to generate favorable conditions for change. The question remains, however, as to whether contracting is the optimal strategy for such a task? Do other clinical strategies accomplish the same goals with either greater efficiency or less risk?

We believe that in many cases contingency contracting is redundant. The clinical procedures which usually precede contracting often accomplish the tasks for which contracting is invoked. The relevant empirical question is stated simply: does the specification of a positive consequence for behavior change increase the probability of that change occurring? When a therapist includes a "reward" for behavior change, whether the format be QPQ or GF, is the likelihood of contractual compliance enhanced? In many instances, we suspect that the answer to this question is no!

Consider a stimulus control model of change in behavioral marital therapy, a model which one of us has already discussed in other contexts (Jacobson, 1978b, 1978c). By stimulus control, we refer to the antecedents of behavior change, conditions prior to behavior change which exert a controlling influence on subsequent responding. A stimulus control model of change in marital therapy assumes that a large proportion of the variance in behavior change is accounted for by the conditions which immediately precede the formation of a change agreement. In the arena of problem-solving, negotiation, and change, the conditions under which the agreement was negotiated have a controlling impact on whether the agreement is successfully implemented. An agreement negotiated under favorable conditions will carry with it a high probability of compliance, whereas an agreement negotiated under unfavorable conditions is likely to be subverted. Compared to the importance of these negotiating conditions, the stimuli which are specified as consequences for change in the contract are often of minor importance.

Although there are probably a great many factors that influence compliance with a behavior change agreement, in many cases the negotiating session itself prompts partners' initial behavior change efforts; positive problem-solving sessions serve as discriminative stimuli for compliance, and negative problem-solving sessions minimize the likelihood of compliance. To illustrate this point, consider two hypothetical negotiating sessions between Amy and David where the problem under consideration is David's behavior in the presence of Amy's parents, adapted from Jacobson (1978c):

> Amy prefaces her request for change by emphasizing and expressing appreciation for David's previous efforts to interact positively with her mother, whom David despises. She also offers to present him with feedback during the evening which will inform him as to whether or not his performance is satisfactory. David, on the other hand, admitting that he is guilty of the transgression which Amy has identified, expresses a willingness to change. The couple remains on task throughout the discussion and focuses on the pros and cons of various possible solutions. After fifteen minutes of concentrated problem-solving an agreement is reached: David agrees to ask his mother-in-law at least five questions during the course of an hour's conversation, and further promises to remark positively both in regard to her physical appearance and in regard to the meal she has cooked. Amy promises to reinforce David with a back rub and verbal

> appreciation contingent upon compliance; noncompliance will result in negative feedback on Amy's part as well as three nights in which David must vacuum the rug (a job that is usually Amy's).

In the second hypothetical situation, Amy begins the problem-solving by requesting that David stop "acting like an ass in front of my mother":

> David responds by denying his wife's assertion and insisting that her mother deserves his remarks. Amy reminds David that she behaves politely in the presence of his parents despite her distaste for his father's "arrogance." She continues by accusing David of being selfish and narcissistic, and she attributes this behavior to the fact that he was "pampered and coddled" as a child. Finally, after ninety minutes of put-downs, criticisms, and sarcastic remarks, they reach an agreement identical to the one in the above example.

In contrasting the two hypothetical problem-solving sessions, it is a good bet that no matter what stimuli are specified as reinforcers in the final change agreement, compliance is more likely to result from the former negotiating session than it is from the latter. Thus, the antecedents of change agreements reduce uncertainty about the likelihood of the agreement being successfully implemented. Compared to the predictive power of these antecedent conditions, the supposed "reinforcers" specified in the agreement itself are often trivial.

The argument here is not that the environmental consequences of behavior change are unimportant. On the contrary, we have already indicated that behavior change will not occur in the absence of a supportive environment, which in most cases constitutes an altered environment. The contention here is that negotiating sessions themselves produce changes in the environmental cocoon which envelops behavior change. Negotiating sessions not only produce change agreements; they also affect the context in which an agreement is implemented. This impact is often more profound than the alteration in the environment produced by programming "rewards" and "punishments" into the change agreement. First, the negotiating session generates cognitions on the part of both partners which accompany initial change efforts. David, for example, is not only changing his behavior toward Amy's parents; he is also saying certain things to himself in conjunction with those behavior changes. He might be voicing positive expectancies regarding the likelihood of his behavior change being reciprocated by Amy. Or more generally he may be reminding himself that, "This change will make Amy happy." Following the second negotiating session quoted above, David would probably be emitting self-statements of a different quality, such as

"I'm going to get back at her for making me do this," or "What am I getting out of this?" Although it is problematic to refer to these self-statements as reinforcers or punishers, they do represent different contexts for the occurrence of behavior change, at the very least by mediating between the spouse's own responses and long-term contingencies, which ultimately determine whether behavior changes will be maintained. In any case, change is going to be more immediately reinforcing for a spouse when accompanied by positive expectancies and other positive self-statements.

The contingency contracting model is justified to the extent that important marital behaviors are a function of specific discrete environmental reinforcers; extending this notion to other areas of marital interaction, the model implies an array of marital behaviors, each of which is maintained by its own discrete, circumscribed reinforcers, each behavior-environment sequence being independent of the other. As we suggested in Chapter 1, it is probably more accurate to think of couples as summating and integrating all relevant information over an extended period of time; entire temporal classes of behaviors are either strengthened, weakened, or maintained depending on cumulative satisfaction levels. These complicated reinforcers are derived from a pool of salient environmental stimuli, including behaviors emitted by the partner not simply in response to Behavior A, but in response to a variety of behaviors which have occurred over a given period of time. Thus, when David exhibits politeness toward Amy's mother, she not only gives him a back rub and expresses verbal appreciation, but she also is nicer to him in other situations; perhaps she is more responsive to him sexually, and she is reciprocating his behavior changes by making certain changes in her behavior to comply with his requests. They also continue to have negotiating sessions, which collectively figure into David's reinforcement equation. Finally, during all of this, David is saying things to himself about the relationship. All of this information is being collected and totalled by David, and his tendency to behave in a polite manner toward Amy's parents is a function of all of these happenings, in addition to the particular negotiating session that produced the agreement. Compared to these factors, the importance of one specified stimulus in a change agreement will play a small role.

In the context of marital therapy, environmental changes are occurring at a particularly high rate. Many change agreements are negotiated within relatively close temporal proximity to one another. Whether or not these changes are explicitly formalized in the form of quid pro quos, implicit exchanges are occurring. These opportunities simply add to the likelihood of cumulative reinforcement of behavior change. This is why the techniques discussed in Chapter 6 are often so effective, despite the fact that explicit contracts are not negotiated. The fact is, these increases in positive behavior, although initially induced by the therapist's instructions, will be maintained only by a receptive environment; and, as the effectiveness of these procedures suggests, the environment is often made receptive by the increases in positive behavior which are being simultaneously made by the partner.

CLINICAL HAZARDS OF CONTINGENCY CONTRACTING

To the extent that contracting is unnecessary, we believe that it should be avoided. This belief stems from potential clinical liabilities inherent in its use. In this chapter, we have already alluded to the difficulty in specifying effective reinforcers in GF contracts. To this we now add a further caution, which is equally applicable to QPQ contracts: Even when it is possible to pinpoint effective reinforcers for their utilization in a contingency contract, the mere act of specification may eliminate their reinforcing power. This danger exists because many spouse-provided stimuli in a marriage are reinforcing only when they are accompanied by certain attributions on the part of the recipient. In arguing this point, we are extrapolating from relevant research in social psychology in the areas of attribution theory and extrinsic versus intrinsic motivation (Jones, Kanouse, Kelley, Nisbett, Valins, & Weiner, 1972; Levine & Fasnacht, 1974; Notz, 1975).

There is probably some consensus that for many spouses behavior which is thought by the receiver to reflect "caring" or concern is likely to be reinforcing. However, for such an act to function as a reinforcer, an interpretation on the part of the receiver is required. The identical act, for example, hugging, will serve as a reinforcer in some situations and not in others, depending on, among other things, the inferences drawn by the receiver as to the giver's intent. If the receiver infers that an act such as hugging signifies caring, that act will serve as a reinforcer; however, that same act might be ineffective if the attribution on the part of the receiver changes, that is, if an alternative, more plausible explanation for the action is available. Attempting to use such behavior as a reinforcer in a contract may be fruitless since the receiver is likely to view the act as caused by the exigencies of the contract rather than, e.g., "because he cares about me."

It is likely that partners will *attribute* such changes to *extrinsic* motivation on the part of the other, and therefore value such changes less than these same changes without the occurrence of specified consequences.

From this line of reasoning, it follows not only that contingency contracts are unnecessary, but potentially self-defeating. Changes which would otherwise be well-received and attributed to internal factors such as the partner's "desire" to improve the relationship, or his "caring," might be attributed to the fact that the spouse was forced to change because of the contract.

In our experience, many couples have voiced this concern. At times it is possible, through cognitive restructuring, to debunk them of these notions. But this is a difficult task, given the tenacity with which people insist that environmental explanations for behavior somehow make that behavior less "worthy" (Skinner, 1971). It is more advisable as a clinical strategy to avoid power struggles with couples over their tendency to dichotomize "internally-motivated" and "externally-motivated" behavior. For couples who devalue change attributable to a contingency contract, contingency contracts should be avoided. If the above critique is correct, contracts are often dispensable anyway since the functions they serve are also served by other clinical strategies.

Our critique of contingency contracting has focused on its redundancy with other procedures, as well as its possible clinical liabilities. It is an entirely speculative view at present, although research is currently underway to examine predictions derived from this formulation. Let us emphasize that we are not casting aspersions on the clinical utility of contracting *per se*. Written change agreements, as the end production of a negotiation (problem-solving) process, are a vital cog in the behavioral marital therapist's armamentarium. Our concerns are confined to the "contingency" emphasis in behavioral contracting. We urge therapists not to throw out the baby with the bathwater. In addition to all of the advantages we have already mentioned in support of the utility of written change agreements, a contract is a public agreement to institute beneficial relationship changes. The art of reaching noncoercive agreements, augmented by a public commitment toward their implementation, is at the core of the behavioral treatment strategy. Whether or not the specification of contingencies adds to the power of this procedure remains an unresolved issue.

SUMMARY

This chapter discussed the formation of written change agreements in marital therapy. Contingency contracting is a systematic way to create an environment which fosters behavior change, and is consistent with a behavior exchange model of marital interaction. Quid pro quo exchanges may be preferable to parallel or good faith contracts in most cases, both because of their relative efficiency and their ability to circumvent the problem of uncovering effective reinforcers. Although contracting can serve as a valuable adjunctive clinical procedure, its technology is often unnecessary since contingencies which support behavior change are often generated by other clinical procedures. Due to the potential liabilities of contingency contracting, it is probably wisest to avoid it when less costly interventions prove sufficient.

CHAPTER 9

Treatment Strategies for a Variety of Problem Areas

AS CHALLENGING as marital therapy is under the best of circumstances, it is made even more difficult when the marital problems are accompanied by other types of problems. In this chapter we take a brief look at the following situations confronted by the marital therapist that require strategies beyond the scope of the general framework presented in Chapters 6-8: sexual dysfunctions, child problems, depression, spouse abuse, affiliation-independence discrepancies, jealousy, and separation or divorce. We explore how brief interventions for these situations might complement or be incorporated into a marital therapy program. We also make recommendations as to when it may be best to dispense with the marital therapy and focus exclusively on the other issue.

Sex Problems

The distinction between marital therapy and sex therapy that exists in the professional literature contradicts what is found in clinical practice. Because many couples experience both marital and sexual problems, it is quite natural for therapists to practice marital and sexual therapy simultaneously. While we are aware of no data that reveal the incidence of overlap between marital and sexual problems, it is easy to understand why couples' presenting complaints often encompass both areas. Couples with widespread marital difficulties are likely to have less than optimal sexual interactions. Similarly, the frustrations of a sexual dysfunction may jeopardize other aspects of the marital relationship.

A couple's sexual relationship holds a unique place in the total marriage because of the potential gratifications from sex coupled with the exclusive nature of the sexual relationship. Not only do sexual intimacies carry a high reward value but, according to many spouses, such rewards should be forthcoming only from the marital partner. In contrast to other areas of interaction, spouses' mutual dependency in sexual gratification may be absolute. When a husband's enthusiasm for skiing is not shared by his wife, he pursues that interest with someone else. Only an unusual and unconventional relationship permits the same solution when one spouse does not wish to engage in sexual activity with the other. Thus, when faced with a relationship that does not provide anticipated sexual rewards, a spouse may find himself or herself questioning the very basis of the marriage.

In addition to sexual gratification per se, spouses' perceptions of sexual functioning can generate a multitude of impressions regarding the relationship as a whole. A good sexual relationship can foster feelings of being attracted to and valued by the other person; a poor sexual relationship can raise doubts about one's appeal and worth. Due to a lack of education and communication regarding sex, couples who see no solutions to their sexual "difficulties" may translate these into sexual "incompatibilities" and conclude that their differences are irreconcilable.

Another factor contributing to the overlap between sexual and more generalized marital problems is the importance of good communication in satisfactory sexual relationships. Communication skills, such as the ability to initiate interaction and give feedback, are as essential in sex as in other arenas of marital interaction. However, in light of some couples' limited experience and embarrassment in talking about sexual matters, whatever communication deficits already exist may be exacerbated when it comes to discussing sex.

Finally, it must be remembered that sexual interactions do not occur in a vacuum. Sexual attraction that is experienced in an evening may be closely related to a variety of other interactions of the couple that occurred throughout the course of a day. Feelings of resentment and anger from unresolved conflict during the day may interfere with feelings of tenderness and caring usually associated with lovemaking. As one wife concluded after describing an argument she and her husband had, "After I've been chewed up one side and down the other, I'm certainly in no mood to make love. But this causes Bill to rant and rave all the more." The fact that Bill demanded sex after arguments despite his wife's disinterest exacerbated their problems. Since sex, without feeling affectionate, was foreign to the wife's view of lovemaking, the husband's advances while she was still reeling from an argument caused her to feel even more estranged from him.

Over a longer period of time, certain spouses accommodate to the pain of a distressed relationship by becoming inattentive to all emotions, or as described by another woman, "going dead to all feelings." To reawaken these emotions through physical intimacies involves reexposing oneself to the possibility of emotional pain. Highly distressed spouses often are not ready to take such a risk.

Treatment of Sexual Dysfunction

In this section we consider different strategies to use with couples who, in addition to other marital problems, also present specific sexual dysfunctions, i.e., impotence or premature ejaculation for the male, or primary or secondary orgasmic dysfunction for the female. We distinguish these specific dysfunctions from sexual dissatisfactions, due to different sexual preferences or sexual boredom, which are discussed in the following section.

Fortunately, the most widely utilized therapeutic programs for sexual dysfunctions (e.g., Kaplan, 1974; Lobitz & LoPiccolo, 1972; Masters & Johnson, 1966) are highly compatible with behavioral marital therapy. These treatments offer a combination of education and corrective experiences that foster the acquisition of satisfying sexual behaviors and combat the anxiety that interferes with sexual performance. However, the obvious quandary when working with couples experiencing both a sexual dysfunction and more generalized marital problems is where to begin the therapeutic intervention. Usually it is not a question of offering one therapy to the exclusion of the other but rather what to focus on first. It is felt by some marital and sex therapists that this decision rests on whether the marital incompatibilities preceded or resulted from the sexual dysfunction (e.g., Masters & Johnson, 1966; Sager, 1976). When it appears that the sexual problems have preceded and triggered the marital disharmonies, sex therapy is often recommended. However, when sexual problems are the by-product of other relationship tensions, marital therapy is the preferred treatment.

In our view, the decision of how to begin treatment reduces to a question of efficacy. The therapeutic intervention should be chosen on the basis of what will provide the quickest benefits and have the more profound overall effect on the relationship. Offering sex therapy first makes sense under the following conditions: (1) there is an obvious sexual dysfunction that is contributing to the marital dissatisfactions, (2) the sexual problem can be treated through established sex therapy procedures, (3) the partners are not so turned off to one another that they are unwilling to engage in sexual activities, and (4) they are eager to embark upon a sex therapy program. According to these guidelines, one would begin with sex therapy when it appeared that such a program could readily improve the sexual relationship and perhaps even dissipate other marital dissatisfactions.

Obviously, the couple's readiness to pursue sex therapy is a major consideration in deciding between sex therapy and marital therapy. Consider the following couples seen for therapy. Judith portrayed her situation in the following manner. "I've never been able to have an orgasm. I don't know if it is *my* problem or *our* problem, but I do know that it's taking a toll on our marriage. We're so tired of trying and failing that we hardly ever have sex anymore. And both of us are real edgy and uptight with each other. The smallest thing can set us off. I don't know what we'll do if this doesn't get any better . . ." From this description it appeared that the marital dissatisfaction was a by-product of the sexual dysfunction. Over the five years Judith and Tom had been married, they had grown increasingly frustrated at their inability to resolve this problem. Tom began to attribute Judith's inability to have orgasms to his own failings (e.g., "Maybe something's wrong with me"), while Judith's questions about her own sexuality led her to wonder whether they both should be exploring new relationships. Although their desperation caused these spouses to consider separation, this course of action was more a forced choice than a desirable option. They were unwilling to accept the status quo and, at this point, saw no alternatives to separation if the problem continued.

Several factors led the therapists working with this couple to believe that sex therapy was the most efficient way to intervene. It appeared that the sexual dysfunction rather than other spheres of interaction was largely responsible for the marital tensions. Secondly, the spouses' sexual withdrawal from one another was due to frustration rather than a lack of attraction. Both partners did, in fact, desire sex with one another and were willing to engage in sexual activities under the therapists' guidance. They simply wanted to avoid further failure experiences and, for lack of a better solution, had resorted to abstinence.

A second couple came in for therapy demonstrating more serious signs of marital distress but requesting sex therapy. After 15 years of marriage, Don and Heidi had just learned about a sex therapy program and sought treatment for their combined sexual problems of premature ejaculation and primary inorgasmia. A thorough assessment of this couple revealed a stable but unsatisfactory relationship in which each partner's dissatisfaction was well masked. Although there were several longstanding marital problems, the spouses verbalized that everything would be better as soon as the sexual problems were alleviated. These spouses' eagerness to begin sex therapy and apparent reluctance to work on other aspects of their relationship were instrumental in the therapists' decision to begin therapy by focusing on the sexual relationship. While it was clear that the couple needed communication training, the therapists felt that that aspect of therapy would be best received under the rubric of sex therapy. Furthermore, since the treatment of this couple's sexual problems appeared to be relatively straightforward, the therapists felt that sex therapy would offer them a success experience in the one area they viewed as most important. Momentum from such a success could then be used to bridge the transition to other areas of the relationship if that were still necessary.

However, not all couples are ready to work in the area of sexual intimacy. Albert and Lydia, for example, held very different perceptions about their sexual relationship. Albert felt that their marriage would be much improved if only Lydia could experience orgasms and desired sex more frequently. Lydia, too, wanted to have orgasms but viewed this goal as secondary to establishing a relationship that was more conducive to sexual intimacy. Lydia, in fact, exhibited her reluctance for sexual contact by consistently switching the topic of discussion from sex to the lack of trust in the relationship. In this case the therapist decided that making sex the immediate focus would offer unilateral support for Albert. Furthermore, such a focus was bound to fail since it rested heavily upon being able to elicit Lydia's cooperation. The therapist did not diminish Albert's hope that Lydia would become a more responsive sexual partner but made the establishment of a "more trusting" relationship the initial therapeutic aim. This focus was certainly in line with Lydia's goals and, in fact, was complementary to what Albert wanted.

In general, sex therapy is not recommended when there is so much animosity between the partners that they do not view one another as attractive, desirable sexual partners. There are obvious risks in asking such couples to put themselves in a highly vulnerable situation demanded by sex therapy exercises. Even in the beginning stages of therapy, during sensate focus exercises (Masters & Johnson, 1970), spouses are instructed to communicate tenderness and affection through touch. Certainly it would be difficult to convey or receive such expressions if the spouses do not experience those feelings. The overall success of sex therapy depends upon spouses' experience of pleasure and sense of mastery at each step in the program. Thus, what a therapist wants to avoid is having spouses engage in situations that foster anxiety or discomfort, or increase the partners' ill-will towards one another.

Since there are no tested guidelines on when to begin with sex or marital therapy, the therapist must make the decision on the basis of presenting information, and then evaluate that decision by monitoring the couple's progress after a course of action has been initiated. We view a decision to begin with the sex therapy as more risky and yet potentially more powerful. The risk is whether the spouses can put aside their negative interactions and attain the level of cooperation necessary to work on the sexual dysfunction. While failures in this area are diagnostically meaningful, they can postpone the attainment of benefits and can intensify the couple's despair. Yet, if successful, sex therapy can offer a potent source of reinforcement as well as provide a success experience that will motivate a couple to work on other problem areas.

Treatment of Sexual Dissatisfaction

In addition to offering sex treatment for specific sexual dysfunctions, marital therapy can play an important role in enhancing general sexual functioning. Through the assessment procedures described in Chapter 4, the therapist learns whether the partners are satisfied with the quality and quantity of their sexual activities. Data supplied by continuous use of the SOC contain a detailed index of the pleasing and displeasing aspects of the couple's sexual interactions and can clue the therapist as to what type of intervention might be useful.

Range of activities. Over the years spouses often fall into sexual routines that offer little variation or change. Given such a situation it is not uncommon for partners' interest in sex to diminish and their frequency of sexual activities to decrease. It is essential that couples who have become bored with their sexual routines consider new sexual activities and communicate previously unstated preferences to their partners. Many couples find sexual manuals or pornographic materials helpful in expanding their range of sexual options. Then, to help relieve some of the anxiety associated with trying new sexual activities, the therapist can build an expectation that the first attempts are not always perfect.

Difficulties can arise when the two partners disagree on the types of activities they wish to incorporate into their sexual repertoires. The problems are particularly acute when one partner requests a behavior, such as oral sex, that the other finds repugnant. A therapeutic strategy when confronted with contradictory preferences is acceptance of the different positions, detection of the common denominator that is agreeable to both partners, and exploration of new options that both spouses might find acceptable (Heinrich, 1978). The therapist initially wants to communicate that each partner is entitled to his/her preference and to indicate that such disagreements between partners are not uncommon. Secondly, it is useful to find out what aspect of the activity is offensive, i.e., the odor, the wetness, the sensation? Through such exploration, the therapist models how to discuss such objections and perhaps discovers that only certain aspects, rather than the entire activity, are distasteful. From there the two partners can brainstorm what modifications of this particular activity might make it more acceptable, e.g., masking the odor with a body lotion, oral caressing of body parts other than the genitals. Hopefully, this procedure will illustrate to the couple how they can utilize alternatives and avoid becoming stymied when their initial viewpoints appear diametrically opposed.

Frequency of sexual activities. Spouses' sexual preferences may also vary in terms of how often they desire sex. Discrepancies in this area can introduce tension into the sexual relationship and reduce the enjoyment for both partners. The partner who feels under pressure to engage in sex more frequently may come to dread the other's advances and go to great lengths to avoid situations that may lead to sex. Confronted with such behavior, rather than straightforward communication, the other partner may become confused and angry over the frequent rejections.

In one couple seen for therapy, the husband wanted sex at least five times per week while the wife found three times to be plenty. During their problem-solving phase of therapy, the husband asked that sex occur more frequently and also be more enjoyable. The wife's predictable reaction was to balk at what she experienced as an unreasonable demand. The therapist intervened at this point to restructure the situation:

T: Stu, while your requests for more enjoyable and more frequent sex represent understandable and desirable goals, you must recognize the contradictory nature of those two requests. Given Sue's reaction, even if you get her to agree to engage in sex more frequently, the chances are good that the quality will go down. At this point, I think you need to make a choice between quality and quantity.

H: Well, humm. Yeah, I guess so. I guess I choose quality. But I don't want to give up on the other.

T: I'm not saying to ignore your request for more frequent sex. But for right now, I think your decision is a good one. Perhaps by making sex more enjoyable, Sue might accept the request for more frequent sex in the future. What could Sue do to enhance your enjoyment of sex?

The husband went on to specify how he wanted Sue to arrange for the children to be gone and to have leisurely sex with him on a weekend afternoon. While it appears that the therapist intervened on the wife's behalf, this intervention seemed necessary to avoid a deadlocked battle over sexual frequency.

All differences in sexual frequency will not be amenable to the solution adopted by this particular couple. Sometimes these preferences reflect differences in spouses' sexual drives and cannot be resolved with an exchange-type intervention. In such cases, there are several alternatives. The couple may wish to try a straightforward compromise in which they have sex four times a week or alternate weeks so that they have sex three times one week and five times the next. Other possibilities include the exploration of ways to increase the arousal of the partner with the lower sex drive so that person is more receptive to sex, or to respond to the needs of the other partner without having intercourse. The couple may simply decide that it is best for the person with the high sexual drive to relieve his/her own needs through masturbation.

Initiations and refusals. While it is not unusual for couples to develop a ritualized means of communicating their desires to have sex, the ritual may not be entirely satisfactory to one or both partners. In asking couples how they initiate lovemaking, we encountered the following complaints: "Well, it just happens every Sunday afternoon, like clockwork," "That's the only time he's affectionate with me," and "In our entire married life, she's never taken the lead." As illustrated by these responses, sexual initiations suffer from being (1) unidirectional, (2) demands rather than requests, (3) habitual rather than conveying a spontaneous desire for sex, and (4) turn-offs instead of turn-ons. Since the initiation often sets the tone of the whole interaction, there can be great benefit to a couple in discussing and rehearsing new ways to initiate sex. Often the woman who rarely or perhaps never initiated sex may be both pleased and intimidated by her husband's request that she assume this role. This woman needs a great deal of support as well as some specific direction as to how she might communicate her desires for lovemaking.

As initiators, both partners can benefit by expanding their repertoires of initiations and learning what types of stimulus conditions make the partner more responsive to sexual overtures. Partners may need to tap into their own sexual fantasies and share these with one another. Couples may find that they can enhance sex by "setting the scene" through special music, a favorite cologne, particular articles of clothing, candlelight, dancing for the partner, or whatever fulfills individual pleasures. The element of surprise or change may also be an important factor. Initiating sex at a different time of day or different location can heighten the excitement.

Knowing how to refuse sex is crucial to relationship well-being, for an insensitive refusal usually counts as a significant displeasure. The key in this area is differentiation between rejections, which communicate a categorical "I'm not interested" or "You don't turn me on" and refusals, which communicate "I really don't feel like it right now but will be more in the mood a little later" or "I'm not really in the mood but maybe you can help me get in the mood." If spouses have particular difficulty accepting refusals, it is helpful to have them practice refusals in the session and then go home with the assignment that, during the upcoming week, they must refuse at least one initiation of sex. Through such an exercise, couples learn that refusals are not devastating to a relationship and can, in fact, enhance lovemaking when it occurs.

Withholding sex. A distressed spouse who feels powerless to change his/her partner may choose the sexual arena to act out the disappointment and frustration occurring in other marital spheres. While the withholding of sex can function as a very powerful form of coercion, it also signals a partner's desperation. We have found it important to develop an aura of good faith between the partners and trust in the therapists before attempting to reverse someone's decision to forego sex. Eventual success in this area depends upon discovering what would make it possible to abandon the sexual prohibition and then assisting both spouses to make the necessary changes. However, when one partner decides to continue withholding sex, in spite of some positive changes in the relationship, the other is forced to choose between accepting a nonsexual relationship and terminating the relationship.

In a case seen by one of us (Margolin, Christensen, & Weiss, 1975) the wife, who felt powerless in the area of financial decision-making, refused to engage in sexual activities until the husband shared financial control. The initial phases of therapy helped the couple to share more positive events and engage in fewer conflicts, but then it became evident therapy could go no further in these directions until major problem areas were attacked. Furthermore, unless the spouses went ahead and approached these avoided areas, they would backslide from the progress they had already made. As the couple approached the session in which they knew they would be confronting these issues, they had a large argument and the wife demanded separation. Even after the husband responded by meeting a request of the wife and establishing separate checking accounts, the wife continued to talk about separation. Viewing this crisis as reluctance to abandon the strongholds of power, the therapists recommended that the couple remain together at least long enough to share some of the essential gratifications of married life. The therapists and clients then wrote the following contract in which the wife actually negotiated for consideration rather than for more financial changes.

CONSIDERATION AND SEX

Wife	*Husband*
Accelerate:	Accelerate:
1) Initiates sexual intercourse with husband one time.	1) Initiate and engage in one 20 minute conversation with 6 positive statements, e.g., "I never thought of that," "That is a good idea," "That is a new way of looking at it."
2) Engages in sexual intercourse with husband one time.	2) Initiate and engage in one 20 minute affectional period which will include behaviors like foot rubs and touching and patting.
Reward:	Reward:
1) One album of wife's choice.	1) $6 of clothing.
2) Reduction by $2 of therapist penalty.	2) Reduction by $2 of therapist penalty.
Penalty:	Penalty:
Do dishes for 3 days.	Make lunches for 3 days.

We the undersigned agree to the conditions of the above contract. We further agree to accept the partner's initiation of the above activities or suggest a more convenient alternate time.

Wife .... *Husband* ....

Therapists

....

Date ....

The decision to write this contract contradicts our earlier statement about the inadvisability of sexual contracts, but was felt to be strategically important in this case. Having made such a contract, the wife could engage in sex without losing face. She readily complied with the contract but verbalized her motives as an attempt to avoid the contract penalty.

An important component in the success of the above case is that the wife's refusal to have sex was a manipulative gesture motivated by pride and desperation. She did, in fact, enjoy sexual intercourse with her husband. But what if the prohibition reflects that one partner, for whatever reason, finds sex aversive? In that case, the therapist must rely on some of the same options as when one partner wants sex at a very low frequency. It is necessary to explore what aspect of the sexual relationship is aversive, and to determine how sex could at least be tolerable, if not enjoyable. If the aversion is simply the general feeling one partner has towards the other, it is important to identify what the other person does to create that feeling. Based on that information, the other partner can decide whether it is worth it to try to change those behaviors. At the same time, it is necessary for the therapist to explore why the partner experiencing this aversion desires to stay in the relationship. Either the aversion is transitory, offset by more positive feelings, or the person is clinging to an irreconcilable situation. Perhaps the withholding of sex is, in fact, an expression of the person's desire to terminate the relationship.

Well-Functioning Couples

Therapists who are fortunate enough to be working with a couple having a satisfying, active sexual relationship are advised to use the couple's strength in this area as a stepping stone for growth in other relationship areas. If the couple has a strong sexual relationship but problems with affection, the assignment of pleasuring activities (e.g., massages, foot rubs) can get the couple to expand their repertoire of physical intimacies to nonsexual activities. Couples learning new communication skills can practice these skills (e.g., making requests, giving feedback, sharing expectations) by discussing their sexual relationship. Even couples who are requesting no changes in their sexual activities can utilize education about sex to dispel myths and to renew sexual experimentation and excitement. This education may be particularly useful to aging couples who are experiencing changes in their sexual functioning and lack the information needed to put these changes in perspective.

Summary

It is our opinion that marital therapists must concern themselves with a couple's sexual functioning. For couples experiencing sexual dysfunctions, the marital therapist must directly address these problems or else refer the couple for additional therapy. Dissatisfactions regarding the range or frequency of sexual activities can be handled by procedures, such as brainstorming and negotiation, which are described in more detail in earlier chapters. Finally, education regarding sexual functioning is recommended for all couples to enhance the sexual relationship, which, in turn, is likely to have a positive impact on the relationship as a whole.

CHILD PROBLEMS

A great deal of speculation exists about the relationship between child problems and marital discord. Sometimes couples in marital therapy wish to devote a good deal of time discussing the problems they are having with their children. Similarly, in many cases when the child had been the presenting problem, the therapist quickly sees a need to refocus the therapeutic endeavor onto the marital relationship. Although switches between a marital to family focus are quite common, they could be determined more rationally by having the initial evaluation include assessment of parent-child dimensions (Weiss & Margolin, 1977).

Proponents of family systems theory view the relationship between marital and child problems as predictable and even inevitable. Since all family members have an investment in preserving the status quo, intrusions that threaten change are responded to by adjustments that maintain old ways. According to this theory, the deterioration of a marital system can be stabilized by a child who has a problem. The child's problems may postpone marital decision-making, may deflect marital conflict, or may even strengthen the marital bond as the parents unite to protect a sick or weak child (Minuchin, 1974; Satir, 1967). Although the disturbed interaction can exist anywhere in the larger family unit, it is generally assumed that the parents' relationship has great influence on the children. While Framo's (1975) claim that "whenever you have a disturbed child, you have a disturbed marriage" (p. 22) may be a rather extreme statement describing this relationship, other systems theorists assume marital involvement in most child problems. Minuchin (1974), for example, illustrates how parents' interactions can affect their youngsters by measuring the children's physiological stress responses in a family interview. The family consisted of two parents and two diabetic adolescent daughters. The children initially watched their parents engage in a stressful interaction from behind a one-way mirror and then joined the parents in the interview room. During both the observational and interactional phases, the daughters' blood was monitored for plasma-free fatty acids (FFA), a biochemical indicator of emotional arousal. Both children showed significant increments over baseline FFA levels when just observing their parents and then even higher levels when in the same room as the parents. The FFA levels of the one daughter who was consistently used as a pawn between the parents showed the highest elevations and the longest interval to recovery.

There is some empirical support for an association between marital discord and child problems. Examining only a clinic sample, Johnson and Lobitz (1974) found a moderate correlation between marital adjustment and rate of deviant child behavior. Patterson, Cobb, and Ray (1973) found marital problems in at least half of their sample of children referred for behavior problems. More importantly, a number of studies have shown less marital satisfaction in parents of referred than in parents of nonreferred children (e.g., Love & Kaswan, 1974; Oltmanns, Broderick, & O'Leary, 1977). Oltmanns et al. (1977) noted, however, that there was overlap between their referred and nonreferred samples and that all parents of referred children did not show marital problems. Furthermore, the level of marital discord was not related to the degree of positive behavior change demonstrated by the child at the termination of therapy.

Although these studies do indicate an overlap between marital and child problems, the findings are quite limited. Thus far, there have been no comparisons made between distressed and nondistressed couples for possible differences in the incidence of child problems. In addition, no conclusions about causality can be made from any of the studies mentioned above. Although family system theory suggests that marital dissatisfaction may precipitate behavior problems in the child, it is equally plausible that the child's problems place untoward stress on the marital relationship. It must also be noted that the association between child and marital problems offers the therapist no particular guidelines in terms of treatment planning. Even if the problems are causally related, there is no reason to suspect that treatment for one problem alleviates the other problem.

What does the marital therapist do regarding child problems? When couples report that they are having problems with their children, it is important to evaluate the severity of those problems. Generally we have found it useful to make some progress on the marital front so that the couple can join forces in dealing with the child's problems. However, upon occasion we have encountered child problems so severe that they demanded immediate attention. When parents demonstrate their anger with one another through their children, they may end up neglecting or even abusing the children. In a family seen by one of us, the children became the major battleground for the spouses' arguments. The spouses never divided up child-rearing responsibilities and used them instead as leverage to secure a desired behavior change from the partner, e.g., "I'll stay home with the kids Friday night if you call off your fishing trip." However, since compromises were not always reached, the children were sometimes neglected. Furthermore, child-rearing took on the quality of "one more chore" rather than an activity in which either parent took delight. The therapist on this case set up a precondition for marital therapy: The spouses had to clarify and carry through on their child-rearing responsibilities before being seen for marital therapy. Whenever the therapist encounters instances of child abuse or neglect, it is time to disrupt the ongoing therapy and treat the situation as a crisis needing immediate intervention. Whatever steps are necessary to insure that the child will no longer be neglected or abused should be taken.

A more common situation is that the spouses are aware that their children are having problems and they are eager to alleviate those problems. When marital therapy is the primary focus but the spouses indicate that they have particular concerns about a child, the therapist might agree to work with the family either immediately or after the couple has demonstrated a certain degree of progress in the marital relationship. In either case, expansion into the family arena necessitates the formulation of a new treatment contract.

Both behavioral and reflective parent training, the two most commonly used approaches for disturbed parent-child relationships (Tavormina, 1974), dovetail quite nicely with the marital treatment we have described. Therapy for the parent-child problems often consists of helping spouses to generalize their listening, conflict resolution, and negotiation skills to interactions with their children. This redirection can be supplemented with bibliotherapy on contingency management with child (e.g., *Families: Application of Social Learning to Family Life,* Patterson (1971)) or on parent-child communications (e.g., *Parent Effectiveness Training* by Gordon (1970) or *Between Parent and Child* by Ginott (1965)). Some couples transfer their newly learned skills from marriage therapy without any assistance from the therapist. For example, one client, who complained that her teenage daughter was disrespectful and belligerent with her, found she could engage her daughter in much more pleasant conversations by employing the listening skills she developed in marital therapy. When working with other families, who need more direct assistance, it is helpful to bring the children into the therapy sessions and work with the family unit. The therapist might initially play a very active role in encouraging each family member to share what she/he wants from other family members and directing the discussion so that it is evident that the requests had been heard. The therapist can also be instrumental in modeling how parents can interact differently with their child. For example, parents of adolescents may need a demonstration of how to grant autonomy when it is appropriate and yet maintain a certain degree of authority. Lastly, problem-solving plays as important a function in the resolution of family problems as in marital problems. When family problem-solving is done within the therapy session, the therapist can assist the family in formulating a mutually beneficial contract. It is important, for instance, that the parents do not pick the wrong issue to push, such as what friends Johnny should associate with, and ignore the more significant concerns, such as his stealing. Similarly, it is important that the child does not set unrealistic goals for him/herself.

An additional issue related to child-rearing that frequently comes up in marital therapy is one partner's dissatisfaction surrounding the other partner's parenting. Usually these problems are best handled by having the dissatisfied spouse negotiate for changes in the partner's child-rearing behavior. A wife who wanted her husband to relieve her of some of the responsibilities of caring for their four-year-old daughter requested that he pick up the daughter from day care on Monday, Wednesday, and Friday afternoons, and that he stay home with the daughter Monday evening while she went to class. These types of managerial child-rearing functions are usually contracted far more easily than qualitative changes that reflect values about how to parent. Related to this second category, another wife complained that her husband paid very little attention to the children, and that when he did interact with them, he was too critical. After some work on changing this complaint into a request, it finally took the following form: Each evening the husband was to tuck the children in bed. Additionally, during his two hours to babysit on Saturday morning, he was to play with the children rather than just be in the house with them. The husband initially complied just to please the wife, but then reported some weeks later that he saw improvement in his interactions with his children.

Summary

Family therapists suggest that child problems are often a function of faulty marital relationships. There are no data that directly support this assumption, nor does marital therapy necessarily relieve the child problems. However, the similarity in the skills necessary for effective marital functioning and effective parenting makes for a smooth and easy transition from marital to child-rearing problems.

DEPRESSION

There is increased recognition that depression and marital maladjustments may be related (e.g., Cammerer, 1971; Overall, Henry, & Woodward, 1974; Weiss & Aved, 1978; Weiss & Birchler, 1978). Interestingly, the empirical evidence supporting an association between marital dissatisfaction and depression is strongest for males. Two studies that examined outpatient clinic populations (Coleman & Miller, 1975; Johnson & Lobitz, 1974), found strong correlations between husbands' depression ratings and marital maladjustment ratings but the correlations for wives on the same two ratings were not significant. In their examination of a nonclinic population, Weiss and Aved (1978) found that for wives marital satisfaction and depression were related primarily through the uncontrolled variance in physical health status; for husbands, the significant relationship between marital satisfaction and depression remained even when physical health status was parceled out.

A number of well articulated and well documented theories of depression provide a context for understanding how depression may be related to marital discord. According to Seligman's (1975) learned helplessness model of depression, when individuals learn that their outcomes are independent of their responses, they refrain from emitting adaptive responses and evidence salient features of a depressed state. These individuals believe they have no control over what will transpire in response to their behaviors, much like the spouse who perceives no relationship between his/her action and the partner's response. Beck's (1967) cognitive model of depression suggests that depressed persons view themselves as deficient and inadequate, and construe their experiences as evidence of personal failure. These perceptions engender feelings of guilt and self-blame, much like the partner who has low self-esteem because she/he is sexually rejected by the partner. Finally, Lewinsohn's (1974) behavioral theory of depression proposes that low rates of response contingent positive reinforcement elicits depressive symptomalogy. The amount of response contingent positive reinforcement that an individual attains is a function of several factors: (1) the number of events that are reinforcing for the individual, (2) the availability of those reinforcers, and (3) the individual's ability to attain those reinforcements. For example, spouses who lack skill in attaining reinforcement for being effective marital partners may resort to dysfunctional, noncoping behaviors as a way to obtain the spouse's attention and concern.

When working with a couple in which one of the spouses is depressed, the therapist must evaluate whether the depression is maintained by variables within the relationship or external to the relationship. The question to ask is whether or not the partner provides antecedents or consequences that affect the occurrence of the depressed behavior (McLean, 1976). Depression that is relationship specific can often be identified by its circular pattern (Feldman, 1976; Weiss & Birchler, 1978). The depressive behavior relieves that partner of responsibilities and elicits sympathy or solicitous attention by the nondepressed partner. That attention, in turn, increases the high rate of self-deprecating thoughts, which further reduce the depressed person's coping responses. Sometimes, when the depressed partner finally does attempt to change, the nondepressed partner suddenly withdraws attention, thereby punishing these positive efforts. This pattern can be examined systematically if a daily measurement of depression is obtained in conjunction with daily SOC data. A pattern of high rates of spouse pleases when the partner is experiencing a high level of depression, and lower rates of pleases at other times, signals that relationship factors may maintain the depressive behavior.

On the possibility that the depression is relationship-maintained, we suggest seeing partners together for the intake session whenever the referral problem is one spouse's depression. Conjoint therapy is recommended under the following conditions: (1) the depression is related to marital problems; (2) the nondistressed partner is behaving in a manner that sustains the depression, whatever its cause; or (3) the nondistressed partner is experiencing dissatisfaction due to the other person's inability to function in the relationship. Although this final condition includes situations in which the depression is unrelated to the marriage, we recommend that the nondepressed partner participate to stabilize the relationship. Otherwise the relationship may continue to deteriorate, contributing still another factor to the depression. Individual, rather than couples, therapy is recommended when none of the above conditions exists.

When a decision is made to work dyadically with a problem of depression, the therapist must clearly state what marital therapy can offer, and how that will affect the presenting problem of depression. Consider the following explanation given to Frank and Sally:

T: Now Frank, when you first called me, you talked about your feeling depressed and wanting to get some help with that. You also mentioned that you wanted to learn to express yourself and that you had gotten some help in that regard through an adult education course. And yet, as we talk today, most of what you're upset about concerns your relationship with Sally and her threats to leave if you don't make some changes.

H: Yeah, but I want these changes for me too.

T: Right. They'll be important to you no matter what transpires between the two of you as a couple. And Sally, if I've heard you correctly, you're still interested in making a go of this relationship but only if Frank starts communicating more and stops locking you out of his life.

W: Yeah, I'm real tired of feeling like I don't exist or that my feelings don't matter.

T: What I really need to know, Sally, since I originally asked you to come in just this one time, is if you would be willing to help out in the process of getting the two of you to communicate better.

W: I've done everything I know how, but if you have some ideas . . .

T: The way I see it, Frank's work has got him down, but the relationship between you has got you both down. In my experience, it may be easier and quicker to make some changes in the relationship than to find a new career for Frank, particularly in light of your financial situation. So I recommended that we start with the relationship and then move into the area of Frank's career. What that means is that in the first phase both of you can expect to be actively involved in making some changes.

The therapist then went on to describe what was involved in marital therapy and to acknowledge how it differed from what the couple initially requested. While it may appear heavy-handed to redefine therapy in this manner, there are several reasons why the therapist felt obliged to have this couple consider a type of therapy they had not requested. It appeared that Frank's depression was related to a variety of factors, such as financial problems, dissatisfaction with his job, and concerns about his children from a previous marriage. Yet, his most pressing concern was his fear that he might lose Sally. Furthermore, the relationship with Sally, in contrast to the other problems, was modifiable in the immediate future and was in great crisis. The other problems also demanded attention but would take some time to change. On Sally's part, the relationship had become so intolerable that she was seriously contemplating leaving Frank, which, as her final alternative, was better than "being dragged down with him." Over time, it became increasingly evident to the therapist that Sally was maintaining Frank's depression. Sally only spoke of leaving when Frank became slightly less depressed; when he was least able to cope, she did not dare to mention separation.

It was critical to this case that the therapist negotiated a treatment contract in which the relationship, rather than Frank, was the therapeutic focus. Otherwise, Sally's role would have been one of "assistant therapist" with Frank continuing as the "identified patient." However, when the partner is sustaining the depression but the depression is not formulated around relationship issues, this distinction is not as clear. We find it useful to describe how spouses are so interdependent that when something troubles one spouse, it also affects the relationship. Examples of this dependency can usually be found in what the couple has said just in their first session. However, we do not recommend pushing the notion of the problem being relationship based beyond what is plausible to the clients. Initially, it is enough to elicit a verbal commitment from the nondepressed spouse; she/he is usually willing to cooperate. Sometimes, in fact, the nondepressed person is so eager to be helpful that she/he starts to assume control of therapy for the depressed partner just as she/he was compensating for the depressed person in other contexts. The therapist must actively discourage this by having the nondistressed partner focus on changing his/her own behavior.

Below we describe some ways that behavioral marital treatment can be modified when one partner exhibits depressive behaviors that are related to or sustained by the relationship. References continue to be made to the therapy received by Frank and Sally after they negotiated for a 10-week course of marital therapy.

Increase Awareness of Spouses' Control over One Another

That spouses exercise a huge amount of control over one another is a particularly important message for depressed partners who tend to view themselves as powerless. Unfortunately, depressed spouses are often exercising their control in a negative way. Frank's unresponsiveness, for example, was a very effective way of making Sally conclude that he was unavailable to her and causing her to seek supportiveness elsewhere. Thus, it was important for Frank to recognize the negative impact of his depressive behavior. It was equally important for him to become aware of ways he could have a positive impact upon Sally. These goals were realized by having Frank monitor the relationship between his behavior and Sally's reactions to him. Self-monitoring, (cf. Ciminero, Nelson, & Lipinski, 1977), rather than spouse monitoring, was the intervention strategy since Frank needed confirmation about his own worth as a husband and did not need to reinforce his belief that he was incapable of reciprocating her generosity. This exercise illustrated for Frank that he was able to elicit a wide range of responses from Sally and resulted in his focusing more attention on her. Moreover, it enabled Frank to become more realistic and accurate in his self-evaluations, thereby contributing to the second objective of reducing negative self-statements.

Combat Negative Self-Statements

Frank's personally demeaning and blaming statements played an important role in maintaining his relationship with Sally. Statements such as "I know I don't deserve such a good wife" functioned as public acknowledgments of Frank's indebtedness to Sally. These statements were congruent with Sally's expectations of herself under these circumstances, and compensated for the fact that she was not getting much in return for all the support she was showing Frank. Statements such as "Those are my hangups" signalled Frank's helplessness and caused Sally to reduce her pressure for him to change. These statements were particularly effective in dissipating Sally's anger and resentment. After repeatedly observing these interaction patterns in the sessions, the therapists helped the couple to see how the exchanges contributed to the dysfunction in their relationship. In addition, Frank's perception that he was an "inadequate" husband was dealt with through cognitive restructuring (cf., Ellis, 1962). The therapist asked Frank to define his requirements for being a "good" husband and then explored the meaning of not meeting those requirements. By operationalizing "good" husband, it became clearer to Frank that his goal represented incremental steps rather than a "good vs. bad" dichotomy.

Increase Pleasant Events

Since depressed people usually receive and emit few reinforcing behaviors, an increase in the exchange of pleasing behaviors is critical for couples in which one or both partners is depressed. A major focus of Lewinsohn's (1974) treatment program for depression is the identification of rewarding activities and the restoration of an adequate schedule of positive reinforcement. Marital therapy simply approaches these objectives with a dyadic focus, as described in Chapter 6. In light of the fact that spouses typically function as the major source of reinforcement for one another, it is often the case that the nondepressed spouse is also experiencing a low rate of positive reinforcement. Sally, for example, frequently bemoaned the fact that she and Frank never had fun anymore. Unless the two of them began to engage in more pleasant activities together, she was ready to seek these rewards elsewhere. However, when working with a depressed couple, it is important that pleasant activities be introduced in gradual steps (Weiss & Birchler, 1978). Although it is necessary to arrange for activities that are incompatible with depressed behavior, initially it is advisable to avoid activities that demand a more cheerful spirit or energetic demeanor than the depressed person can possibly muster.

Establish Appropriate Contingencies for Depressed and Nondepressed Behaviors

Since depressed feelings and behaviors do not maintain a uniform intensity, careful observation of these events provides useful information about what intensifies or lessens the depression. When focusing on the relationship, it is important to look for relationship related events that affect the depression. What can the nondepressed spouse do that makes the depressed person more or less depressed? Does the depression typically divert the couple's attention from some other issue?

For the most part, Sally maintained and compensated for Frank's depression by becoming more active as he became more withdrawn. However, when he began to behave more normally, she immediately increased her expectations of him and became more critical. This was vividly demonstrated during one therapy session when, while practicing communication skills, Frank assertively expressed some views about disciplining their daughters. Halfway through the communication exercise, Sally stopped paying attention to Frank, and announced, "I can't handle it, I just can't handle being gentle with Frank." The pronouncement angered Frank and also squelched his attempt at straightforward communication.

Further familiarity with this couple revealed that Frank and Sally actually alternated in the role of rescuer and responded best when the other person was in crisis. In accordance with the initial picture of this couple, when Frank behaved depressed Sally coped quite adequately. However, when something negative happened in Sally's life, she implored Frank's support with statements such as, "I can't go on this way. I'm going under." At such times, Frank rallied and came to her aid with support and understanding. This seesaw pattern was predicated upon the fact that Frank and Sally commanded the most attention from one another when they were experiencing problems. A therapeutic goal for this couple was to substitute interactions around positive experiences for their current mode of crisis intervention with one another. The scheduling of time to talk about what interested them or what was going well for each of them was an initial step towards this goal.

Skills Training

Depressed spouses may need training in specific skills, such as assertiveness, sociability, or problem resolution, to make them better able to elicit reinforcement. Since Frank felt indebted to Sally, he had a difficult time assertively expressing requests or opinions. This, of course, only frustrated Sally because she was aware of vague demands but was uncertain about what would please Frank. Frank's unassertiveness was also expressed through a tendency to acquiesce verbally to each of Sally's requests but to follow through on very few of them. During the course of therapy, Frank learned to make clear requests and to negotiate for specific changes. He found, for example, that Sally did not resent his request for independent time, as long as she knew about it in advance. Together, they engaged in constructive problem-solving around financial issues. It had been Frank's habit to hand his paycheck over to Sally and then ask her for cash as needed. Since Frank was dissatisfied with this pattern, he recommended that he keep a portion of his checks and deposit that money in a separate checking account for his own use. This plan fulfilled two aims: Frank obtained control of a portion of his paycheck and Sally knew exactly how much money was available to her for household expenses.

Setting Therapeutic Contingencies

The low response rates which are characteristic of depression are likely to affect these clients' compliance with therapeutic assignments. If one of the client's presenting problems is a difficulty accomplishing what she/he sets out to do, the therapist does the client a disservice by sanctioning the noncompletion of therapeutic tasks. In working with such clients, it is necessary to take this problem into consideration and make sure that the homework assigned is manageable. If, even then, it becomes obvious that one or both spouses are not carrying out the agreed upon assignments, the therapist should consider establishing contingencies to increase the couple's therapeutic efforts. Likewise, the therapist needs to be cognizant that the completion of agreed upon activities represents an achievement for depressed clients that is not to be minimized.

Summary

When working with depressed clients, the therapist must evaluate whether the depression is maintained by relationship variables or extra-relationship variables. In our view, conjoint therapy is the recommended treatment mode when depressive behaviors are elicited or maintained by relationship processes. Such therapy can be used to gain the support of the nondepressed spouse, to diffuse cycles that maintain depressed behavior, to resolve marital problems that may be the source of the depression, and to stabilize marriages that are deteriorating in response to one person's depression.

SPOUSE ABUSE

Although there appears to be a growing awareness and concern about family violence, marital therapists have not been particularly vocal about such matters. In some instances of physical abuse, the most therapeutic course may be for a couple to terminate rather than to treat the relationship, and a marital therapist may be in an opportune position to assist a couple in making that decision. The situation must be viewed as critical when one partner, most likely the wife, is in danger of physical harm that cannot be contained through stopgap measures directed toward the couple. In such cases, it is the therapist's ethical responsibility to abdicate the role of "relationship advocate" and help that person find protection. However, in other cases in which the threat of physical harm is not quite as intense, a couple may wish to use marital therapy to explore whether they should end the relationship or whether they can learn to control their abusive patterns. It is our view that marital therapy can also play a preventative function with couples whose conflict patterns are becoming increasingly intense and having an erosive effect on overall marital adjustment. The therapist can help these couples explore the potential danger in their conflict patterns and offer them some alternative means of handling anger.

A number of programs recently developed by feminist groups direct their attention towards providing emergency housing and care for battered women and their children (Higgins, 1978; Martin, 1976). The underlying assumption of these programs is that the husband perpetrates his aggression upon the wife, who, as a victim, is unable to extricate herself from this destructive relationship. Very often the function of these programs is to assist in the termination of abusive relationships. The programs provide physical facilities in the form of refuges or safe houses as a source of shelter and protection for battered women. They also provide psychological support for women who have experienced abusiveness, regardless of whether they are in the process of dissolving the abusive relationship. Although the services are directed primarily towards women, occasionally the programs also offer therapy or counsel for the abusive husbands. These programs serve the important function of providing a source of safety for battered women but they vary in their sensitivity to dyadic issues.

As marital therapists, we must consider ways to assist abusive couples who do not want the protective services described above and are not choosing to terminate the relationship. It is our experience that the majority of partners seeking marital therapy periodically inflict intense levels of emotional pain upon one another through brutal words and vindictive actions. A notable, albeit low, percentage of these couples have experienced incidents of physical abuse. Based on the findings that marital conflict tends to escalate over time (cf. Straus, 1974), a greater percentage may be headed towards physical abuse. With some modification and expansion, the therapeutic procedures described in previous chapters are applicable to the abusive couple who elects to remain in the relationship and who is willing to put forth efforts towards stopping the pattern of abusiveness.

According to the social learning formulation of marital violence, the mismanagement of anger and frustration can be the breeding ground for emotional and physical abuse. In contrast to the view that aggression is an innate tendency that needs periodic discharge to avoid a more destructive explosion, research has shown that engaging in aggressive activities tends only to produce greater subsequent levels of aggression and violence (Berkowitz, 1970; Straus, 1974). Unfortunately, once spouses begin to exhibit violence they often learn that violence is a powerful mechanism in getting the partner to comply. Very often the victim also recognizes that violence is a particularly effective means of controlling behavior and that person may reciprocate with similar or equally coercive behaviors. With both partners engaging in such behaviors, conflict can escalate quickly and continue on to great intensity. Thus, the common "therapeutic" injunction to ventilate anger can have serious repercussions, particularly for the couple who is already experiencing high conflict levels. The most important goal for those couples is that they learn to avoid, or dissipate, the early stages of anger, and thereby avoid the escalation of conflictual interactions (Ellis, 1976; Mace, 1976).

A written account by a woman who had a particularly violent conflict with her husband on the previous day illustrates how quickly an argument can escalate from angry words to violent actions. The tension had been brewing between Tim and Margie since the previous evening when the husband had hurriedly left the house after a phone call from another woman. Margie's initial method of coping with the problem was to avoid any discussion of it with Tim. Finally, when she could no longer postpone interacting with him, the following transpired.

> . . . I got up again, I couldn't relax, and I went and stood in front of the heater for awhile because it was really cold. Tim got up and

came out and sat on the couch. I was feeling very negative. I didn't want to deal with him but he was forcing me to. I cannot hide it when I'm unhappy. He asked me if I'd seen his bank book and I said "no" and went in the bathroom. So he said, "Well you're in a good mood, the day's already shot behind your negativity." I told him (that) he knows me better than to think I could pretend everything was okay when I was still pissed off from the night before. I could tell he was working up to an angry (mood), so I went in the bedroom to get dressed. I wanted to split before it got to be a scene. He came into the bedroom and started asking me what the matter was, my negativity was inexcusable and I should tell what my problem was. I got *scared* because he had that wild look in his eyes I'd seen before. I just wanted to get AWAY from him. He was suddenly beyond reasoning with. I told him I could talk to him about it now but I had no words because I was scared and upset and arguing with him can get so out of hand. Besides he *knew* what I was upset about and why did *I* have to confront him with words that could only make him angry. He insisted that I could not leave or anything else until I said something, so I told him I was disgusted and upset because he was lying to me and sneaking around behind my back. Well, he now had his words and accusations so he screamed at me for being so stupid and jealous and possessive and making something sordid out of his friendship with a girl. The next thing I knew he hit me on the side of my head and when I tried to get away from him he hit me again and pushed me into the closet and slammed the door on me. Now I was *angry*, my neck had gotten wrenched again and I thought my glasses were broken and I was just consumed by total anger. I wanted to go out and kill that son-of-a-bitch for abusing me so I jumped up, forgetting everything, slammed the closet door open and in a blind rage went out to . . . I pounded him for a second with my fists and screamed, "How dare you abuse me! If you ever hit me again I will kill you!" But then I caught a glimpse of his face and it suddenly hit me that all I was doing was removing any control from the situation at all. Suddenly I was terrified and I ran into the bathroom to get away. He followed me there and saw I was hysterical and panicking. He was yelling at me and trying to get a point across, but I was so terrified all I could think of was "God help me. He's going to kill me." I couldn't talk to him so he hit me again (twice) I fell on the floor afraid to move. I screamed. I was afraid someone would call the police so I tried to calm down and tried to calm Tim down. "Please relax and talk it out, okay. Please?" But he wouldn't calm down. He hit the wall once because I couldn't say anything coherent—all I could do was stare at him. The power of his anger and frustration just turns him into another person. I was afraid to speak because I might make it worse. Then I told him that if he came near me ever again I would call the police. I think maybe that made him aware a bit of where he was—he said "Hell, I'll call them for you" and he went and picked up the phone. I saw his attention was diverted so I ran out the door into the rain.

In spite of the intensity of this episode, this was the first instance of physical abuse between Tim and Margie. A previous battle between them had included verbal rage but then ended when Tim put his fist through a wall. After the current episode, Margie briefly acknowledged that she "should get out of the situation before he really does kill me some day," but in no way committed herself to that course of action. Although Tim explained his temper as "something he was born with, just like his dad," his abusive behavior could be readily traced to his family history. Tim's father used physical punishment to discipline Tim and his younger sisters. Then, when his Dad died and Tim was made "man of the house" at age 15, he found that threats, slaps, and occasional beatings kept his sisters in line. In a critical incident, one sister was planning to drop out of school but then changed her mind after Tim beat her. Since Tim viewed his anger as beyond his control at times, he feared that he might get into trouble with the law or cause someone permanent harm. Yet, he also felt that anger was acceptable, and even necessary at times, and just hoped to avoid any irreparable incidents.

In addition to the fact the relationship between Tim and Margie was to be ongoing, there were two reasons why relationship therapy was used to deal with this couple's problem of abusiveness. Based on the assumption that violence may be a desperate but unsuccessful attempt at dealing with problems, one reason for including both partners was to help the couple acquire effective problem-solving skills. A history of this couple's relationship revealed that they had experienced little success in resolving disagreements. While they could temporarily settle arguments by becoming overly conciliatory, they never resolved the basic issues behind the arguments. In this particular incident, neither partner knew how to initiate a discussion of the problem that was confronting them. Margie's attempts to remain silent, in hopes that the whole incident would disappear, clearly communicated her dissatisfaction. When she finally broke her silence, she came forth with a series of accusations that touched off Tim's anger. Tim dealt with his feelings of guilt and remorse by being confrontive and goading Margie to attack him; he then responded angrily which completely side-tracked them from the problem at hand.

The second reason for offering conjoint therapy was to contradict their notion that Tim possessed a trait-like propensity towards aggression; this belief only absolved both partners of their responsibility for letting the abusiveness occur. While it is true that some persons who abuse their marital partners display other signs of emotional disturbance, there are no data to suggest that these persons are disproportionately represented in the population of violent spouses. There is evidence, however, that individuals who were on the receiving end of violence as a child are more likely to engage in violence as an adult; furthermore, individuals who observed violence between their parents are more apt to engage in conjugal violence as adults (Gelles, 1972). It was felt in this case that couples therapy could be used to instill the notion that anger is a learned interactional pattern and thus could be changed. In this abusive relationship there were stimuli that elicited abusive behaviors and responses that maintained those behaviors. The identification of those patterns could increase this couple's chances of controlling violence.

Treatment Components

In addition to the treatment strategies discussed in previous chapters, there are several procedures to employ that have been explicitly designed for enhancing spouses' anger management skills and reducing abusiveness (Margolin, in press).

Identify the cues that contribute to angry exchanges. The first step to anger control is learning what cues elicit and maintain the anger responses. Assuming that anger progresses in intensity such that an individual is not instantly enraged, that person can learn to use early signs of anger as a discriminative cue for coping responses that are antagonistic to the anger. However, it takes practice for spouses to become careful observers of their own anger so that they are actually aware of very subtle reactions that register anger. Behavioral diaries and the Anger Checklist, described in Chapter 4, often prove useful. In addition, spouses can sometimes help each other by identifying cues that go unperceived by the person emitting them.

In the process of identifying anger cues, spouses can gain greater appreciation for how their behaviors affect the partner. It is not uncommon for spouses to learn that the strategies they had employed to avoid anger work counterproductively and actually increase the partner's anger. Ed and Harriet provided such an example. Harriet, who had previous experience in individual counseling, dealt with upsetting situations by demanding immediate discussion of the problem and uncensored expression of feelings. However, Ed, who had previously hit Harriet and feared the full potential of his anger, typically reacted to an upsetting situation by withdrawing and refusing to discuss the troubling issue. Although Ed withdrew in an effort to avoid a major blowup, Harriet interpreted his behavior as a rejection of her. She then would become incensed at his inaccessibility and berate him for avoiding her. The more he withdrew, the more angry Harriet became, eventually goading Ed into an overt display of anger. When anger was finally expressed, it had built to such an intensity that it inevitably resulted in physical abuse. On the day following an angry explosion, both partners would be overcome with remorse and extremely conciliatory to one another. However, the consequent high level of positive exchange only reinforced and perpetuated the cycle of conflict. Careful tracing of this pattern was necessary to help this couple realize why their strategies to avoid anger were failing.

In the process of identifying abusive patterns, it may become evident that both partners have contributed to the escalation of anger. This places both partners in the role of abuser and victim. The therapist can use this information to acknowledge each partner's pain and confusion as a victim as well as help each partner accept responsibility for any actions that accelerated the abusiveness. Spouses should be encouraged to view as problematic responses that were not in themselves abusive, but that aggravated rather than diminished the partner's rage.

Establish some ground rules. Due to a variety of cultural and societal values, the belief that spouses have the right to hit each other is not uncommon. Yet, in work with abusive couples it is necessary to establish a ground rule that abusiveness is unacceptable under any circumstances. To give this ground rule meaning, it is important to set up a consequence if the rule is violated. While the most logical consequence is that the spouses will separate, this cannot be an empty threat. Once the ground rule and consequence are established, the partners must be willing and prepared to follow through.

Develop a plan of action to interrupt the conflict pattern. Once the partners have adequately identified anger provoking circumstances and their angry reactions to those situations, they can then proceed to develop response repertoires that interrupt the conflict patterns. The new behavior patterns must incorporate two components: (1) immediate actions to disengage from the conflict; and (2) a plan to reunite to deal with the problem at a later time. Since couples who have long histories of arguing quickly escalate to high intensities of conflict, they must act immediately if they are to terminate conflict. The first spouse to observe an anger cue should acknowledge the anger with a neutral, nonblaming statement. In recognizing anger, spouses should refrain from acting anger out with behaviors that are destined to inflict pain, such as being critical or threatening. Since spouses are unaccustomed to acknowledging and deciding how to deal with their anger, it is necessary for a couple to practice these procedures under the therapist's supervision and at a time when they are not angry. As the actions to interrupt anger become more familiar and automatic, spouses are better able to utilize them in a moment of anger.

When the recognition of anger does not suffice to mitigate the conflict and the argument progresses to the stage when either spouse is no longer thinking rationally or censoring anger provoking responses, it is best for the spouses to separate from one another. Simply going to opposite ends of the house or outside for a walk may work, particularly if both spouses understand the purpose of that behavior and know they will reunite at a later time for further discussion. However, spouses also need to recognize when more definitive action is needed. Spouses who may be confronted with this later situation should plan for it in advance, by arranging for a place to stay for an extended period of time, and becoming familiar with community shelter facilities.

As mentioned previously, violence can be a particularly effective means of getting a person what she/he wants and, for this reason, certain partners may prefer not to control their anger. In such cases, the therapist can have the abusive spouse explore the potential consequences of continued abusiveness and can demonstrate that there are equally effective and less dangerous ways to exercise control. However, when dealing with a person who remains unwilling to cease his/her use of violence, the therapist's efforts are best directed towards the recipient of the violence. Although it is extremely difficult, that person can diminish the effectiveness of the other's anger by not responding in a compliant manner. How to carry through on such a strategy obviously depends upon the intensity of the violence and may entail: (1) simply avoiding being drawn into an argument, (2) temporarily getting away from the abusive partner, or (3) permanently terminating the relationship.

Modifying faulty cognitions regarding relationship functioning. Spouses with problems in anger management tend to maintain unrealistic expectations and assumptions about relationships. Some beliefs inhibit problem-solving discussion, e.g., "You won't love me if I disagree with you," or "It is best for me to hide my feelings and go along as though nothing is wrong." Others keep spouses engaged in arguments that should be terminated, e.g., "The future of our relationship rests on being able to resolve this argument now" or "I know I'm right and I've got to prove that to him." Spouses who subscribe to any of the above assumptions or other faulty suppositions need education about the role of anger and disagreement in a relationship. The therapist must make it clear that while angry feelings occur in every relationship, anger does not need to develop into a frightening or uncontrollable situation.

The modification of cognitions also applies to the restructuring of expectations and perceptions that spouses hold for one another. Expecting one's partner to be able to mindread unspoken desires or always to be logical is likely to result in many disappointments. Spouses sometimes translate such disappointment into anger. To avoid this problem, therapy time can be used to examine the feasibility of spouses' expectations, to explore the effects of these beliefs on the relationship, and to modify unrealistic expectations.

Express rather than act out dissatisfaction. One of the reasons that couples have problems with anger is that instead of confronting issues at an early stage, they deal with issues only after they are blown out of proportion. This pattern compounds over time since the couples' lack of success in resolving issues only makes them more hesitant to bring up new issues. These spouses need communication skills that permit them to express problems or feelings in language that is descriptive rather than vindictive. They also need to be able to identify and take responsibility for their own feelings by stating "I feel angry when you're late" rather than yelling "You make me angry when you're late." Practice with these new skills and the problem-solving strategies discussed in Chapter 7 will help the couple realize that dissatisfaction can be a stimulus for change rather than a stimulus for unproductive confrontation.

Summary

We are advocating relationship counseling for only a portion of cases involving spouse abuse. It is recommended only in those instances in which: (1) the couple is committed to improving the relationship; (2) the abusiveness does, in fact, have a relationship basis, and (3) the couple gains immediate control over the physical abusiveness so that the risk of physical harm is quickly diminished. The specific procedures described are appropriate for couples who have trouble controlling their anger even if their anger has not reached the point of physical abuse. Many couples in therapy experience their anger as an ever deepening wedge driving them further apart. The expressions of anger are repetitious and unproductive and only increase partners' feelings of hurt and distance from one another. The procedures to be used with these couples should help them terminate or avoid angry exchanges and then work constructively on their problems.

CONFLICTS REGARDING AFFILIATION AND INDEPENDENCE

In one of the case examples in Chapter 5, a couple was discussed in which the husband was overly dependent on his wife, and the wife was repelled by her husband's excessive affiliative behavior. This example typifies a fairly common style of relationship conflict (cf., Napier, 1978). One partner (Partner A) relies on the other (Partner B) for an inordinate proportion of his/her reinforcement. Partner B, on the other hand, seems to be reinforced by a much broader array of stimuli, a substantial proportion of which fall outside of the relationship. Consequently, A is much more dependent on relationship-derived reinforcers than is B. A seeks more contact with B, and contact of a more intensive nature than B desires. B, in contrast, seeks more contact outside of the relationship than A. This in itself can lead to relationship conflict. The potential for conflict is often exacerbated by the way each partner responds to the discrepancy. B is likely to find A's efforts for intimacy aversive, since A seeks a level of contact beyond that which is optimal for B. In response to A's demands, B may withdraw further from A, which in turn will be extremely punishing to A. A may then redouble his/her efforts to increase the frequency of intimate contact with B, which will then result in further withdrawal by B. This vicious cycle can be quite refractory to spontaneous reversal, and the most likely outcome is a gradual decrease in relationship satisfaction.

Stan and Carol were in their late twenties and had been living together for five years. He earned money as a craftsman by day, and was also a successful painter. She was in her final year of Ph.D. training in public health. Both were highly intelligent, engaging, physically attractive people. There were two precipitants to their request for couples therapy. First, Stan had recently admitted to an affair with another woman. Second, Carol, who had a very successful graduate career, was facing the prospect of applying for jobs. Her success created numerous opportunities for her in desirable locations; yet it also created the necessity for a decision concerning whether the two of them would remain together in the event that her job plans dictated relocation in a new city.

The evolving pattern in their relationship conformed precisely to the model presented above. Stan enjoyed his work and was also a musician. He had a circle of friends connected to his avocations, and had met the other woman in the context of his participation in an amateur band. Most of his social life was conducted independently of Carol. Despite Carol's involvement in graduate school, she did not seem to derive much satisfaction from it. She had no avocations, and, although she had some friends of her own associated with graduate school, these friends were not very important to her. Stan determined when the couple would spend time together and when he would engage in activities outside of the relationship. When he left home to spend time with his friends, Carol would stay at home. She seldom left him alone, except to attend classes. Stan encouraged Carol to engage in outside activities; thus, even on those few occasions when Carol did initiate independent actions, she did so at his request, and she was still acting as a relatively passive force in the relationship. Even her behavior in regard to her career was under Stan's control. She was awaiting his directive regarding where to apply for jobs.

Ron and Cheryl exhibited a strikingly similar pattern to the one described above. Both in their mid-thirties, they had been married for eight years. Their major conflict revolved around Cheryl's frequently expressed desire to socialize with her own friends without Ron. Ron objected to the frequency of her independent socializing. In his view, couples should spend their leisure time primarily together. He had few friends of his own, and thus was more dependent on the relationship for his social activity. The conflict had worsened over time, as Ron's increased protests and demands interacted with Cheryl's preference for contact outside of the relationship. The more he objected, the more attractive her other options became.

Two perspectives can help elucidate the malignant nature of this particular relationship conflict. The first is social exchange theory, which would predict relationship conflict as a direct function of the attractiveness of alternatives to the present relationship. Although the availability of attractive options outside the relationship has no *direct* effect on the attractiveness of the relationship *per se*, it certainly affects a partner's tendency to seek outcomes only through the relationship. Given the potential for positive outcomes outside of the relationship, the relationship itself will have to be that much more gratifying for the partner to choose it in lieu of these alternatives. However, we have already seen that the conflict centering around this issue renders the relationship *less* attractive, and thereby increases the tendency of partner B to prefer outside contacts. Ultimately, termination of the relationship may result. From the perspective of A, who has few opportunities for positive outcomes outside of the relationship, the standards for the relationship itself will be lower. Termination by A is therefore less likely. However, as relationship satisfaction plummets, there may reach a point where, despite these relatively low standards, the alternative of being alone will eventually be preferable to the agony of remaining with a withholding partner. Thus, either A or B may initiate separation in such a situation.

The other perspective which sheds light on this relationship conflict is one which emphasizes power and control. In virtually every way, partner B is in control of the relationship. It is B who determines when and to what degree the couple will have contact, and when and to what degree contact outside of the relationship will occur. A assumes a reactive, passive position. Since powerlessness and uncontrollability are highly undesirable for one who is so afflicted, A is unhappy. Yet power and control in no way insure satisfaction even for the one in charge. *The hypothesis that we will entertain in the paragraphs below is that a balance of power on the dimension of affiliation-independence produces the most stable, as well as the most satisfying, relationship for both participants!* It is our belief that the key to successful treatment of such relationship conflicts is to facilitate a balance of power by inducing A to assert more control in the relationship.

There are two ways to accomplish this balance of power, at least in principle. One is for the behavior of B to change in the direction of increased affiliation with the primary relationship; the other is for the behavior of A to change in the direction of increased independence from the relationship. The former alternative is unlikely to be feasible in most cases, since any behavior change in the direction of affiliation is likely to be aversive, and contrary to B's personal goals. Since increased affiliation must be produced at the cost of decreasing engagement in attractive outside activities, the outcome is likely to be unsatisfying to B. We recommend the latter alternative, that of focusing on A's behavior; if A can be influenced to become more independent and assume more control of the relationship, not only is B likely to be more satisfied, but B is also likely to alter his/her behavior toward A in such a way that A is likely to be more satisfied with the relationship.

Although any initial attempt to alter A's behavior is likely to be met with a protest from A, an appropriate explanation for the treatment strategy is likely to mitigate or assuage such concerns. The protest is likely to be generated as a result of the short-term costs of deflating the degree of intimacy in a relationship which, as far as A is concerned, is already hovering at less than the desired level. If the goal of a more intimate, satisfying relationship is clearly identified, and the behavioral suggestions are depicted as strategies to achieve this end, A is likely to be more accepting of such a treatment regimen.

This type of conflict may represent one of the rare contraindications for conjoint treatment. Treatment of the more affiliative spouse alone possesses the following advantages. First, it facilitates efforts to extricate A from B's control, since therapy is conducted at a safe distance from B's direct influence. Second, it presents the therapist with the opportunity to form a special relationship with A, and thereby provide the necessary support to ameliorate the stress of the therapeutic directives. Such an alliance would be untenable if the therapist were treating both partners regularly and conjointly. Third, the initial impact of A's behavior change on B is likely to be greater if B is not present during the sessions since the new behavior will be more surprising and the attributional source will be ambiguous. With a readily identifiable cause for the new behavior, that is, the therapist's instructions, the impact may be attenuated since B will have doubts about the permanence as well as the motivation for these changes.

On the other hand, couples usually enter therapy with a complex web of conflicts, rather than one which can be reduced to the affiliative-independence discrepancy which we have been describing. It is a mistake to focus exclusively on this issue, and conduct sessions solely with the more affiliative partner, when there are other salient issues which would be better treated in a conjoint context. Moreover, it is difficult to monitor the impact of an intervention on a partner who is not participating in the sessions. The marital therapist works partly in the dark whenever only one partner attends the sessions; the costs entailed by creating uncertainty through individual sessions should be weighed against the potential benefits. A compromise may involve a combination of two modalities where, on alternate weeks, individual sessions with the affiliative spouse are conducted.

The reversal of affiliation-independence discrepancies involves four basic steps, illustrated in the treatment strategy adopted for Ron and Cheryl:

Step One: The affiliative spouse (A) must temporarily accept the partner's (B) independent behavior without protest. The verbal protests from Ron increased the attractiveness of relationship alternatives for Cheryl, and exacerbated the internal aversiveness of the relationship itself. Therefore, Ron's remarks were actually negatively reinforcing Cheryl's avoidance behavior. Since Cheryl was seeking "distance" from the relationship, Ron's entreating and cajoling impeded Cheryl's efforts and led to a spiraling of Cheryl's attempts to escape from the relationship. When Ron followed the directive to cease his efforts to deter Cheryl, she experienced immediate relief and found the relationship more rewarding. Although she initially increased distance from Ron, the stage was set for a reversal of this process.

Step Two: The affiliative partner should greatly reduce, again temporarily, the rate at which she/he rewards his/her partner in an attempt to seduce him/her out of his flight from the relationship. Relationships that exhibit this dysfunctional pattern often include a highly undesirable pattern of the affiliative spouse using positive control in an ineffective, self-defeating way. Ron attempted to present Cheryl with an unusual number of rewards in an effort to compete with her solitary or independent activities. For example, he began to buy presents for her and when this did not curtail her independent behavior, he tried cooking gourmet meals and completing her domestic tasks for her, all to no avail. Cheryl found these alleged rewards punishing because they were viewed as attempts to impede her quest for distance. Thus, eliminating them had the paradoxical effect of increasing her satisfaction with the relationship. In addition, by reducing this noncontingent gift-giving, Ron's costs were lowered, and the relationship was more satisfying to him also. Both steps one and two decreased Ron's direct efforts to seduce Cheryl back into the relationship. The irony that is suggested by the next two steps is that the relationship will improve only when Ron can begin to direct his attention toward what will make his life more satisfying, both within and outside of the relationship.

Step Three: The affiliative spouse must pursue a more independent life by cultivating or resuming activities and interests alone and outside the relationship. The affiliative spouse is often so dependent on the partner for reinforcement that all other reinforcing activities have been greatly reduced. By directing Ron to "reaffiliate" with extrarelationship interests and activities, he gradually became less dependent on Cheryl to provide all sources of gratification. Since he was successful in this endeavor, the affirmation derived from such activities reinforced such pursuits, and reduced the pressure on Cheryl. In addition, Cheryl became more attracted to the relationship as Ron became a more self-sufficient, competent person outside of the relationship. As he moved away from her, he acquired the resources that accentuated his capacity to be reinforcing to her. Thus, by moving away from Cheryl, Ron achieved the initial treatment goal, increasing intimacy.

Ron cultivated relationships as well as activities. His new sources of interpersonal reinforcement served a powerful healing function, since his self-esteem had suffered a series of blows at the hands of his withholding spouse. Ron felt less desperate, and behaved with less desperation in his primary relationship, once his interaction with Cheryl no longer embodied a struggle for his self-affirmation. We are not advocating new sexual relationships, but simply an investment in other relationships.

One crucial element in Ron's redirection is that it occurred on his own terms, rather than in response to Cheryl's requests. Ultimately, Ron had to assume control of his own life; if he had responded to Cheryl's suggestion that he "develop outside interests," he would have been continuing the pattern of living his life as a passive reactor to Cheryl. Ideally each spouse had decision-making power regarding when independent activities would be pursued. But in the past Ron had acted independently only after he learned of Cheryl's plans to do so. Ron had to assert some control by initiating such pursuits, regardless of Cheryl's plans. He began to decide when and how to direct his activities outside the relationship. This task was facilitated by encouraging Cheryl to stop urging Ron to develop extrarelationship behaviors: When she said "I want you to be independent," Ron's options were greatly constrained, since even independent behavior became just another response to Cheryl's controlling actions.

Step Four: The affiliative spouse must state his/her desires for relationship change directly to the independent spouse. Despite the prohibition against pleading for more affiliative behavior from Cheryl, Ron did seek increased satisfaction from the periods of time when they were together. Initially, he had feared that total acceptance of Cheryl's relationship behavior was necessary to prevent her from withdrawing even further. Yet just the opposite was true. His very acceptance constantly signaled dependency, and fed into the rigid pattern of power and control. By saying, "This is what I want from you when we are together . . .," Ron began to take control of the relationship. Cheryl responded positively to such requests for change. These requests were distinguished from the prohibitive pleas for excessive contacts in that they did not signify dependency, but were simply an assertive, legitimate statement of what Ron wanted from Cheryl in order to be happier in the relationship.

Summary

This set of steps, if enacted appropriately, will often reverse a deteriorating process created by an affiliation-independence discrepancy. The effectiveness of these four steps may be limited in a relationship where the pattern has been addressed at a very late stage in the cycle; when the process has been underway for a long time, some independent spouses do not respond to A's behavior changes by becoming more attracted to the relationship. In this case, if A has successfully achieved a broader array of reinforcement opportunities outside of the relationship, he will often be happier despite the lack of change on B's part. The relationship, however, may be in greater jeopardy than it was prior to therapy. Or, the couple may continue to function as both partners become comfortable with a less enmeshed, relatively independent life-style.

This intervention strategy will not always be effective. If A's capacity to achieve reinforcement outside the relationship is limited, and efforts directed toward independence are likely to be punished, the plan becomes less viable. This intervention strategy presupposes sufficient skills on the part of A to make success in Step 3 likely. Also, to the extent that the affiliation-independence discrepancy results from factors extrinsic to the current situation, factors based more on individual differences between the spouses which exist above and beyond this particular relationship, the situation will never be entirely satisfactory to both parties. One spouse may always desire more interpersonal distance than another, or a relatively intense focus on one primary relationship.

Finally, caution is indicated lest the therapist diagnose an affiliation-independence discrepancy in situations where the apparent pattern is merely a veneer, masking a more complicated reciprocal pattern of exchange. Stan and Carol were a case in point. A thorough behavioral analysis of the historical development of their present pattern suggested that Stan's preference for reinforcers outside the relationship was triggered by Carol's self-preoccupation and subsequent withholding of benefits. Her involvement in graduate school and excessive concern with her performance therein led her to stop tracking Stan, and she became, in his words, "insensitive" to him. Her love and concern for him would surface only when he exhibited preferences outside the relationship. What had initially appeared to be a straightforward pattern of conflict over affiliation and independence turned out to be a mutual pattern of withholding, where the role of prime withholder shifted from one partner to the other. Since Carol's withdrawal had served as an antecedent for Stan's, it would have been a mistake to simply focus on increasing Carol's independence. This couple needed to learn new strategies for maintaining reciprocity, and as a result a more standard marital therapy program was indicated.

Jealousy and External Threats to the Relationship

Jealousy is a complex phenomenon. To some degree it exists in all relationships. It is often thought of as an emotional state, much like anxiety, but it actually can be defined in terms of at least three different response modalities: Jealousy can be inferred on the basis of a physiological (emotional) state, a characteristic set of cognitions, or an overt behavioral repertoire. Jealousy is usually described as a combination of anxiety and anger, apparently elicited by a stimulus to which one's partner seems to be attracted. Cognitively, jealousy takes the form of a preoccupation with losing the partner, either totally or partially. That is, the threat is either that the partner will terminate the relationship for the new external stimulus, or that there will be some reduction in benefits to the jealous partner as a result of the new stimulus. Behaviorally, jealousy is inferred from emotionally-charged outbursts which apparently constitute attempts to compel or coerce the partner into redirecting his/her attention away from the external stimulus and toward the jealous partner. They can be pure expressions of feeling ("I'm really scared; what if she leaves me?") or threats and demands ("I'm going to walk out on you forever unless you promise never to see him again").

The stimulus for jealousy is usually a third person, often but certainly not always of the same sex as the person afflicted with jealousy. However, jealousy may also occur in reaction to the partner's greater involvement in any extrarelationship activity, such as overdedication to work or the single-minded pursuit of a new hobby. The common element in these situations is that one partner's comparison level of alternatives has shifted, with that partner experiencing increased reinforcement from nonrelationship activities. For example, consider Linda's jealousy regarding David's expressed attraction to another woman, Liz. Although Linda was jealous of Liz, she was not concerned about ultimately losing David; that, she felt, was unlikely. But if David and Liz were to be sexually involved, Linda would not be with him as frequently nor would she be the sole provider of his sexual pleasures. Her jealous thoughts resulted from the anticipation of a reduced rate of reinforcement as well as doubts about her own desirability. Another husband, Rex, exhibited a very similar reaction to Judy's increasing tendency to work late at night. Here the reaction was directed toward the partner's work, rather than toward a third person. He too felt deprived of his partner's reinforcers and wondered whether her affinity for work was subsuming greater importance that her attraction to him.

Although both Rex and Linda displayed similar reactions, jealousy because of the intrusion of another person is often based upon factors that are not present in the other situation. Sexual involvement with another person may be viewed by the jealous partner as a violation of a basic tenet of the marriage. The violation may be interpreted as willful disregard of the jealous person's values and/or evidence of a discrepancy in the partners' beliefs about marriage. The jealous partner may also feel deceived if the extramarital relationship had been going on for some time without his/her knowledge. These factors can arouse a great deal of uncertainty and confusion about what is to be expected from this relationship.

Overinvolvement with one's occupation or avocation may also mean being less accessible to the partner but the explanation for this situation is usually less threatening. Working late to advance a career, earn extra money, or satisfy workaholic tendencies is not a direct reflection on the partner. Jealousy in this situation may be mediated by the same factors we described earlier in reference to affiliation-independence preferences.

Jealousy seems to contain both respondent and operant components. The emotional experience which is often labeled "jealousy" is elicited by the presence of the new stimulus along with evidence of the partner's attraction to that stimulus. The emotional response is probably cognitively mediated, since most often the situation which elicits jealousy is ambiguous and requires an interpretation on the part of the observer. The emotional reaction does not automatically produce any particular set of responses, but it does provide strong signals for some sort of unusual action. In addition to the behavioral signs of the emotional experience (crying, trembling, etc.), the behavior which follows is usually a set of operants designed to eradicate the situation producing the reaction. In an example presented in Chapter 5, the wife's pouting and sullen facial expression were reinforced by the husband's predictable suggestion that the couple leave the problematic social situation.

Considering jealousy as a respondent, a reaction elicited by a situational constellation, we do not mean to imply that the response is automatic or natural. There is no evidence that particular situations inherently provoke jealousy in individuals; rather, it makes more sense to view the reaction as one that depends on the subject's interpretation of the situation. Most prominent among the many cognitions that can mediate a jealous reaction are labels attached to the situation which make the new relationship threatening. Even in an extreme situation which would evoke a jealous reaction in most people, the role of cognitive labeling is clear. Consider, for example, a man who has just learned that his wife has taken a lover. If he were to tell himself that "All she wants from him is sex; I can understand why a new partner would be exciting after being with one person for 15 years; I'm sure that it won't last very long," the reaction would be mild. If, however, he were to say "Oh my God, she's going to leave me; she doesn't find me attractive anymore, I can't stand it," the reaction would be far more pronounced. To the extent that someone anticipates a loss of reinforcement resulting from the partner's attraction to a new person, an emotional reaction is not surprising.

Yet there is more to jealous reactions than fear of losing reinforcement from the partner. The cognitions which produce jealous reactions often involve the loss of self-esteem tied to the implications of the partner's new attraction. It is not uncommon for an individual's self-worth to be based in large part on the attention and apparent regard in which she/he is held by the partner. When another person finds us attractive, loveable, and important, we often use that positive regard to perceive ourselves as loveable, attractive, and important. When the subject is provided with evidence that his partner finds another person loveable, attractive, and important, more is at stake than simply the continuation of the relationship and the current level of reinforcement which it provides. The basis for the person's positive self-regard is being challenged. Deducible from a jealous reaction are thoughts such as "I am unattractive," "I am not worth much," or "I am nothing." Since a person's tendency to derive self-esteem from the attention and regard she/he receives from another person is not identical to his/her attraction to that other person, jealousy is not necessarily proportional to the degree of love felt by the jealous person for the partner. This is an important point, because it is commonly assumed that jealousy stems from feelings of love and caring, and is an inevitable, even a positive response to the partner's attraction for other people. This is not necessarily true. A client named Dan was, by all counts, about to terminate his marriage; he found little reinforcing value in his current partner Ava. Yet, when he learned that she had slept with another man he became extremely upset and depressed. The explanation for this apparent contradiction can be found in his dependence on Ava for his positive self-regard. This dependence continued despite the low rate of rewards which she provided him.

There is also an operant component of jealousy which is not directly elicited by a particular stimulus situation. Throwing books, violence, verbal threats, and the like are not automatic responses. Explanations for these behaviors, such as "I couldn't control myself," or "I was not responsible for my actions" are misguided and inaccurate. Spouses choose behaviors to express their jealous feelings. These behaviors can be thought of as instrumental attempts to restore the status quo ante jealousy or to reciprocate the misery experienced by the jealous person.

Treatment Considerations

When considering how to treat problems of jealousy, it may be evident from the discussion thus far that there are at least four domains on which the intervention may be concentrated. First, the situation may serve as the locus of intervention. Thus, the therapist may help the couple modify the situation so that it no longer evokes the various manifestations of jealousy. Second, the cognitions that mediate jealousy may be the main targets for therapeutic intervention. A cognitive restructuring treatment would be indicated were this the case. Third, the emotional component of the jealous reaction may be directly treated, for example, by an extinction procedure such as systematic desensitization. Fourth, the focus of intervention may be on the operant or instrumental component of jealousy, using a reinforcement procedure to try and shape alternative behavioral responses. The case example in Chapter 5 illustrates such a focus, although cognitive restructuring was also used in this situation. The treatment strategy chosen will depend in large part on the unique characteristics of each particular situation, as evaluated by a thorough assessment.

Consider the case where one partner is currently engaged in an extramarital relationship. Here the jealous reaction is clearly provoked by actual threatening events, although depending on the jealous person's interpretation of the situation the reaction will be either restrained or highly emotional. In any case, if marital therapy is indicated, we strongly believe that the extramarital relationship must be suspended, at least for the duration of therapy. This does not imply a moralistic stand on open marriage, but rather a practical position which reflects our assessment of the likelihood of successful therapy. One problem which would almost inevitably follow from the continuation of the extramarital relationship is the imbalance of power. With one partner alternating between two relationships, the two spouses are not beginning therapy on equal footing. The partner without a lover is likely to be perpetually jealous and on the defensive. More importantly, marital therapy, as we have outlined it in this book, is an intensive experience, which requires a full-time commitment from both partners. It is virtually impossible to devote the time and effort which are required for marital therapy to be successful, while concurrently maintaining a second sexual relationship. Clients simply have to decide whether or not improving their primary relationship is worth the cost of temporarily terminating the other relationship. Such termination is the only way to give the marriage a fighting chance. Marriages are hard pressed to compete with affairs, which have all the advantages usually seen in a courtship period without any of the liabilities which usually accumulate over time (e.g., habituation).

Often, couples thrown into a state of crisis because of an extramarital affair will enter therapy as the partner decides to end the affair. Entering therapy constitutes a renewed commitment to the relationship on the part of the transgressing spouse. However, this does not necessarily result in an end to the jealous reaction from the partner. In one case, a wife stated that "I don't think I can ever trust him again. He could go five years without seeing anyone else and I still couldn't be sure that it wouldn't happen again. After all, he went seven years this time." The therapist reassured her that her mistrust was not surprising, and that a continuance of those feelings was expected for a period of time. Both partners should be told that residual mistrust need not be viewed as a catastrophe, and that they should not wait for the mistrust to disappear before taking steps to improve their relationship. In the meantime, mistrust will have to be tolerated. In the case of the couple from whom the above quote was taken, the husband, in his efforts to reassure his wife that he was trustworthy once again, was committing himself to goals which would have eventually proven unworkable, such as limiting himself to friends of the same sex. This excessive reassurance sets a dangerous precedent: When a partner commits him/herself to changes which will later prove unsatisfactory to him/her, the other's mistrust will simply be perpetuated by the violation of the renewed promises.

Once decisions about terminating extramarital relationships have been reached, therapy will resemble the treatment programs already described in this book, depending on the nature of the problems. But what about instances of "irrational jealousy," where infidelity has not occurred, but nevertheless the jealous person experiences frequent jealous reactions? The example presented in Chapter 5 illustrates one often-viable approach to the problem: intervening on a behavioral level, and structuring the environment in such a way that "non-jealous" behavior will be reinforced. Jealous behavior is similar in some respects to a conditioned avoidance response; both are highly resistant to extinction because the very act of carrying out the response prevents the responder from discovering that the situation which is being avoided does not present any real danger. In the case of some jealous rituals, the subject seems to be acting as if the ritual itself prevents any actual illicit action from occurring. If she/he can be persuaded to desist from such activities in order to test the hypothesis that the partner will continue to be faithful without demonstrations of jealousy, the tendency to react strongly will often gradually dissipate. It is necessary that the partner reinforce the non-jealous behavior, as in the Chapter 5 example.

Cognitive restructuring is often the preferred treatment emphasis for people plagued by irrational jealousy. A form of rational-emotive therapy (Ellis, 1962; Goldfried & Davison, 1976) is often helpful in counteracting the self-defeating thoughts that mediate jealous emotional reactions. Common among the irrational ideas of jealous people are fantasies that they must be able to provide their partners with everything the partner needs from life. If someone views this utopian ideal as a prerequisite for positive self-regard, it is hardly surprising that he/she would be prone to misinterpret a partner's legitimate desire for alternative friendships and/or interests. When the jealous reactions seem to be more a function of the person's negative self-image rather than a response to anything in the relationship, it would be advisable to conduct the cognitive restructuring in the context of individual as opposed to conjoint therapy. Therapy, in that instance, would be directed towards the individual's gaining control of his/her obsessional jealous thoughts.

Summary

Jealousy is a common phenomenon in relationships but can become destructive to a relationship when frequent displays of jealousy disrupt positive aspects of the relationship. Jealousy can be treated like any other undesirable couple interaction. Through a thorough analysis of the jealous reaction, a decision can be made whether to direct treatment towards the stimulus situation, the mediating cognitions, the emotional reactions, or the overt jealous behavior.

SEPARATION AND DIVORCE

Throughout the book we have been discussing treatment strategies which presuppose that the current relationship will continue. Despite our preoccupation with relationship enhancement and maintenance, at times dissolution and separation are preferable treatment goals. In other instances, despite the stated goals of an improved relationship, the outcome of therapy will be separation, either because sufficient changes have failed to occur in therapy, or because one or both partners remain insufficiently satisfied even after apparent, positive changes have occurred. Not only is it erroneous to assume that preservation of the relationship is always the optimal therapeutic path, but it is foolish to automatically regard any therapeutic endeavor which ultimately produces a divorce as a failure.

Consider the case of Noel and Anna who entered therapy with the acknowledgment that their relationship had been deteriorating for the past seven years. Noel had recently acquired various somatic complaints that were related to anxiety and, he believed, were exacerbated by the marital tensions. For this reason, plus almost constant dissatisfaction with the relationship, he had begun to think about a divorce. Anna, too, was not happy with the relationship but did not see sufficient cause to break up their family. During the interpretive meeting, the couple decided that they wanted to try marital therapy and temporarily postpone making a decision about divorce. Over the next few months of marital therapy, progress was made but setbacks were frequent. On two separate occasions,

Noel came to the sessions despondent over what he saw as both partners' lack of commitment, but he still was not entirely willing to discuss divorce.

Finally, after about twelve sessions, it became evident that this couple would progress no further. The partners decided that they wished to independently sort out their reasons for staying together and for separating. In the next session, Anna stated she wanted to stay together. However, her reasons for continuing the relationship were as follows: (1) to provide a unified family for the children; (2) to maintain the smoothly running household they had achieved; and (3) to avoid disappointing their parents. Not one reason was offered that was a direct reflection upon Noel and Anna's marital relationship. Noel's reasons for remaining together were an assortment of relationship ideals that, upon further reflection, he realized were unattainable within the context of this relationship. With this evidence before them, Noel and Anna decided upon a trial separation.

Unfortunately, therapists sometimes conduct themselves as if divorce was the enemy, and maintenance of the couple's life together was the only viable path. Behavior therapists may be particularly prone to assume this posture because their empirical orientation requires that they operationalize the "success" and "failure" of therapy. This tendency for bias in our view of positive outcome is reflected in the outcome investigations discussed in Chapter 10 where success is universally defined in standardized manner across couples, and the standard of an *improved*, implicitly a continuing, marriage is universally designated as synonymous with successful therapy. To the extent that marital therapists align themselves with the perpetuation of marriages regardless of the particular interests of the individuals involved, their effectiveness is vitiated.

Beyond the mere acknowledgement that separation may be an inevitable and at times desirable outcome of marital therapy, there are virtually no well-accepted or empirically verified guidelines. When is separation indicated? Who is to render the all-or-none verdict regarding a couple's ultimate status? Given such a verdict, how is a therapist to proceed? These are exceedingly complex questions which contain ramifications for any conceptual or theoretical doctrine of the successful marriage, as well as one's tactical approach to marital therapy itself. Most importantly, these questions have ethical implications which encompass both the inevitability of the therapist's influence, and the potential for abuse of this powerful position, a position which cannot be abdicated without a cessation of contact with the couple.

There is a tendency for marital therapists to become tacit advocates of the institution of marriage. This is certainly not true of all marital therapists; moreover, clinicians vary in the stridency of their advocacy. Yet it is important to recognize the ramifications of even subtle predilections on the part of the therapist for perpetuation of their clients' marriages. Consider the twin states of confusion and ambivalence accompanying the entry of many couples into therapy. Often at least one partner is uncertain not only about whether the relationship should continue were its present state to remain unaltered, but also regarding the desirability of maintaining even a greatly improved relationship with the current partner. When such ambivalence accompanies couples' initial tentative approach behavior toward a marital therapist, it must be respected by the therapist, and caution must be exerted so that such individuals are not induced into therapy for the wrong reasons.

These wrong reasons include both guilt and the desire to please the therapist. If the therapist emphasizes the desirability of committing oneself to improving a relationship, and by implication condemns the option of separation as "giving up," an ambivalent spouse is constrained in his decision-making leverage. When the deleterious effects of divorce on children are blithely added to the guilt induction, an ambivalent spouse may experience even greater difficulty in opting for nonparticipation in therapy without extreme guilt. Similarly, when the therapist communicates a strong desire for commitment to therapy rather than separation, his/her zeal, with its inevitable reinforcement of protherapy decisions, creates the danger that a couple's ultimate decision may be influenced to an unwarranted degree by these therapist prompts.

One might argue that there is little danger in a commitment to a therapy regimen, regardless of the stimuli which prompt such commitment. The worst possible outcome is a failure to improve the relationship, in which case the couple would be in the same position that they were in just prior to entering therapy, except for the additional information that therapy was unable to significantly change the marital situation. Now the couple is better equipped to render an informed decision regarding the question of separation. Unfortunately the ramifications of unsuccessful marital therapy are not always that straightforward. If an ambivalent spouse has undergone considerable emotional discomfort as a result of a distressed relationship, one adaptive response is to reduce the frequency of costly approach behaviors toward one's spouse. These costly behaviors increase one's vulnerability to the partner's punishing responses. Marital therapy requires the renewal of such costly transactions, and thereby increased vulnerability. The failure of the therapy venture can have negative consequences for both partners. The partner who reinvests may find it more difficult the second time to reconcile him-self/herself to the futility and perhaps even danger of emitting costly relationship behaviors. Even if the reattainment of the status quo ante therapy is possible, a great deal of suffering inevitably accompanies the process of regaining this protected position. In the process of reinvest-ment, hopes are also raised in the person who is less inclined to separate. For that person, unsuccessful therapy may entail enduring a second rejection. Thus, with couples who appear to be serious candidates for divorce, the possible benefits of renewed commitment to the relationship must be weighed against the possible costs of such an endeavor to the individuals involved.

It should also be noted that a therapist can display the opposite bias and be an advocate of divorce. It is not uncommon to work with a couple in such high distress that one wonders why they are putting themselves through this misery. If the therapist feels a particular affinity for one spouse and views his/her suffering as the fault of the other person, there may be predilection to see the preferred partner rid of the other person. A bias towards divorce can also be the product of having gone through a successful divorce oneself and having learned that, in certain instances, divorce is the correct decision. Caution against a bias towards divorce is especially crucial with couples who talk about divorce more than they mean to act upon the idea. Spouses may use "divorce talk" as a meta-communication to express their dissatisfaction. By responding to these comments more seriously than the spouses themselves intend them, the therapist can inadvertently promote divorce as an inevitable outcome.

Ultimately, of course, the decision regarding separation and divorce belongs to the couple. However, this caveat is not always a particularly useful guideline in the early stages of therapy, since the feasibility of the couple reaching a decision independent of the therapist's influence is open to question. Consider the stance adopted by many spouses when they seek the services of a "relationship expert." Among other things, it is not uncommon for couples to seek advice from the expert, as a supplement for or at times even in lieu of therapy. The partners want an informed comment on their relationship and its prognosis. Thus, they are primed to be influenced by the therapist and are quite sensitive to the cues which the therapist provides concerning his/her opinions about the relationship.

To this advice-seeking posture, add the inherent influence provided by the therapy milieu and its accoutrements. One might reasonably question the feasibility of a nondirective posture regarding the issue of therapy versus separation. The dilemma for the therapist is how to best help the clients in this situation, given the extraordinary capacity for influence, and the practical impossibility of *not* influencing. This dilemma is compounded by the subjective nature of this decision, and its dependence on values which bear little relationship to any theoretical perspective. That is, the therapist will inevitably *react* to the couple, not only as a professional but also as an individual with beliefs about a proper course of action for the couple. Although these beliefs do not necessarily influence the therapist's behavior in this situation, it is a good bet that the independence of these two modalities will be safeguarded only upon a conscious effort to maintain such a schism.

Unfortunately, theoretical systems of psychotherapy are not much help in generating a professional opinion on the advisability of therapy versus separation. One appealing solution to this dilemma involves the therapist's renunciation of all personal convictions and confining them to the private sphere while focusing exclusively on facilitating the couple's choice of what, for them, is the optimal path. This appealing goal turns out to be easier to state than it is to implement, and it may reflect a naive view of the therapy relationship. To the extent that the therapist cannot *not* influence the client, implementation of this plan will be difficult indeed.

An antithetical solution to this dilemma is to explicitly and directly offer one's personal opinion to the client (Halleck, 1971), while simultaneously admitting that this opinion is a very personal one rather than a reflection of professional expertise. The appeal of this strategy lies in its honest acknowledgment of the therapist's covert yet transparent beliefs, so that at least the clients will be aware of the factors impinging on the final decision, and the influence process will not be quite as insidious.

The optimal path probably lies somewhere in between these two extreme positions. As Chapters 4 and 5 indicate, the behavioral approach devotes at least the first two weeks of couple contact to evaluation and assessment. During this time the couple remains uncommitted to therapy, and they have the opportunity to delay their final decision until they have accumulated considerable information. For ambivalent spouses vacillating between separation and marital therapy, this relatively protracted assessment period can be extremely useful and reassuring. For one thing, the evaluation process itself provides feedback about the relationship, including an emphasis on positive aspects which often have not been tracked by distressed couples for months or years. Secondly, the effort expended by spouses provides them with an indication of what commitment to therapy might mean. This often helps couples assess the behavioral costs of entering into an intensive treatment program to improve the relationship. Finally, when, in the interpretive meeting, the therapist outlines the treatment program, along with, hopefully, a realistic appraisal of the probabilities of benefit and the arduous effort required to attain these benefits, a couple can make an informed choice regarding the desirability of such a commitment.

During the period of assessment, it may become evident that divorce is a consideration but the partners themselves are very hesitant to mention it. This reluctance may be due to the fact that one partner has already decided to divorce but does not yet want to reveal this decision. It could also reflect a partner's fearful overgeneralization that his/her thoughts about divorce portend no hope for the relationship. In either case, it is helpful to acknowledge that, given the circumstances of the spouses' dissatisfaction with the relationship, thoughts of divorce are to be expected. As a matter of fact, it would be more surprising had they not considered divorce as an option. To put divorce in perspective for these spouses, it is helpful to assess where the partners stand on a continuum that ranges from "divorce as a last resort if the relationship continues to deteriorate" to "divorce as a foregone conclusion, regardless of what takes place in therapy."

Our conclusion is that it is wise to develop a conservative posture on questions concerning the decision of whether to separate or to commit onself to therapy designed to improve the relationship. The spouses should be respected as individuals, and a spouse leaning toward terminating the marriage should not be cajoled into therapy. Given our position on the pervasiveness of therapist influence, it is incumbent upon therapists not to ignore their potential for biasing couples' decisions, and to adopt a strategy which is, as much as possible, unencumbered by their personal views about the desirability of therapy or separation.

If a final decision to separate has been made, and the therapeutic task is to help one or both spouses cope effectively with the decision, there is little to be gained by treating the couple in a conjoint setting. Conjoint separation therapy simply reinforces couples' ambivalence about implementing their decision, and prolongs their inability to function independently of one another, an inevitable goal of separation counseling. The primary tasks of separation counseling usually involve helping individuals engage in the behaviors necessary to function adequately as single people, and thereby to overcome the emotional discomfort inherent in the loss of a partner. First, newly separated people are often depressed either as the consequence of the loss of reinforcement provided by the partner, the self-statements they repeatedly engage in to explain the separation to themselves, or the loss of discriminative control which the partner provided for many aspects of their behavior. Therapy often becomes a combination of strategies for correcting faulty self-statements, for reducing anxiety generated by the transition from the coupling state to the state of being alone, and for the training of specific skills designed to overcome deficits which interfere with effective functioning as single people. These skills can be either instrumental (cooking, balancing a budget, planning free time) or social (interacting with friends as a single person, meeting new people). Virtually all of these therapeutic goals are more easily and efficiently attained if spouses are treated individually.

Perhaps an exception to the principle of individual rather than conjoint treatment lies in those instances where certain unresolved divorce-related issues need to be negotiated between the couple. Although many of these questions are typically handled through attorneys representing each spouse, negotiation and problem-solving skills of the variety discussed in Chapter 7 may in some instances facilitate agreements on such critical issues as visitation, custody, division of property, future contact between spouses, and the like. One limiting factor in the potential of problem-solving with separated couples is their ability to adopt a collaborative set. In a treatment program designed to improve an ongoing relationship, the adoption of such a negotiating stance is in the interests of both partners, for reasons elaborated in Chapter 5. When each spouse is no longer trying to build a satisfying, harmonious relationship, but is instead seeking the best possible settlement for himself/herself, the rules of problem-solving are not always applicable. Accommodation, compromise, and reciprocity may not be in each spouse's best interest when negotiating a separation agreement or divorce settlement. The potential benefits of overcoming past resentments and building a new life provide the *raison d'etre* for the collaborative posture in an ongoing relationship, whereas the incentive for such a posture is often absent in spouses who have decided against continuation of their relationship. Problem-solving training in a conjoint context, as an adjunct to legal negotiations, is probably best reserved for those relatively rare amicable separations where collaboration is a viable option.

It is our view that, once the decision to terminate a relationship has been made, therapeutic strategy must deviate fundamentally from the tactics outlined in this book; therefore, a detailed exploration of therapeutic strategies designed to help people cope with separation is discontinuous with and lies well beyond the scope of our endeavor. On the subject of divorce counseling, the reader is referred to Johnson's

(1977) thoughtful book written to the recently divorced or separated person.

SUMMARY

This chapter has surveyed a potpourri of problems which couples bring to the attention of therapists. Sexual problems, child behavior problems, depression, physical abuse, discrepancies between spouses in their desire for independence, jealousy, and separation-divorce were all briefly discussed. All of these problems can be handled within a social learning or behavior exchange framework; yet each requires some unique considerations, and will, more often than not, require specific deviations from some of the more standard techniques discussed in previous chapters.

One aspect of the model presented in this book is reflected in the survey of these various areas: Behavioral marital therapy is far from a monolithic approach to marital problems. For every couple, there is a somewhat unique treatment plan, although the treatment plans are alike in their theoretical underpinnings and their procedures for analyzing the problem situation.

CHAPTER 10

Empirical Status

IN ORDER TO WRITE this book, it has been necessary to speculate well beyond available data. We have based many of our suggestions on such nonexperimental sources as clinical experience and deductive reasoning. Although a substantial number of testable hypotheses can be abstracted from our manuscript, few of them have already been tested. Although the overall efficacy of a broadly-defined behavior exchange approach to treating couples is fairly well-established, the specific, fine-grained suggestions in this book have not been isolated as effective interventions. The conflict between science and clinical demand is painfully evident in our endeavor. Science, although inexorable, is a slow, painstaking process. The alacrity with which experimentally documented facts about marital therapy are produced does not come close to keeping pace with the information required by the practicing clinician in his/her everyday practice. It would be a wonderful world if counselors and therapists could postpone their interventions until the data were in. Unfortunately, they must proceed and, as the recent divorce statistics suggest, the demand for their services is irrepressible. Thus, this book has been written, replete with our beliefs and convictions about the subtleties of clinical work with couples.

Ultimately, however, the continued development of behavioral marital therapy depends on the evolution of empirically-based technology and a thorough understanding, based on controlled experimentation, of the mechanisms by which positive changes occur. In the current chapter, we explore in detail what is *known* regarding the clinical effectiveness of a behavior exchange approach in the treatment of relationship problems. In the first section, some of the criteria for evaluating outcome research in marital therapy will be considered. Then the outcome literature is reviewed, including uncontrolled, controlled, analog, and comparative outcome studies. It will become clear that our optimism regarding behavior therapy with couples is not based simply on blind adherence to a model, but rather on an impressive array of preliminary data. Unfortunately, the review also indicates that a great deal of empirical work remains to be done, to establish the generalizability of current findings as well as to answer other crucial clinical, methodological, and conceptual questions.

As recent comprehensive reviews of the marital therapy literature have indicated (Gurman & Kniskern, 1978; Jacobson, 1978b), behavior therapy has been the only school to rigorously assess the effectiveness of its procedures. It should be clear at the outset that no other therapeutic approach has received any replicated empirical support in well-controlled outcome studies (Jacobson & Weiss, 1978). Since rigorous self-scrutiny and critical evaluation have been among the major strengths of behavior therapy from its inception, we hope that other approaches use behavior therapy as a model in at least this one respect. If marital therapy is ever to become a science rather than simply an art, all approaches, not just behavior therapy, must put themselves on the line in the empirical arena.

REVIEW OF OUTCOME RESEARCH

Methodology of Outcome Research

Literature abounds on the methodology of psychotherapy outcome research (Bergin & Strupp, 1972; Campbell & Stanley, 1963; Paul, 1969; Hersen & Barlow, 1976; Sidman, 1960), yet perhaps it will be useful to preface our review with a few remarks on the minimum requirements of such research. The *only* substantive difference between outcome research and anecdotal speculation is that the former allows for unbiased statements to be made about the effects of a given treatment. To the extent that sources of bias are eliminated in an evaluation of a therapy procedure, that evaluation approaches the standards of outcome research. A supposed outcome study which fails to eliminate potential sources of bias is a misnomer. Our task here is to consider the important sources of bias in marital therapy research, and how to eliminate them through research design.

One very important source of bias in anecdotal accounts of psychotherapy procedures is inherent in the assessment of whether or not positive changes have occurred. Subjectivity abounds in this endeavor. For one thing, goals in marital therapy are usually poorly defined, which allows much room for doubt at the conclusion of therapy. If couples enter therapy complaining of poor communication, and they are taught to express anger more directly, but in other ways their communication remains the same, has therapy been successful? If a couple has been aided in their child-rearing, but the husband's erectile difficulties have remained untouched, have they been helped? Since an almost infinite number of changes are possible in therapy, without the prospective specification of goals, any change—even if inadvertent—can be used to support the effectiveness of therapy. Secondly, unless goals have been specified, anecdotal accounts usually rely on very unsystematic methods of assessing whether or not the goals have been attained, thus allowing for biased evaluation. Bias can occur here either due to inadequacies in the *measuring process* or inherent weaknesses in the *measurement source*. The former is exemplified by global measures of change, such as a dichotomous judgment as to "improved" or "unimproved," without explicit criteria or decision rules for rendering that judgment. The latter is typified by judgments of outcome rendered by the therapist him/herself. With the therapist's inevitable investment in the outcome of his therapy, and given the impossibility of ruling out the therapist's potential bias, therapists' assessments of change occurring in their own therapy are unacceptable as primary dependent measures in *outcome research*. However, they are the most common assessment source in anecdotal accounts of psychotherapy procedures. Recent studies have confirmed our suspicions regarding therapist bias (Sloane et al., 1975): Therapist ratings of outcome do not correlate with either client self-report ratings or the ratings of objective observers, although the ratings of the latter two groups *are* highly correlated. The difference between therapist ratings and those of the other groups is that therapists overestimate their effectiveness, relative to clients and objective assessors. However, therapist ratings are unacceptable not so much because of the inevitability of bias, but because such bias cannot be ruled out.

If the therapist ratings of outcome are one source of bias present in anecdotal accounts but unacceptable in research, how about client self-reports? Clearly they are also potentially biased. Any one of a number of factors may result in clients presenting biased estimates of their degree of improvement. They may suddenly "feel better" at the conclusion of therapy as a way of justifying the effort and expense. This hello-goodbye effect, to the extent that it is responsible for such reports, is a spurious basis for success, and is unlikely to endure once therapy has terminated. However, since practicing therapists seldom follow up their patients, they do not discover the spuriousness of such apparent success stories.

The client may also simply wish to please the therapist, and thus may report improvement. These demand characteristics tend to be very difficult to rule out when relying on self-report instruments. Thus, findings can be artificially inflated, and real differences between treatments can be disguised by this demand effect.

Yet self-report measures must be utilized in outcome research, since the client is the consumer, and his satisfaction level must ultimately determine the viability of our product. Thus, the research design must take steps to minimize the bias inherent in client self-reports. Standard psychometric considerations, such as reliability and validity, are important concerns. Notice that the validity issue is inversely related to the demand problem. Demand characteristics are plausible to the extent that the self-report instrument is undisguised. When the way to answer in the "healthy" direction is obvious to the client, the potential for demand effects is greatest. Yet it is in these instances where the validity question is least problematic, since direct questions regarding the client's current functioning have obvious *face validity*. If the test attempts to assess marital satisfaction in a disguised or indirect way, demand effects are less likely, but now face validity has been lost. It must now be demonstrated that a score on a particular instrument is predictive of, or related to, some accepted measure of marital functioning. Validity and demand questions must both be adequately addressed in an outcome study. Self-report measures should be of demonstrable validity. Demand suspicions can be allayed either by the inclusion of alternative measures which are impervious to demand effects, or by controlling for such effects in the experimental design through appropriate comparison groups.

Self-report measures must also be supplemented by more objective indicators of change. Direct measures of the clients' presenting problems by objective third parties are the ideal objective outcome measures. Clients usually come into therapy with specific complaints, although they are often hidden under a veneer of abstraction. Couples have complaints about communication, affection, sex, and the like; ultimately the success of therapy will be predicated on positive changes in these areas. Although at first glance this seems like a simple solution, it becomes very difficult to obtain such direct *in vivo* measurements. Observers in the home can produce reactive behavior on the part of spouses; such measures cannot be considered objective. If the spouse becomes the assessor, no matter how quantifiable or objective the recording becomes, a reliability problem is introduced, which can be monitored only by bringing an observer back into the home, which in turn might change the behavior being monitored. Clients cannot be trusted with data collection gone unverified; there is evidence that they do not record accurately, particularly while in the distressed state (Robinson & Price, 1976).

Finally, couples can be observed in the clinic or lab, and the level of functioning can be determined by an otherwise uninvested observer. Coding systems such as the MICS (Hops et al., 1972) or Gottman's CISS attempt to eliminate the problem of bias by leaving the rating to a neutral trained observer. This can be done reliably. The unanswered question related to these instruments is, what relationship do behavioral rates tabulated in the lab have to either presenting problems or general levels of marital satisfaction? Although both the MICS and CISS have shown themselves to differentiate between distressed and nondistressed couples to a statistically significant degree (Gottman, Markman, & Notarius, 1977; Vincent, Weiss, & Birchler, 1975), recent studies have found that observer-coded data do not correlate highly with spouse-recorded data (Margolin, 1978b; Robinson & Price, 1976). The meaning of these findings is presently unclear. But it is clear that given the current tenuous state of marital assessment, as many different dimensions should be tapped as possible; one measure should never be exclusively relied on. Multidimensional assessment, including observer-coded behavior, spouse-coded behavior, and self-reports, is necessary.

The second major source of bias in anecdotal accounts of psychotherapy procedures is the attempt to attribute changes that occur during the time in which the patient was attending therapy sessions to the content of those sessions. Any one of a myriad of events or variables could be responsible for such changes. The difference between such anecdotal accounts and psychotherapy research is that the latter carries with it the possibility of attribution of causality to the treatment program itself, either by including appropriate control groups, or by proper within-subject controls. We reserve the term *internal validity* for those studies which allow for such probabilistic cause-effect statements to be made. Internal validity is a minimum criterion for outcome research; it is the characteristic which most clearly differentiates science from anecdote.

Once a treatment package has been demonstrated to be effective relative to some control baseline, two areas of extension and elaboration become the primary focus of investigators—the identification of active ingredients within the treatment, and the generalizability of the findings. The question of active ingredients probes the various explanations for why the treatment might have an effect, in addition to the factors which the theory emphasizes. Control groups can be designed which rule out competing explanations for change, such as nonspecific control groups or placebo control groups (Jacobson & Baucom, 1977). Control groups can also determine the relative contribution of various active ingredients within a treatment package.

Generalizability is a generic term for any extension of the findings from a particular study to other relevant stimulus or response dimensions. For example, do behavior changes occurring in therapy generalize to the real world? Marital therapy is obviously of little use to couples unless changes that occur in the behavior of couples while in the therapist's office transfer to the home. Similarly, questions regarding *maintenance* of treatment gains beyond the time interval in which the couple is in therapy are vitally important; such questions can only be answered through rigorous collection of follow-up data. More subtle, perhaps, but equally important, are questions relating to *external validity,* that is, the extent to which the findings from one study apply to other couples, treated by other therapists, in other therapy settings.

As the research on behavioral marital therapy is evaluated, let us keep in mind the different possible conclusions one can derive from a given set of data. First, some uncontrolled pioneering studies will be mentioned. Then controlled studies will be evaluated in some detail. Finally, analog and comparative outcome studies will be reviewed.

Uncontrolled Studies

In the early years of behavior therapy with couples, reports consisted primarily of replicated case studies. Only the most seminal of these reports will be reviewed here. Other review papers discuss these uncontrolled studies in detail (Greer & D'Zurilla, 1975; Jacobson, 1978b; Jacobson & Martin, 1976). Data reported by Stuart (1969), Weiss and Patterson (Patterson, Weiss, & Hops, 1976; Weiss, Hops, & Patterson, 1973), and Azrin, Naster, and Jones (1973) will be discussed because of their impact on the field. It should be remembered that none of these studies allows for the establishment of a casual relationship between treatment and outcome, since proper controls were not included in their experimental designs.

Stuart (1969) reported the first application of a behavior exchange model to the treatment of distressed relationships. He evaluated a quid pro quo contracting procedure with four distressed couples, each of whom presented similar complaints. The four wives all complained that their husbands participated in insufficient amounts of conversation with them. The husbands, in turn, were desirous of a greater frequency of sexual activity with their wives. QPQ contracts were formed in each case, introducing a token economy program in the home. Husbands received tokens for increasing their time spent in conversation with their wives; these tokens could be redeemed for sexual favors from their wives (e.g., three tokens for kissing, 15 tokens for sexual intercourse). To evaluate the effectiveness of these procedures, couples recorded rates of conversation and sexual activity during a pretreatment baseline, throughout treatment, and after treatment for at least six months. All four of the couples indicated substantial desirable changes in both conversation and sexual activity, changes which were maintained through the follow-up period. Greater general satisfaction was reflected in a self-report inventory administered to couples prior to, immediately following, and between six months and a year following treatment.

Stuart's study has been widely cited and has lead to a widespread misconception that behavior therapy with couples is a mechanical exchange procedure in which couples routinely exchange conversation for sex (tit for chat). From a methodological standpoint, it is not clear whether or not couples' reported changes are due to treatment *per se,* since proper controls were not utilized. Stuart's exclusive reliance on self-report data also limits the interpretability of his findings. QPQ contracting has been a widely used therapeutic strategy. However, token economies have been used rarely; in fact no other published reports include the use of tokens as part of their treatment strategy. Moreover, as we mentioned in Chapter 8, sexual activity is hardly an ideal target behavior in a contract; nor is it clinically wise to utilize it as a reinforcer for behavior change.

The most influential of the early papers were those published in the early and middle 1970's by Robert L. Weiss, Gerald R. Patterson, and their associates. The modular treatment package which they created included a number of tactics designed to increase positive marital behavior, communication and problem-solving training, and contingency contracting. Treatment was evaluated by client self-reports (e.g., Locke-Wallace MAT, Areas of Change Questionnaire), observations of behavior recorded in the home by spouses (Spouse Observation Checklist), and observations of communication in the lab, coded by trained observers using the MICS, (see Chapter 4 for a description of these assessment instruments).

The outcome data reported by Weiss, Patterson, and their associates are based on ten uncontrolled case studies. The couples were young, well-educated, and mildly distressed. Based on the MICS, as a group the couples exhibited higher rates of facilitative behavior, and lower rates of disruptive behavior after therapy than before therapy. These data were collected in laboratory-based problem-solving interactions, coded by observers who were both blind to experimental conditions and sufficiently trained to code the behavior reliably. Eight of the ten couples improved on these two observational measures. Regarding the data collected by spouses in the home, husbands and wives both reported significantly more "pleasing" behavior after therapy; only wives reported a corresponding decrease in "displeasing" behavior after therapy. Of the eight couples on whom complete data were available, six improved on these quasi-observational measures. Self-report measures also indicated significant, positive changes from pre- to posttest.

These investigators deserve credit both for presenting follow-up data (posttest measures were collected 3-6 months following therapy termination), and for their use of multiple, well-validated outcome measures. Unfortunately, the absence of control groups prevents the unequivocal attribution of changes to the treatment program. As a result, these findings were merely promising and suggestive rather than definitive.

Azrin, Naster, and Jones (1973) reported data on twelve couples who each received four weeks of treatment designed to increase positive marital behavior through procedures similar to those described in Chapter 6. Prior to this treatment, each couple received a placebo procedure for three weeks. Every night from pretreatment through termination, and then at one-month intervals following termination, couples completed a Marital Happiness Scale (MHS), which served as the only outcome measure in the study. This measure required couples to rate their degree of marital happiness on a scale of 1-10 for each of nine problem areas as well as a 10th category of general happiness. Eleven of the 12 couples reported greater "happiness" at the conclusion of therapy than at the conclusion of the placebo procedure. Couples continued to improve up to the one month follow-up, as evidenced by the fact that 88% of the spouses reported more happiness at that point than immediately after treatment termination. No consistent changes occurred during the placebo procedures for couples as a group, although some couples responded positively during this phase. At the one-year follow-up, eleven of the twelve couples remained together.

Although Azrin et al. reported impressive gains resulting from a relatively simple intervention procedure, their study remains uncontrolled despite the initial placebo phase. Their within-subject design amounts to a series of A-B manipulations, and there is no way to rule out the variety of competing interpretations of the positive changes which occurred. One wonders, in addition, whether their placebo was perceived as bona fide and credible by couples, and no data are reported which elucidate this. The behavioral treatment included numerous nonspecific tactics which might account for reported changes in and of themselves, yet were not incorporated into the placebo procedures. As an example, we quote from a prior critique of the study (Jacobson & Martin, 1976, p. 550):

> . . . although the couples initiated the completing of the MHS at the beginning of the placebo procedure, it was only during reciprocity counseling (behavior therapy) that they were instructed to exchange their forms each evening subsequent to rating their degree of happiness for that day. It is conceivable that simply exchanging their rating sheets each night significantly altered the ratings; since these ratings constituted the criterion measure of marital happiness, it would have been desirable to rule out this extraneous source of change by instructing the couples to exchange their rating sheets during the placebo treatment.

In addition to the above criticisms, Azrin et al. must be faulted for relying on a single self-report instrument as their only dependent measure. The instrument they used was not empirically derived, and appears to be devoid of psychometric properties.

Collectively, the uncontrolled studies reported here, as well as others not discussed (e.g., Carter & Thomas, 1973; Goldstein, 1971; Margolin, Christensen, & Weiss, 1975) paint a promising picture of the efficacy of a behavioral exchange approach. It remains for the controlled research discussed below to establish a cause-effect relationship between a behavioral approach and improved relationship functioning.

Controlled Studies

Jacobson's studies. Jacobson (1977a, 1977b, 1978a; in press, b) has completed three studies investigating the effectiveness of behavioral marital therapy. Two of them evaluated a treatment containing training in problem-solving and contingency contracting. The third looked at problem-solving training in comparison to a control procedure which consisted of instructions for couples to increase positive behavior.

The initial pilot study (Jacobson, 1977a) evaluated a standard eight-session treatment package by comparing it with a baseline established by a waiting list control group. Ten couples were randomly assigned to one of the two groups, and compared on the basis of observational measures ("positive" and "negative" behavior rates derived from the MICS) and a self-report measure (MAS).

In addition to the between-group comparisons, couples receiving therapy were each analyzed as separate single-subject experiments involving the collection of multiple baseline data. That is, each spouse recorded problem behaviors emitted by the partner on a daily basis, from the initial interview until the end of therapy. As therapy progressed, treatment strategies (problem-solving and contracting) were directed on one target behavior at a time. The rationale behind a multiple baseline design is that if behavior changes occur only upon a specific treatment intervention, and if other behaviors remain stable until the treatment is applied directly to them, the treatment itself must be responsible for the behavior change (cf. Hersen & Barlow, 1976). A multiple baseline design for a couple who participated in the study is depicted in Figure 1 below. The wife recorded both the time her husband spent interacting with the children, and the frequency of his engagement in household tasks. The graph provides evidence not only that positive changes were occurring, but that the treatment itself was responsible for the changes.

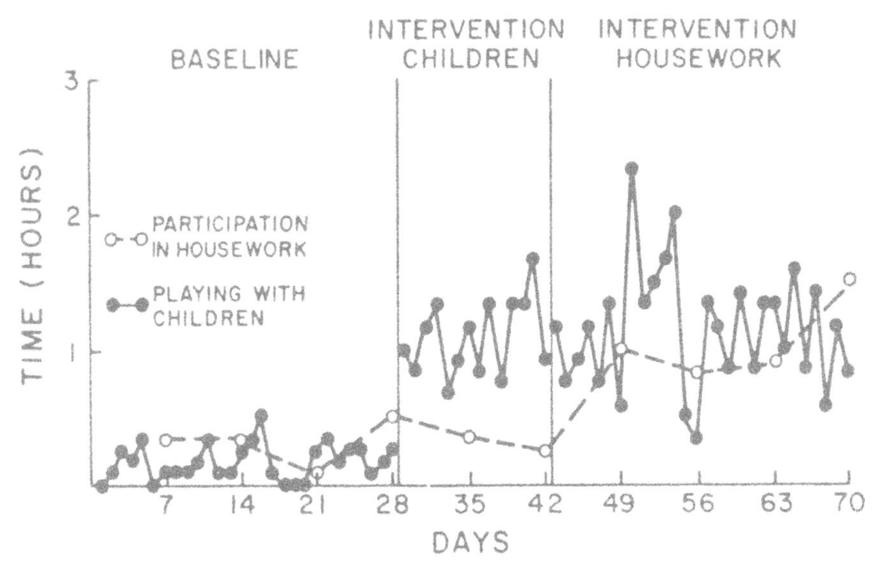

FIGURE 1. Wife's daily record of time spent by husband interacting with children and participating in housework (Couple 2).

On all between-group measures, couples in the behavioral treatment improved substantially, and the superiority of treatment to the waiting list baseline was statistically significant. Copies of the MAS were sent to all spouses who received treatment one year after the termination of therapy; the positive changes in their level of satisfaction were maintained. In all, 90% of the spouses reported scores within the normal range of marital adjustment after therapy, whereas prior to therapy only

20% reported scores within normal limits. Within-subject measures, based on data collected by spouses at home, corroborated the between-group comparison.

Since this study involved only one therapist (the principle investigator), and since the sample size was small ($N = 10$), one purpose of the second study was to replicate the findings of the first study with a larger sample ($N = 32$) and additional therapists (Jacobson, 1978a). A second purpose of the second study was to control for nonspecific or placebo factors which potentially compete with the theoretical "active ingredients" as explanations for change. A nonspecific control group was designed to hold these nonspecific factors constant, and the groups differed from the experimental treatment only in that problem-solving and contingency contracting were absent; on all other therapist variables (e.g., activity level, extent of directiveness) and procedural variables (e.g., structure of treatment sessions, use of home work assignments) the groups were identical. Manipulation checks undertaken during the study confirmed the credibility of the placebo manipulation. Finally, the study compared the relative effectiveness of good faith and QPQ contracting, by including two behavioral treatment conditions which combined problem-solving and contracting: one group formed GF contracts, and the other, QPQ contracts.

Using the same between-groups measures as did the first study, the findings of the latter were replicated: Treatment couples improved significantly relative to a no-treatment baseline. Furthermore, the behavioral conditions proved superior to the nonspecific group on these measures. However, there were no differences between QPQ and GF conditions. The discrepancies between behavioral and nonspecific groups were maintained as of a six month follow-up, based on MAS scores.

Thus, the effectiveness of problem-solving and contingency contracting was not due simply to nonspecific aspects of the treatment setting. However, on one additional self-report measure, a measure which may have been highly susceptible to demand characteristics, couples in the nonspecific condition reported improvement commensurate with that of behavioral couples. Thus, there is some evidence that couples in this condition perceived their relationships as having improved as a result of therapy. Yet the results suggest the inadequacy of nonspecifics alone; the behavior exchange technology was necessary in order to yield substantial benefits for most couples. Unfortunately, the generality of these findings was limited by a number of factors. First, the study was conducted in a university community, and the participating couples were young, only moderately distressed, and acquired through newspaper and radio advertising. Whether or not behavior therapy would be effective with a self-referred, severely distressed clinical population remained an open question. Second, the standardized, structured nature of the treatment intervention limited its applicability to the practicing clinician, who typically designs treatment strategies to fit the needs of individual clients, as we have advocated in this book.

A third study was designed to mollify both of the above criticisms (Jacobson, 1977b). Couples were treated by the investigator in an urban psychiatric hospital setting. Not only were they all experiencing severe relationship difficulties, but many of the spouses presented histories of individual difficulties, with diagnoses ranging from "schizophrenia" to "manic-depressive illness." Six couples were studied as separate single-subject experiments, using multiple baselines comprised of data collected by spouses in the home, as in the first study. The baseline against which problem-solving training was compared consisted of three to four weeks of instructions to increase desirable behavior (and decrease undesirable behavior). Here the relativity of the term *control* should be emphasized, since the condition consisted of an approximation to the procedures enumerated in Chapter 6 of this book. However, the instructions remained somewhat general, and specific behavior changes were not recommended. Depending on methodological and/or clinical considerations unique to each case, problem-solving was eventually applied systematically to one target behavior at a time.

Five of the six couples showed unequivocal evidence of improvement from the beginning to the end of treatment. For the sixth couple, improvement was reported on self-report measures and substantiated by observational measures (MICS), but because they did not consistently collect data in the home, functional relationships between treatment and outcome were not documented. Of the five couples helped by therapy, problem-solving training was demonstrably necessary and facilitative for four of them. One couple did not respond favorably to problem-solving, but did respond favorably to a more intensive focus on increasing positive behavior, using procedures similar to those discussed in Chapter 6. On the basis of follow-ups varying from six months to a year, all of the five couples had maintained their treatment gains.

Jacobson's research strongly supports the general effectiveness of behavior therapy with couples, with some suggestion that even severely distressed couples can derive considerable benefit. Furthermore, the technology seems to be therapeutic; it is not simply the generalized, nonspecific accoutrements of psychotherapy that are accounting for the positive changes. There is also some evidence that problem-solving training can be an effective treatment even without contingency contracting, as we intimated in Chapter 8. Furthermore, the equivalence of GF and QPQ contracting justifies our assertion in Chapter 8 that QPQ is the preferably contracting form, due to its relative efficiency. However, it should be noted that the equivalence of the two forms could be interpreted as support for the redundancy of contracting *per se,* since much of the variance in outcome may have been due to the problem-solving training which was common to both groups.

Lest one overgeneralize from the results of these studies, some cautions should be mentioned. First, the investigator served as at least one of the therapists in all three of the reported studies. There is pressing need for independent replication in an experimental setting with other therapists. Second, there is no definitive information to be derived from these studies regarding the relative effectiveness of various techniques within a behavioral framework. It is clear from the third study that different couples respond favorably to different types of intervention. Third, not all couples improved their relationship while undergoing behavior therapy. Furthermore, couples who do improve do not always maintain the level of improvement subsequent to termination. Unfortunately, as of now there is no empirical basis for determining whether or not couples would have responded more favorably to another treatment approach. Whether variables exist that either indicate or contraindicate the use of behavior therapy remains an empirical question. Finally, the data leave unresolved a more philosophical question, namely whether or not the couples who ended their relationship following therapy should be considered *treatment failures* (cf. Chapter 9).

Tsoi-Hoshmand's study. A multifaceted behavioral treatment package was evaluated by Tsoi-Hoshmand (1976) in comparison to a no-treatment baseline. She confined her assessment to three self-report measures which, although well-validated, leave open the possibility of demand effects accounting for group differences. She served as the therapist for all couples. The three measures consistently favored the behavioral condition over the control condition, and follow-ups of one to four months indicated improvement in 70% of the cases. These are impressive statistics, corresponding favorably to those reported by Jacobson (1977a, 1977b, 1978a) as well as the Oregon group (Patterson et al., 1976; Weiss et al., 1973). Unfortunately, couples were not randomly assigned to treatment conditions, thus leaving open the possibility that the two populations, treatment and control, differed in ways which influenced outcome independently from any treatment effects. Moreover, as one of us reported elsewhere (Jacobson, 1978b), Tsoi-Hoshmand used questionable statistical procedures to analyze her data. Thus, despite her rather impressive findings, methodological deficiencies preclude any definitive conclusions.

Turkewitz' study. O'Leary and Turkewitz (1978) report a study by Turkewitz, unpublished at the time of this writing. Her study is possibly the best-designed outcome investigation to date. Couples receiving communication training alone were compared to couples receiving communication training plus an informal contracting procedure. In the latter condition, couples were taught skills in exchanging and increasing positive behaviors without an explicit focus on written contingency contracts. Results at posttest on some self-report measures indicated that both treatment conditions improved significantly more than a waiting list control, but did not differ from one another. However, Turkewitz found a most interesting age treatment interaction: Young couples benefited more from the combined program than they did from communication training alone, whereas older couples responded more favorably to communication training alone. Although any interpretation of these findings is pure speculation, perhaps younger distressed spouses still retain a significant amount of reinforcing power vis-à-vis their partner, whereas older couples have been more affected by satiation. Since behavior exchange procedures rely heavily on the ability of each spouse to provide positive behavior as a reinforcer for the other, the still significant capacity of more recently acquainted couples to accomplish this could account for their positive response to such exchange training.

On the one self-report measure which was also included in Jacobson's studies, the MAS, Turkewitz found no significant differences among her three groups. Although trends favoring the two treatment groups relative to the control group were apparent, response to treatment was sufficiently variable to preclude statistical significance. Moreover, on a modified version of the MICS (only verbal categories), no differences were apparent between the three groups on measures of pre-post behavior change in a conflict resolution task.

The findings of this study are considerably more equivocal than Jacobson's, and are difficult to interpret due to the inconsistent results across measures. Discrepancies between findings in the two laboratories may reflect differences in client populations, differences in the sensitivity of the dependent measures, or differences in the nature of the treatment. Turkewitz derived her own version of the MICS for this study, and her codes may not be as sensitive to changes in marital distress as the somewhat different codes used by Jacobson. In addition, Turkewitz relied exclusively on a conflict resolution task requiring couples to resolve disputes regarding how a hypothetical couple should handle a particular problem. She included no assessment of the couple's ability to solve salient problems from their own relationship. This task used alone may have been less sensitive to change than the tasks in Jacobson's study.

Another plausible explanation for the discrepancies are differences in the treatment procedures. Neither of the treatment programs evaluated by Turkewitz included systematic problem-solving training of the type emphasized in Chapter 7. Her communication training procedures were eclectic, and more closely related to the methods used by Bernard Guerney Jr. than they were to the problem-solving approach emphasized in this book. We have found problem-solving training to be the most powerful and most widely applicable component of behavioral marital therapy, a contention supported by two of Jacobson's (1977b, 1978a) studies. Perhaps Turkewitz' findings would have been stronger had she included this treatment approach in either or both of her therapy conditions.

Analog Studies

Given the practical constraints which often limit our capacity to study psychotherapy in a naturalistic setting, analog studies often serve as desirable alternatives (cf. Kazdin & Wilson, 1978). Analog studies allow for the controlled investigation of specific, discrete therapy interventions in simulated settings, settings which are analogous but not identical to naturalistic settings. Analog studies can be designated as such either on the basis of their procedures or on the basis of the subject population. In the former case, discrete, usually brief interventions are studied in a highly controlled experimental setting. These investigations can produce very powerful demonstrations of the effects of certain independent variables, effects which are often difficult to isolate in naturalistic settings due to the number of extraneous factors not under the investigator's control. The "error variance" accompanying the presence of such factors often obfuscates findings, and precludes a powerful test of a particular therapy variable. However, it is often hazardous to generalize from findings obtained with analog procedures to the clinical milieu of the practicing therapist. Thus, external validity is sacrificed for internal validity.

In the case of studies which qualify as analog studies by virtue of their client populations, usually either mildly distressed or nondistressed subjects are utilized. The obvious advantage of normal subjects is their availability. Large-scale group investigations can be conducted more efficiently, since the requirement of waiting for clients to present themselves at a clinical setting is removed. However, the external validity problem again rears its ugly head. One aspect worth noting is the problem of a ceiling effect. Since nondistressed couples enter therapy with scores already within the normal range on the outcome measures, any treatment is relatively limited in the quantitative impact it can have on posttest performance. Thus, change can be difficult to demonstrate. This problem is particularly acute in comparative outcome studies, where two treatments are statistically compared. The ceiling effect decreases the likelihood of demonstrating reliable differences between treatments.

Harrell and Guerney (1976). In this investigation a group format involving both communication training and contracting was evaluated. Each group included three couples and one therapist. The groups each met for eight weekly two-hour sessions. Sixty nondistressed couples were recruited through advertising, and randomly assigned to either the treatment group or a no-treatment control group. On a series of observational change measures (including both MICS-derived measures and ratings on a conflict negotiation task), treated couples improved significantly more than did untreated couples. However, none of the self-report instruments (which included the MAS) discriminated between the two groups.

What are we to make of this behavioral vs. self-report discrepancy? Perhaps behavioral marital therapy in groups has its limitations. These results suggest that group therapy was effective in bringing about changes in couples' laboratory problem-solving behavior. However, the treatment yielded no impact on couples' overall reports of marital satisfaction, which might reflect a lack of generalization of these new behaviors to the real world. Couples receive less individual attention in a group setting, and perhaps the limited individual attention precludes the consolidation of skills necessary for their adaptation to the everyday life of the couple. This interpretation is highly speculative, and is only suggested as one of many possibilities. Another possible explanation lies in the ceiling effect which may have been created by the authors' use of nondistressed couples in their sample.

Margolin and Weiss (1978b). Margolin and Weiss assigned distressed couples to one of three analog treatment conditions: a behavioral (B) condition, a behavioral-cognitive (B-C) condition, or a nondirective (N) condition. All received feedback from an undergraduate or post B.A. therapist regarding their communication in conflict-related areas. N couples were told to focus on their spouses' reactions and feelings. The therapist modeled expressiveness and understanding, in addition to using therapy techniques such as reflection. B spouses were shown how to reinforce their partners for "helpful" communication by pressing a button which controlled the onset of a pleasant tone. Unless at least one helpful remark was acknowledged within a specified period of time, an aversive noise was presented. The B-C groups could avoid the aversive tone only by agreeing on the presence of a helpful remark on the part of one of them; agreement was defined as the simultaneous depression of the respective "helpful" buttons, while each person labelled both his and his partner's remarks. B-C couples also differed from B couples in that the therapists attempted to restructure their cognitions about the relationship; specifically, B-C couples were told to attribute their difficulties to behavioral deficits in communication rather than to defective personality traits on the part of the spouse.

Couples in all three conditions produced statistically significant reductions in negative behavior from pretest to posttest, on the basis of both observer coded behavior (MICS) and data on "displeasing" behavior recorded in the home. However, on both observer-coded positive behavior and on the MAS, B-C couples changed significantly more than did couples in the other two conditions. Finally, on self-reports of "pleasing" behavior in the home, B and B-C couples improved on an equivalent degree, and their improvement was significantly greater than that manifested in N couples.

These findings are impressive, given the distressed nature of the sample and the relatively brief two-session intervention. However, it is somewhat difficult to interpret the differences between the B and B-C conditions, because they differed not only with respect to the presence of the cognitive manipulation, but also on a number of procedural dimensions. The standard behavior therapy treatment described in this book includes the cognitive restructuring components of the B-C condition (cf. Chapter 5). Thus, the findings are consistent with our belief that the technology of behavior therapy must be augmented by the subtle clinical considerations interspersed throughout the book. One final interpretive dilemma in the study involves the finding that all three treatment conditions reduced their negative behavior substantially and to equivalent degrees. Does this mean that a reduction in destructive interaction is a more easily attained product of marital therapy? Or were these findings attributable to demand characteristics common to all three conditions?

Jacobson and Anderson (1978). This study involved a component analysis of problem-solving training to assess the contributions of behavior rehearsal and feedback to the effectiveness of the treatment package. Sixty couples were randomly assigned to one of four treatment groups or to a no-treatment control group: one treatment group received instructional training in problem-solving, without either feedback or behavior rehearsal; another group received feedback but no rehearsal; a third group received rehearsal but no feedback; and the standard condition included both feedback and behavior rehearsal. Treatment was standardized, brief (three sessions), and highly structured. Couples were treated in groups of three by one of four graduate student therapists. Outcome was assessed both by behavioral observations of the frequency of desirable problem-solving behaviors taken before and after therapy, and by behavioral ratings of overall problem-solving efficacy.

On most measures, the group receiving both feedback and rehearsal showed more improvement in problem-solving behavior than all other groups; the full treatment group was the only one to show significant improvement above and beyond the baseline provided by the no-treatment control group. Thus, in order for couples to improve their problem-solving performance, they needed both feedback and the opportunity to practice their problem-solving in the clinical situation. Despite the use of relatively nondistressed couples in a brief, standardized treatment setting, this study suggests that systematic training of the kind discussed in Chapter 7 is necessary in teaching couples to improve their problem-solving performance.

Analog comparisons between treatments. We will briefly mention some unpublished comparisons between behavior therapy and other forms of marital therapy. Unfortunately, the studies suffer from methodological limitations which obfuscate their interpretation. The ceiling effect problem mentioned at the beginning of this section affects all of these studies since analog subject populations were used.

Fisher (1973) compared group behavior therapy with an "Adlerian" group condition and an untreated control. Forty-one couples were assigned to one of these conditions. Each treatment group met for six sessions. On the basis of three out of four self-report measures, behavioral couples reported significantly greater improvement than the Adlerian couples, who improved no more than did control couples. No observational measures were used to evaluate outcome.

A similar limitation plagues Wieman's (1973) comparison of group behavior therapy and conjugal relationship enhancement (CRE). An additional problem in Wieman's study is his use of a behavioral treatment devoid of any communication training. Their intervention was limited to procedures similar to those used by Azrin et al. (1973) and reminiscent of one component in Turkewitz' complete treatment package. Groups met for eight weekly sessions. Between group comparisons found, not surprisingly, both groups to be significantly more effective than a control baseline but not significantly different from one another. Given the potential ceiling effect in this sample of couples, and the use of only self-report measures, interpretation of the results is difficult. Cotton (1976) essentially replicated these findings, and his study is subject to the same criticisms.

Thus, with the exception of the study by Turkewitz, in all of the controlled analog studies, behavior therapy was found to be effective relative to comparison control groups on observational measures. And with the exception of Harrell and Guerney's (1976) study, self-report measures tended to corroborate the observational measures. The comparisons with other treatment approaches were indeterminate, due to exclusive reliance on self-report measures (Cotton, 1976; Fisher, 1973; Wieman, 1973), the use of nondistressed populations (except for Margolin's study) and treatments which resembled clinical behavior therapy only vaguely.

A Comparative Outcome Study with a Clinical Population

Liberman, Levine, Wheeler, Sanders, and Wallace (1976) compared a group of four couples receiving behavioral marital therapy to a group receiving an "interaction-insight" approach. This latter group should probably be thought of as a placebo, since it was devised by the authors (three of whom served as therapists for both groups) who are behavioral in their orientation. The behavioral group received a comprehensive treatment package including communication training, behavior exchange skills, and contingency contracting. Outcome was assessed by a series of measures, including various well-validated self-report instruments, spouse recordings of "pleasing" behavior in the home, and observational measures derived from the MICS. There were no differences between the two groups on the self-report measures, although couples in both groups improved substantially; these improvements were sustained at a one-year follow-up. On five of the six MICS measures, there were significant differences favoring the behavioral group.

SUMMARY AND CONCLUSIONS

Some evidence has accumulated supporting the effectiveness of behavior therapy with couples. When results from controlled, analog, and comparative outcome studies are combined, seven out of nine controlled investigations unequivocally found behavior therapy to be more effective than a control baseline, an eighth study found behavior therapy effective on the basis of behavioral but not self-report measures, and a ninth found support for behavior therapy on self-report but not on behavioral measures. Four studies found behavioral treatments to be more effective than a placebo, at least on a majority of the dependent measures. These latter studies were all conducted with clinical populations (Jacobson, 1977b, 1977a; Margolin & Weiss, 1978b; Liberman et al., 1976). However, results have not been completely consistent across studies, and there is a great need for replication of our procedures (including problem-solving training) in laboratories other than our own.

The technology does not seem to tell the whole story, since in every study there was some evidence for the potency of nonspecific factors in and of themselves. In Margolin & Weiss' study, on many measures there were significant differences between two behavioral conditions that differed primarily in that one included some subtle cognitive manipulations.

Communication training seems to be an often necessary and at times sufficient treatment for many couples. Jacobson's, as well as Turkewitz' (O'Leary & Turkewitz, 1978), data suggest this. In those comparative outcome studies where behavior therapy was no more effective than another treatment, communication training was excluded from the behavioral condition (Cotton, 1976; Wieman, 1973). Ironically, the comparison treatments in these studies were communication training treatments themselves, although derived from a Rogerian theoretical perspective. There exist other controlled studies which support the effectiveness of nonbehavioral communication training (cf. Jacobson, 1978b). To quote from Jacobson (1978b), ". . . it may be that the most effective element of the behavioral approach is the one which is least unique to a behavioral approach."

The data seem to indicate that different couples respond best to different emphases within a behavioral perspective. Jacobson's (1977b) study demonstrated this, as did Turkewitz' (O'Leary & Turkewitz, 1978). There is clearly a need for more parametric research designed to uncover client characteristics which predict their response to various techniques.

Third, there is some empirical basis for doubting the general effectiveness of contingency contracting (Jacobson, 1978a, 1977b; O'Leary & Turkewitz, 1978). In addition, others have reported that contracting is perceived by both clients and therapists as mechanical (e.g., Liberman et al., 1976). An important line of research is suggested by Jacobson (1978d): process research looking at the variables which predict compliance with behavior change agreements. These correlational studies would help shed light on the contributions of contracting, since its primary value is said to reside in its ability to increase viability of change agreements negotiated in therapy.

Finally, from a clinical standpoint it is important to investigate the advantages and disadvantages of group therapy for couples. A suspicion that group therapy may be insufficient to induce generalization was voiced earlier in this chapter. It may be that couples will demonstrate substantial changes in a group treatment setting, but that these changes may be less *persistent* than in the case of couples treated individually.

Behavior Therapy Versus Other Approaches

As of now there is no empirical basis for the assertion that behavior therapy is more effective than other approaches to treating relationship problems. The comparative studies are inconclusive, and replete with methodological limitations. However, it is fair to assert that behavior therapy is the only treatment for relationship problems which is *demonstrably effective* (Jacobson, 1978b; Jacobson & Weiss, 1978). It is time for the rigor of empirical investigation to predominate over the vigor of theory espousal. The problem of conflict between intimate adults is of widespread concern to all of us, and our services are going to be in increasing demand. All approaches to marital therapy should be made accountable both to the consumers that they serve, and to the scientific community's standards of evaluation.

CHAPTER 11

Case Illustrations

THIS CHAPTER OFFERS two case examples that, in our view, depict the difference between a successful and a partially successful outcome of behavioral marital therapy. The two cases were selected to illustrate the importance of designing a treatment that gives the couple strategies to maintain treatment gains. In the first case, an innovative treatment approach contributes to substantial therapeutic improvement, but then a premature termination of the case results in posttreatment deterioration. In the second case, careful planning for the termination precludes a posttreatment relapse. The cases also illustrate how the format and timing for each treatment step described in Chapters 6 through 9 must be determined by the specific circumstances surrounding each case. Rendering a treatment that is well received and effective requires thoughtful integration of a couple's special needs into the overall treatment approach.

CASE 1

H: Now, how do you want to handle arguments?
W: I think I've handled it, I leave.
H: But how would we . . .
W: (*interrupting*) And the best way to do it is to leave permanently! (*both laugh*).
H: Do you think if we were to sit there and say, "Hey look, let's not discuss this now. Let's wait 'til you come back home, or let's go into another room and not drag the kids into it." We could have done that this morning, couldn't we. You could have, couldn't you have approached it differently?
W: I tried to tell you before the kids even woke up.

H: How did you do that?
W: I said I want to tell you about the doctor.
H: Wait a minute, but that's when it was already 7:00 and late.
W: I didn't tell you last night. How much earlier do you want me to tell you?
H: I don't know. Do you think there could be some other way we could have handled that last night, that we didn't do?
W: No.
H: You mean you want to tell it in front of the kids all the time? I don't want it in front of the kids. I don't want them entering those kinds of decision, for the simple reason I told you. I don't get anything but "lose" out of it. I really don't, because I'm the bad guy. Now if you had said "Hey look, when you get through shaving, or if you'd hurry a little bit more, perhaps we can talk this over" or "Gee, before you go down to the office maybe we can sit down and talk about Pam's (the daughter) teeth." There was no need to do it in front of the kids. There was no need to do it in the bathroom. There was no need to do it there at all. And I don't want to have those kinds of discussions in front of the kids. I don't think it's right. I don't think it's fair to them. I don't think it fair to me.
W: I suppose I come out the winner.
H: You do in this case. How do you think you come out the winner?
W: I don't know. That's what you're saying.
H: Okay, I'll tell you.

This conversation is a segment of the pretreatment negotiation discussion on the topic of "how to handle arguments" by Bill and Betty R. This brief segment characterizes several of the Rs' communication problems. The responsibility for carrying out this discussion seems to fall on Bill, who occasionally makes reasonable suggestions but detracts from these statements with his prosecuting attorney-like style. Betty, in turn, responds to the one aspect of Bill's statements that she disagrees with most strongly. Her statements, particularly the threat "And the best way to do it is to leave permanently," convey her desire for the conversation to end. However, the less that Betty responds to what Bill says, the more he takes over the conversation by giving long-winded speeches, repeating himself, and answering his own questions. Since Betty does not validate what Bill says nor contribute any of her own ideas, the conversation persists in this unproductive manner for the entire 10-minute period.

Betty and Bill, both aged 32, have been married 14 years and have two children, a 12-year-old daughter, Pam, and a nine-year-old son, Freddie. Bill is employed as an electronics engineer for a large firm; Betty is a vocational nurse. The Rs entered marital therapy under somewhat disadvantageous circumstances. Their request for counseling was not self-motivated but was the result of pressure they faced from another therapist who was working with Pam. This therapist had made repeated observations that Pam's problems intensified when the parents were embroiled in a particularly bitter marital battle. He thus insisted that marital therapy was a necessary augmentation to his work with Pam. This recommendation was not well received by the Rs in light of their previous experience with couples counseling, which led to intense arguments and ended in a three-month separation for Bill and Betty. Yet, their concern that they might jeopardize the daughter's therapeutic progress was stronger than their desire to avoid marital therapy.

During the first meeting with this couple, it became evident that the Rs were extremely unhappy with their relationship but that they had adopted a stance of minimal resistance. Their verbalized agreement, which was to separate once the children were on their own, functioned to put their relationship into a state of limbo. The threat of separation lost much of its impact since it was at least ten years in the future. However, they saw no point in taking risks to improve their relationship in the meantime if separation were to be the inevitable outcome.

Confronted with the Rs' lack of motivation to change the relationship as well as their lack of enthusiasm for marital therapy, the therapist focused the first meeting on whether or not there was a reason for the Rs to pursue marital therapy. It appeared that this couple's motivation for coming was simply passive compliance to the request of the daughter's therapist. But, from the marital therapist's point of view, this was not an adequate basis on which to begin working with this couple. Thus, the marital therapist's first objective was to ascertain what the Rs themselves felt they could gain from marital counseling. Not taking issue with the notion that, in fact, the Rs would separate in ten years, the therapist inquired what they could do to make these ten years more tolerable. Bill immediately listed some activities, such as playing tennis, that he would like to share with Betty, but he then explained why those activities would never happen. Betty had more difficulty expressing any changes she would like from Bill. Implicit in her message was a reluctance to risk asking for anything. However, in response to the direct question of whether anything could make the relationship better for her, Betty finally conjectured a terse "I suppose."

At no time did the therapist attempt to convince this couple that they belonged in marital therapy. In fact, she agreed with them that it was not at all evident that marital therapy would be beneficial. The therapist did offer to conduct an initial evaluation to explore this question further but stipulated that she would enter a therapeutic relationship with the couple only if there were evidence that it might be of benefit to them. The burden of proof of whether marital therapy could be worthwhile was thus shifted to the couple. With little discussion, both spouses agreed to accept the therapist's offer for the initial evaluation.

The following types of concerns were expressed during the evaluation process. Betty complained about Bill's attitude of being "always right," his quick temper, his inadequate demonstrations of affection and sympathy, and his messiness around the house. She felt that most of their arguments stemmed from his reluctance to grant her any decision-making power. Bill's strengths, from her point of view, included that he held down a job and took her out to dinner every Saturday evening. Bill's complaints included that they did not have sex often enough, and when they did, Betty did not have a "joyous attitude" about making love. He also found her to be a messy housekeeper and critical of his efforts around the house. In Bill's enumeration of Betty's positive attributes, he praised her skills as a mother and financial manager, and described her as "kind, friendly, intelligent, and capable."

The overall pretreatment assessment picture provided by this couple was one of high distress as indicated by Locke-Wallace Marital Adjustment scores of 51 for Bill and 69 for Betty, but relatively high stability. Threats of divorce were frequent but the spouses' separate reports on the Marital Status Inventory indicated that neither spouse had taken any action whatsoever towards divorce. However, the Rs' strategy for survival in their adverse situation was to arrange their lives so that they had minimal contact with one another. Bill worked from 8:00 in the morning to 4:30 in the afternoon. Betty left for work at 4:00 p.m. and did not return until midnight. Thus, aside from occasional glimpses of one another early in the morning or late at night, these spouses saw one another only on weekends. Even with these schedules, the Rs were able to keep their household running quite smoothly through a carefully planned division of labor. While Betty was at home during the day, she did most of the household chores and errands. Bill cooked dinner for the children and himself and also took responsibility for the grocery shopping.

Data from the Rs' precounseling Spouse Observation Checklists revealed that the majority of the Rs' pleasing exchange was in the areas of household management and childcare, and they verbally expressed satisfaction in these areas. However, their overall exchange of pleasing activities was scanty, with a mean rate of 15.6 pleases per day for Betty and 10.3 pleases per day for Bill. As expected, there was minimal exchange in the areas of affection, companionship, communication, and coupling activities. In addition to a low rate of pleasing behavior, the Please: Displease ratios of 5:3 for Betty and 2:1 for Bill suggested a disproportionate number of displeasing behaviors.

INTERVENTION

Treatment was unavoidably limited to a 10-week duration due to the fact that the therapist was leaving town. The following four objectives were proposed for the 10-week period: (A) Restructuring daily interactions to be more positive; (B) Developing ways to express support and understanding to one another; (C) Writing behavior exchange contracts, and (D) Reeducation about how relationships work. Table 1 illustrates how the multiple facets of this treatment program fit together. Each therapeutic procedure included in a particular treatment session is coded A-D to identify it with one of the four objectives listed above. Homework assignments are also indicated to clarify their relationship with the in-session activities.

Restructuring Daily Interactions

The most notable feature of the Rs' relationship was that they had very little time together. Five weekdays would elapse with two daily phone calls being their only verbal contact. Bill characterized the calls in the following manner: "We may talk about making sure that Freddie takes his bath. They (the calls) lack any personal touching . . . It sounds terrible but usually I call up to see if there are some last minute instructions." These business-like telephone calls were certainly insufficient as the couple's sole means of interaction. Since one or the other spouse was always at work, the couple lacked a time for expressing anything intimate or for a leisurely sharing of the day's activities. Bill and Betty were thereby forced to function quite independently, which had several drawbacks for their relationship. In addition to not knowing much about each other's separate life, they simply were not available to one another for support on a daily basis. Furthermore, decisions that needed immediate attention and were simply made by the one partner who was available often proved unacceptable to the partner who was not consulted. This unilateral decision-making frequently occurred in regard to the children and put a great deal of stress on the Rs' parenting relationship.

TABLE 1

Summary of Treatment Procedures for Each Session

Session Number	Activities in Session	Activities at Home
I.	A. Introduction to writing notes; Discussion on increasing companionship activities	A. Notes; Bike ride D. Reading *Families*
II.	A. Improving the quality of the notes; Formulation of 3 requests D. Introduction to reinforcement theory	A. Notes; Carrying out 3 requests
III.	A. Examination of please/displease graphs D. Discussion on shaping and reinforcement; Development of a reinforcement menu	A. Notes; increasing output of pleases to partner. Specifying important pleases
IV.	B. Introduction to paraphrase/reflection skills D. Discussion on how to help partner make desirable changes	A. Notes B. 5-minute audiotaped discussions practicing paraphrase/reflection skills
V.	A. Introduction to "love evenings" B. Communication exercise D. Reattribution of dissatisfaction to scheduling problems rather than spouse	A. "Love evenings" B. 10-minute audiotaped discussions practicing the communication exercise
VI.	D. Demonstration of ways to handle relationship deterioration	A. "Love evenings" B. 10-minute audiotaped discussions
VII.	B. Listening to communication homework C. Identification of problem areas for behavioral exchanges	A. "Love evenings"
VIII.	C. Writing of affection-childrearing contract	C. Carrying out contract
IX.	C. Writing of sex-communication contract	C. Carrying out second contract: Revise and continue first contract
X.	B. Review communication skills C. Review contracts D. Discussion of how to maintain treatment gains	

The therapist decided to introduce a means by which the Rs could communicate more completely and meaningfully within the constraints imposed by their work schedules. The first therapeutic step towards this goal was for Bill and Betty to leave notes for one another. These notes were to become a vehicle whereby the Rs could increase their informational exchange as well as demonstrate caring and interest in one another. While the writing of notes is a relatively typical solution to the problem of limited interaction, it was new for this couple and was not associated with previous failure experiences. Note writing was also chosen by the therapist for its stimulus control properties. Since written notes evoke no immediate response, they convey information without the possibility of a rapidly escalating argument. Furthermore, it was assumed that the forethought required by written communication might improve the overall quality of the communication. However, to guard against these notes being used as another way to punish the partner, the therapist specifically instructed the Rs that their notes were to contain at least one positive statement. The fact that the therapist had access to these communications increased the likelihood of compliance with that particular instruction. Finally, the tangible nature of these communications eliminated uncertainty as to whether or not the communication occurred as well as selective remembering about the content of the message. Overall it appeared that having these partners leave notes for one another could potentially serve as a preliminary, albeit controlled, step towards modification of the Rs' general communication.

The Rs initially balked at the notion of leaving notes for one another. Bill's earlier eagerness for change in the relationship seemed less compelling as he claimed that he "did not have time for writing notes." Betty, it seemed, heard this recommendation as an assignment to write love poems for one another. Fortunately, both partners' objections quickly dissipated when the therapist clarified the assignment and firmly emphasized its importance. To verify that the instructions would not be misinterpreted by this couple, the therapist asked the partners to write and exchange one note right there in the session. In addition, before closing that session, the Rs had chosen a place to leave the notes and a time by which the notes were to be written. Each partner would receive a note upon returning from work; weekend notes would be written by 5:00 in the afternoon. While this specificity might have lessened the excitement for some couples, it was necessary that Bill and Betty be entirely clear about what they might expect from one another. Otherwise, one partner's personalized interpretation of the assignment might prove disappointing rather than pleasing for the other.

The examples below have been taken from the Rs' first week of leaving notes for one another.

Betty	*Bill*
I had fun at the Girl Scout meeting this a.m. Pam received a notice that she's been accepted at camp this summer. I think it will be fun for her.	Betty— Sorry you had such a lousy day at work. Wake me up and we will have a glass of wine together. Bill
I wasted $20 today on my hair. Hope you had a fun day skiing.	Betty— I'm interested in all of you, not just your hair. Wake me up and I'll show you what I mean. Love, Bill
I enjoyed the lunch only next time I hope you pop for it. You'd better practice "Moon River" or Pam will play it better than you.	Betty— I love you! Bill

The messages illustrated in these notes characterized Betty's and Bill's vastly different communication styles. Bill's notes were personal and affectionate but lacked information. Betty's response to these messages was one of frustration. While it was nice to receive an invitation that read "Wake me up and we'll have wine together," Bill was unreceptive when the situation actually presented itself. Furthermore, a note that read "I love you" was difficult for Betty to accept since it was incongruent with her perceptions of Bill's behavior.

Betty's notes, in contrast, were more newsy but contained some obvious barbs. She consistently undermined her one positive statement with a derogatory remark. Her notes were also quite impersonal, lacking even a salutation or closing. Betty explained the negative tone of her notes as her way of expressing the pain she experienced from this relationship. Since, in her view, Bill did not appear to experience the same degree of suffering as she did, Betty sometimes intensified her criticism simply to evoke a reaction from him.

After discussing the inherent dangers in their strategies during the first week of notes, the partners specified for one another what would make the notes more enjoyable to receive. Bill requested more personalization of Betty's notes while she wanted more information and fewer sexual innuendos. Notes from the second week were of vastly improved quality.

Betty

Dear Bill,
I hope all of you have fun at the dinner and show tonight. Wish I were going with you.
Love,
Betty

Dear Bill,
Although I had a terribly busy day I thought of you often.
Hope you do well at the Spanish class tonight.
Loads of love,
Betty

P.S. Please try to remember to leave Freddie some money under his pillow from the tooth fairy.

Bill

Dear Betty,
It was a nice day. Thank you for being patient with me.
Love ya,
B.
P.S. The cartoon was funny.

Betty,
Music teacher said Pam was doing well. Hope your work wasn't too hard tonight as I know you had a busy day and you're tired. Sweet dreams,
Bill

Notes from later weeks were better yet, with spouses using their note writing as a way to reinforce and to provide constructive suggestions for one another.

Betty

Dear Bill,
I sure hope your garden is successful. Are you sure you don't need more coffee grounds? I enjoyed the barbecue steaks for dinner.
Love, Betty

Dear Bill,
I had to fight tooth and nail to get Freddie into the barber. Please compliment him. Good luck cheering Pam up.
Love, Betty

Bill

Dear Betty,
I think your work on the children's project is above and beyond the call of being a mother. Both jobs are really good. I enjoyed last night, and our lunch time together today. And I think of you often and love you very much.
Love, Bill

Dear Betty,
I hope the roads didn't get wet to give you trouble on the way home. I worry about you when the weather gets bad.
Love, Bill

These notes typically were the first contact that the partners would have after a separation of several hours and thus had a strong impact on their moods when they finally got together. Over time, the notes even took on reinforcing properties of their own. This was most clearly demonstrated by the disappointment that each partner expressed when there was no note on a particular day. When writing notes was finally dropped in week seven as a specific assignment, Bill expressed his desire to sustain this procedure on their own.

While the notes were designed to introduce some positive interaction into the periods of time that Bill and Betty were separated, the quality of their shared time also needed improvement. Concurrently with working on the notes, the Rs were also employing many of the strategies described in Chapter 6 to explore whether they could derive more enjoyment from being together. During baseline, their shared activities consisted of going out for dinner on Saturday evening. While both looked forward to those evenings, Betty complained that Bill always chose the restaurant.

To begin the task of expanding their repertoires of pleasing activities, Bill and Betty formulated individual lists of desired companionship activities. Then, choosing from the mutually agreed upon activities, the Rs decided for that first week to go on a 20-minute bicycle ride. Their only point of dissension was whether to go alone or with the children, a question which frequently came up over the next few weeks.

At the end of the second session, each partner was asked to write down three requests from the partner that would be pleasing to receive but that required no planning and elicited no animosity. After these were written, reviewed by the therapist, and modified according to the therapist's suggestions, the spouses put each request in a separate envelope and wrote on the envelope what day of the week the request was to be completed. For the most part these requests signified tasks that were relatively easy to accomplish such as "taking the newspapers out of the bedroom" or "helping Freddie with his homework." However one of Bill's requests was for an afternoon picnic on Saturday, which happened to be an unseasonably dreary and cold day. Much to the therapist's surprise, Betty went ahead and made preparations so that the whole family could picnic on a red checkered tablecloth in the middle of their living room floor.

The third step in the intervention to improve the quality of the Rs' shared time was having both partners work to expand their total output of pleasing activities as recorded on the Spouse Observation Checklist. Graphs of each partner's pleases revealed that spouses exchanged approximately 12 pleases per day across the first two weeks of treatment. Strategies to increase their levels of pleasing events and ways to reinforce one another for engaging in new behaviors were discussed.

The final stage of this intervention was "love evenings," in which one partner was designated to be especially considerate and caring to the other. During the first week that love evenings were assigned, they proved disastrous instead of pleasurable. In Bill's enthusiasm to give the first love evening to Betty, he began his efforts early in the day. However, when he received no acknowledgment from Betty, he no longer felt like continuing his special efforts during the evening, which was the designated time Betty expected him to be particularly considerate. Betty was unaware of Bill's efforts during the day but did sense his negative reaction during the time she had been awaiting as her love evening. Thus, she too was disappointed and was unwilling to offer a love evening to Bill on the following night. The conflict surrounding this miscommunication continued until the time of their therapy session three days later.

After some discussion about how they might avoid conflicts like that in the future, the Rs agreed to try another love evening and decided to limit their efforts to the designated evening hours. In spite of this inauspicious beginning, Betty reported at the end of therapy that the love evenings were the one aspect of treatment she truly enjoyed.

Listening with Support and Understanding

While the notes were designed to increase the informational exchange between Bill and Betty, therapy was also designed to foster more facilitative verbal interactions. Listening skills, such as paraphrasing and reflection, were taught first to slow down the Rs' verbal exchanges and to guarantee that each partner actually heard what the other was saying. Previous to any intervention in this regard, these spouses created havoc in their discussions by responding to misunderstood statements or to statements made in the context of another discussion. The rapid escalation of conflict that ensued when Bill and Betty were not hearing one another caused many discussions to be terminated prematurely and without any sense of closure. The couple thus learned through repeated incidents such as this to avoid all but the most neutral or inescapable discussions.

The therapist initially introduced listening skills in a didactic manner and illustrated their impact upon a discussion by giving examples of good and bad paraphrases. The spouses then rehearsed paraphrasing one another's statements, offering nothing other than a paraphrase even if they violently disagreed with the original statement. For their first homework assignment in this area, the Rs were to engage in five-minute audiotaped discussions in which one partner was the listener and the other was the speaker. The speaker introduced a topic she/he wished to discuss and the listener demonstrated, through paraphrasing or reflection statements, an understanding and acceptance of what the speaker was saying. The listener also was to avoid taking control of the discussion.

After their initial practice with paraphrasing and reflection, the Rs were introduced to a communication exercise suggested by Flowers (1975) that contained procedures to facilitate dyadic exchanges. Flowers' exercise trains partners to focus attention on the process of communication so that they become astute observers of their own and their partners' communications. In a slight modification of Flowers' original exercise, these partners used flash cards to slow down the communication and to give one another feedback on their process observations. Immediately after making a statement, the speaker evaluated that statement as either clear, fairly clear, or unclear. Then the listener also evaluated that statement, using the same three discriminations. A statement that either partner rated as only a "fairly clear" or "unclear" was to be restated so that an entire conversation did not develop on the basis of one misunderstood statement. The second step was for the listener, or receiver of the "clear" statement to state whether she/he agreed or disagreed with the statement, thereby introducing a way to give straightforward feedback. After the original statement had been responded to in this manner, listener and speaker roles would switch and the same procedures were applied to the new speaker's statement. Flowers' original model also trained partners to notice and indicate several common communication faults. The listener was to cue the speaker when his/her statements were too long, off the subject, threatening, or posed as a rhetorical question. The speaker was to indicate when he/she has been interrupted or he/she wanted the listener to repeat the original statement. The Rs practiced these procedures in the session and at home.

Behavior Exchange Contracts

From several of the Rs' homework tapes, it became apparent that they had great difficulty identifying and expressing what they wanted from one another. Requests made in the past had not been met and each partner was convinced that the other was unresponsive to his/her wishes. What they did not realize was that their lack of success in getting change was as much a function of the manner in which the request was made as of the partner's stubbornness.

As homework to follow the seventh session, the therapist asked the partners to identify three types of changes that would contribute to their marital satisfaction. In the eighth session, each partner identified which change would be easiest for the partner to make. Betty indicated that she wanted Bill to demonstrate more appreciation and enjoyment of the children. This request, which had seemed quite overwhelming to Bill in the past, was now reduced to his employing, with the children, the same types of listening skills he had been practicing with Betty. For his part, Bill wanted more affection from Betty. Although he had an array of ideas about how Betty might demonstrate more affection, he settled for a good morning greeting and kiss for this first exchange. A contract was written to make the conditions of these changes absolutely clear. Although this was a simple behavioral exchange, rather than a problem-solving agreement, the format of a good faith contingency contract was used. The therapist had described various types of contractual agreements and the couple chose the parallel format based on their desire to include individualized rewards and penalties to help them carry out the requested changes. In light of the clients' preferences, the therapist went along with this format even though contingency contracts are usually reserved for the more difficult problem-solving agreements. The complete contract, which follows, was carried out in its entirety by both partners.

Betty	*Bill*
Problem Area: Affection	*Problem Area*: Childrearing
Specific Behavior: Betty will greet Bill each morning with a kiss and a pleasant message (e.g., I hope you have a nice day).	*Specific Behavior*: On each week day and Saturday, Bill will ask one child how the day went and follow up with one further question or reflection. At Sunday morning breakfast, Bill will initiate a 5-minute conversation and demonstrate interest through questions and paraphrasing.
Reward: If Betty completes this behavior 6 out of 7 days, Bill provides a 15-minute back massage with lotion of Betty's choice.	*Reward*: If Bill completes the behavior 6 out of 7 days, Betty treats him to lunch at a place of Bill's choice.
Penalty: ½ hour of cleaning under kitchen sink.	*Penalty*: ½ hour work on cleaning windows.

For their second contract, Betty requested more communication and Bill requested that Betty initiate sex. It was interesting that Betty's request, when further specified, took the form of continuing to engage in conversations similar to what had been assigned as homework during the earlier communication training. Operationalizing Bill's request was more difficult since he fervently believed that Betty's "bad attitude" about sex was the cause of their sexual problems. He maintained that if Betty simply changed her sexual attitude the behavioral changes would follow. The therapist helped Bill to see that his impression of Betty's attitude towards sex was, in fact, constructed on the basis of her behavioral performance. Furthermore, his insistence that Betty had a "bad attitude" only defeated his objective of improving sex relations between them. Bill finally specified what he would like from Betty but then implied that she would be unwilling to carry out the request. Much to Bill's surprise, Betty agreed unhesitantly to the request when asked directly. Once again, both partners fulfilled their respective parts of the contractual agreement which appears below.

Betty	*Bill*
Problem Area: Sex	*Problem Area*: Communication
Specific Behavior: Betty initiates sex by expressing her interest in sex early in the day. Then Betty sets the scene for intimacy with candles, a special negligee, perfume, etc.	*Specific Behavior*: Bill initiates two conversations (approx. 10 min. long) during which he reflects, asks for Betty's opinion and gives feedback (e.g., that's a good idea). If the children interrupt, Betty says "We're busy, we'll be with you in a few minutes," and Bill supports Betty with a similar statement.
Reward: 1 hour of "queen" time during which she lounges in the sun.	*Reward*: Purchase a tool (approximately $10)

Their third contract was written in response to the fact that Betty had been asked and agreed to work overtime for the upcoming week. The Rs wrote a contract to assure that they would have some enjoyable time together although they would be even more pressured than usual during the rest of the week. That contract which reads as follows was written as a joint behavioral change without any contingencies.

> Betty and Bill will be together during a four-hour period Sunday. By Thursday Bill will think of three or more alternatives of how they might spend the time together. Betty will choose the alternative that she most prefers of the three. Bill will then arrange for

that evening (e.g., pick up tickets). Betty will take a nap on Sunday prior to the event.

This contract circumvented all the factors that could impede the Rs' actually carrying out their desire to do something fun together. Betty did not want to be responsible for making arrangements although that was typically her role. She also was not at all concerned what the specific activity would be. Bill's worry was that Betty would be exhausted when it was finally time for them to be together.

The behavior exchange contracts offered the Rs a way to request desired behaviors and a vehicle for actually implementing those changes. One benefit for the Rs in learning to write behavior exchange contracts was the realization that the changes requested by each partner were actually quite manageable. Both partners were quite willing to carry out the requested changes once the request had been stated clearly and then formalized into a written contract. Previous informal or vague agreements did not offer this couple the same assurance that a request would be met.

Reeducation

Although the previous sections indicate that the Rs did make changes towards the desired treatment goals, their experience in therapy was by no means a steady uphill trend towards improvement. Weeks four and six marked particularly critical points during their 10-week course of therapy. The difficulties they encountered at these times appeared related to their unrealistic expectations and their faulty ideas about relationship change. Three specific patterns that characterized the Rs' interaction and impeded their progress were: (1) their use of criticism rather than encouragement; (2) their tendency to retreat from one another when the relationship began to slide; and (3) their belief that they could best live together if they had minimal contact with each other. Almost every session during the third through the eighth weeks included some aspects of relationship reeducation to work on these dysfunctional patterns and premises.

Repercussions for Betty's and Bill's use of criticism rather than appreciation were evidenced by the third session. In the week prior to that session, their notes had shown drastic improvements and their three written requests had been met. Both partners arrived for the session in good moods and reported their satisfaction to the therapist. With uncharacteristic enthusiasm and authenticity, Betty claimed, "Bill was fantastic!" Unfortunately, however, neither spouse had expressed that satisfaction to the partner during the previous week. Thus, in this session, both partners raised questions as to whether they had actually fulfilled the others' requests. Since both partners felt that their positive actions had gone unappreciated or, worse yet, unnoticed, the therapist discussed each partner's responsibility in encouraging the other to emit desirable behaviors by acknowledging the behaviors when they occurred.

The discussion about acknowledging one another's efforts proved insufficient since Betty and Bill arrived for the fourth session intensely distraught and angry. Two days before that session they had ceased leaving notes for one another. During the night previous to the session, Bill woke up when Betty came home from work at 2:00 A.M. and they spent an hour accusing one another of being responsible for what was going wrong in their relationship. In the session, the therapist chose to focus on each partner's feelings of being unappreciated rather than letting each partner recount how she/he had been wronged. The latter exchange had already taken place during the spouses' argument at home. Plus, the spouses' feelings of being unappreciated were quite understandable. It seemed that Bill had put forth special efforts to please Betty and she did not adequately acknowledge them. In fact, in the session, Betty had completely undermined Bill's surprise of laundering the entire family's dirty clothes. Likewise Betty had continued to write notes, except for two days, and to do some pleasing activities. Since these efforts did not meet all of Bill's expectations, he had overlooked what Betty had actually done.

In addition to the lack of appreciation, a further problem faced by the Rs was the manner in which they responded once there was a lapse in the expected interaction. Rather than acknowledging when Betty had forgotten to leave a note, Bill treated this as an unmentionable topic. His intention in not mentioning Betty's omission was apparently to avoid irritating her, Yet, he expressed his disappointment indirectly by refraining from writing a note himself. Then, over the next two days, both partners justified their actions by claiming that the other had ceased making any efforts. The therapist tried to elicit from the Rs nonblaming ways to approach the partner immediately when these incidents occurred but found that Bill and Betty were at a loss for ideas in this regard. Thus, the therapist illustrated several strategies for handling this situation, one of which was simply stating, "I have really been enjoying your notes, so I felt disappointed when I came home today and found no note."

The therapist also responded to the despair that surfaced in the fourth session by suggesting that the spouses' daily schedules were contributing to their distress. The fact that the only time they had to discuss their relationship was 2:00 in the morning was indicative of their untenable situation. To attempt such a discussion at that time of the night predicted to a low probability of success even for the best of relationships. The belief maintained by the Rs that their relationship could survive only if they did not see each other was addressed more fully in the fifth session. By this time, enough SOC data had been collected to look at the correspondence between marital satisfaction and time that the spouses spent together. Based upon graphs of SOC pleases, displeases, time together and satisfaction ratings, it was evident that the couple's highest satisfaction ratings occurred on days when they spent a good deal of time together. One Thursday when Bill stayed home from work, both partners reported having a very enjoyable day together. Furthermore, Sunday, which typically was the only day these spouses had together, was often the best day of the week.

Until this time, the therapist had generally sided with the couple in their pessimistic view of the relationship to avoid provoking counterarguments about why the relationship was doomed to failure. Now, armed with data, the therapist felt there was reason for cautious optimism regarding the Rs' potential for relationship improvement. This information made the therapist's assignments, which generally increased contact between spouses, more reasonable. Furthermore, the therapist could offer a rationale for relationship problems. It was their schedules, rather than bad intentions on the part of each partner, that contributed to the stress they experienced in their relationship.

Termination

In the therapist's estimation, it was unfortunate that therapy was limited to the ten-week period. The most conspicuous omission in the therapeutic course was training in problem-solving skills, as described in Chapter 7. While it is possible that problem-solving could have been addressed before therapy ended, the other aspects of therapy seemed equally important to make inroads into the Rs' longstanding destructive patterns. The Rs were offered a referral for further therapy but declined. At that point they were feeling considerably better about the relationship and wanted a rest from therapy. Bill, however, did verbalize his concern that the changes would not maintain. The therapist asked Bill and Betty to spend some time in that final session discussing what aspects of therapy they wanted to continue on their own to guard against that problem. While most couples are eager to relinquish the contingency mode of behavioral exchange contracts for a less structured format, the Rs seemed comfortable with the structure it provided. They also discussed writing notes which they decided were occasionally necessary, and love evenings, which they felt they were now doing on their own.

Outcome at Post-Treatment

After terminating the ten-week treatment, Bill and Betty repeated the battery of assessment procedures. Results of the measurements at pretreatment and posttreatment are found in Table 2; daily fluctuations in Spouse Observation Checklist (SOC) data are presented in Figure 1.

Looking first at the graph in Figure 1, one can see a change in the patterns of pleases and displeases towards the middle of treatment. During the first half of treatment, the daily frequency of pleases fluctuated dramatically from day to day while displeases showed several distinct peaks, particularly for Betty. After the midpoint of therapy, displeases

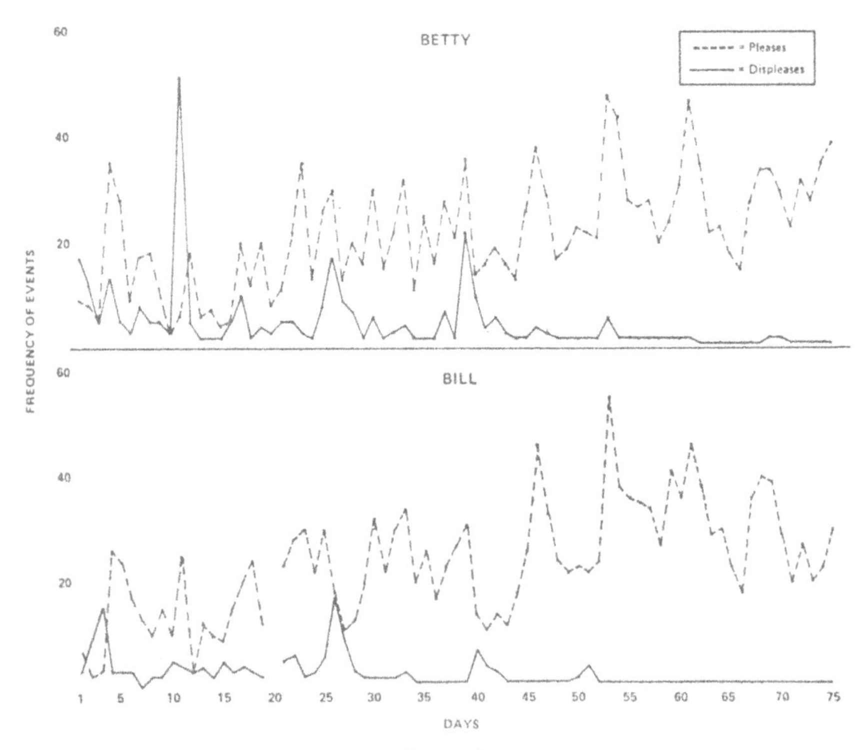

FIGURE 1

TABLE 2

Pre- and Post-Intervention Data Comparison

	BETTY pre	BETTY post	BILL pre	BILL post
Spouse Observation Checklist (SOC)				
Pleases:				
Companionship	.7	6.3	2.0	6.4
Affection	1.5	1.3	.8	2.6
Consideration	2.7	8.0	1.2	7.4
Sex	2.5	1.7	3.0	1.9
Communication process	1.2	2.9	1.3	2.6
Coupling activities	—	.1	—	.1
Child care and parenting	2.3	4.7	.5	2.1
Household management	2.8	4.0	.5	2.7
Financial decision-making	—	.6	.2	.4
Employment education	.2	.3	—	—
Personal habits and appearance	1.3	2.0	.5	2.0
Self and spouse independence	.5	.1	.5	—
TOTAL	15.7	32.4	13.1	26.9
Displeases:				
Consideration	3.2	—	2.5	—
Sex	—	—	.2	—
Communication process	1.5	—	1.0	—
Coupling Activities	—	—	.2	—
Childcare and parenting	1.2	—	.2	—
Household management	—	—	.2	—
Financial decision-making	—	—	—	—
Employment education	—	—	—	—
Personal habits and appearance	3.3	1.3	1.3	—
Self and spouse independence	—	—	.7	1.0
TOTAL	9.2	1.3	6.3	1.0
Daily Satisfaction	4.7	5.3	3.3	5.1
Verbal Communication Behaviors				
Accept Responsibility	1	0	0	5
Approval/Agree	1	8	0	4
Communication Talk	3	0	6	6
Emotional Clarification	2	1	3	4
Mindreading	1	6	6	4
Negative Response	29	6	28	3
Paraphrase/Reflection	0	0	3	6
Problem-solving	3	4	16	4
Sidetrack	8	6	1	4
Self-report Data				
Marital Adjustment Scale (MAS)	69	85	51	80
Areas of Change (AC)	9	9	9	7

leveled out at a very low daily frequency and pleasing behaviors followed a more steady climb with peaks occurring every weekend.

SOC data in Table 2 support this encouraging picture. A comparison of mean daily frequencies at pre- and posttreatment show substantial increases in the number of pleasing behaviors received by each spouse. By the end of treatment Betty was receiving twice as many communication and childcare pleases, which were the two areas she specified in contracts. Results in the areas that Bill contracted for are not quite as positive. There was a three-fold increase from pre- to post-intervention in the area of affection but there was decline from pre- to post-intervention in his receipt of sexual pleases. Both spouses reported large gains in the areas of companionship and consideration. Table 2 also reveals a dramatic decline in mean daily displeasing behaviors from pre- to post-intervention for both partners: By the end of treatment, each partner reported a mean of only one displeasing event per day. Increased ratings of daily satisfaction accompanied the increases in pleasing and decreases in displeasing behaviors.

Communication data that are reported in Table 1 are taken from two pre- and two posttreatment negotiation sessions that were made in the therapy setting. The negotiations were coded according to a modified version of the MICS that included only the following categories: Accept Responsibility, Approval/Agree, Communication Talk, Emotional Clarification, Mindread, Negative Response, Paraphrase/Reflection, Problem-Solving, and Sidetrack. The most notable finding was the reduction for both spouses in their frequencies of Negative Responses, which include criticisms, putdowns, accusations, and complaints, i.e., from 28 to 3 for Bill and from 29 to 6 for Betty. In terms of positive changes, both partners increased Approval/Agree statements. In addition, Bill demonstrated greater willingness to Accept Responsibility. While it appears that Bill actually reduced his frequency of Problem-Solving statements, this finding must be examined in terms of the sequential context of his statements. Out of Bill's 16 Problem-Solving statements at pretreatment, he elicited the following immediate reactions from Betty: 7 Negative Responses, 2 Neutral Responses, and 1 Accept Responsibility. Six times, he himself responded to his original Problem-Solving statement without even allowing Betty any chance to reply. At posttreatment, his 4 Problem-Solving statements were followed by 3 Approval/Agree responses, and 1 Neutral Response. Thus, while there was a decrease in the total frequency of Bill's Problem-Solving statements, his statements at posttreatment carried greater impact.

Examination of the self-report data in Table 2 reveals substantial improvement in spouses' global perceptions of marital satisfaction on the MAS but these scores still indicate a moderate degree of marital distress. According to the AC scores, there was essentially no improvement in the total number of areas perceived as problems. Specific areas that had been problematic at preintervention such as keeping the house clean, disciplining the children, and spending time together had been resolved by the end of treatment, but other issues, such as giving one another more attention, their sexual relationship, and visiting relatives assumed more importance.

The positive behavioral data must be viewed in light of the more ambiguous self-report data. The improvement in global satisfaction most likely reflects the behavioral changes that had already occurred. However, the distance that this couple had yet to go to be satisfied with their relationship indicates that additional behavioral changes were necessary.

Outcome at Follow-up

The 6-month follow-up examination of the Rs' progress was made by asking them to repeat the self-report questionnaires and having them collect one more week of SOC data. Unfortunately, the picture at this time was not nearly as positive as at postintervention and, in fact, was quite similar to the couple's pretreatment level of functioning. The MAS scores had by this time returned to 52 and 66 for Bill and Betty respectively. Similarly, the AC scores returned to 9 problem areas for Bill and increased to a new high of 13 areas for Betty. On the SOC, mean daily pleases dropped from postintervention rates of 32.4 and 26.9 to follow-up rates of 14.4 and 16.9 for Betty and Bill respectively. Only their rates of displeases continued to show improvement over pretreatment levels: Betty reported 4.7 and Bill reported 1.4 mean daily displeases.

DISCUSSION

This case illustrates how the positive gains made during treatment may wane unless there are specific steps to insure their maintenance. It can be concluded on the basis of the posttreatment data that the intervention strategies did effect positive changes in Bill and Betty's relationship. By the end of treatment their SOC records revealed increases in pleasing activities and decreases in displeasing events. In addition, observation of their communication samples revealed that their problem-solving efforts became more productive and less punishing. The effect of these behavioral changes on overall marital adjustment can be best examined through the spouses' ratings of marital satisfactions as measured by the MAS. Although these ratings improved, they did not reach the level of satisfaction expressed by most nondistressed couples.

There were several important cues indicating that the Rs' treatment was insufficient and that future difficulties were likely to occur. Since the Rs did not receive training in problem-solving, they never resolved some of the longstanding disagreements between them. This major shortcoming is reflected in the AC scores which, at posttreatment, remained unimproved over baseline scores. At the time of termination, this couple relied on the therapist to rectify arguments and misunderstandings. In therapy sessions, the therapist still played an active role in monitoring the couple's interaction by interrupting punitive verbalizations and suggesting more constructive ways the spouses could make their points. A couple who were better prepared for termination would be monitoring their own interactions, recognizing and editing punitive statements. It was also evident at termination that these spouses never truly enacted the recommendation to assist one another by reinforcing and prompting efforts toward change. Thus, although their feelings of being unappreciated became less frequent while they were more actively involved with one another during the course of therapy, these feelings were bound to recur.

Overall, therapy helped the Rs to receive more gratification to surmount some immediate conflicts, but they were not left with strategies to evoke when the relationship faltered in the future. By termination conflict had substantially tapered off, but their mastery of conflict management and problem solving was still very much dependent upon the therapist's support and guidance. If there had been no time constraints, the therapist could have promoted more lasting changes by an emphasis on problem-solving strategies, a gradual fading of therapy, booster sessions to work on problems that occurred over time, and the scheduling of crises to occur prior to termination. Strategies to guarantee the maintenance of lasting change are exemplified in the next case example.

CASE 2

Dennis and Pam had been married for three years at the time they sought therapy. They lived with two children: one, a two-year-old son, was theirs; the other, a six-year-old son, had been born to Pam out of wedlock. Both spouses had completed high school. Dennis worked in a factory as an unskilled machine operator, while Pam was a housewife who occasionally earned extra income as an artist.

CONFLICTS PRESENTED

Their marital problems emerged during Pam's initial evaluation at the clinic, where she presented herself as depressed. Since about six months after the wedding, they had been in conflict around a number of issues.

1) *Communication*: Dennis was a very quiet man who preferred a low rate of conversation. Pam was quite verbal and extroverted, and she complained of his unwillingness to engage in conversation with her.

2) *Sex*: Pam desired sex more frequently than did Dennis.

3) *Financial troubles*: The couple was deeply in debt. Each blamed the other for their meager income. Pam wanted Dennis either to undertake a second part-time job or return to school, for which, due to his veteran status, the government would pay him. He was disinclined toward both of these ideas and felt that Pam should increase her freelance work to supplement the income.

4) *Child management*: They often disagreed on when and how to discipline the children. According to Pam, Dennis punished the children only when he was in a foul mood, regardless of whether or not they were misbehaving. According to Dennis, Pam was inconsistent and insufficiently persistent in carrying out punishment.

5) *Household vs. community responsibilities*: Dennis felt that Pam was overinvolved in community activities and devoted insufficient time to her domestic responsibilities.

6) *Lack of shared rewarding activities*: They entered therapy with few common interests.

INTERVENTION

Dennis and Pam attended two assessment sessions and 17 conjoint therapy sessions over a 34-week period. Sessions lasted between 1-2 hours and occurred approximately biweekly. The substantial clinical changes which they manifested are depicted both in Table 3 and in Figure 2. Initial pretesting revealed both spouses to be severely dissatisfied with the current state of the relationship (see Marital Adjustment Scores, Table 3), although only the wife was seriously considering divorce (Marital Status Inventory Score for Wife = 6; for Husband = 0). The high score on the "Areas of Change" Questionnaire reflects the fact that both of them desired a variety of types of behavior change from the other. Their low rates of "positive" and high rates of "negative" behavior on the MICS reflected poor problem-solving; Pam tended to dominate their conversations, and Dennis, on those rare occasions when he talked, was generally derogatory and uncooperative.

Sessions #1-4

During this initial phase of therapy, the focus was on increasing positive relationship behavior. The first session was the interpretive session. Dennis and Pam are the couple on which the interpretive transcripts in Chapter 5 are based. They immediately began to manifest positive changes on the SOC during the week following session #1. Their first homework assignment was simply to study the other's SOC each night after completing their own forms. As Figure 2 suggests, most of the behaviors that each was tracking began to change in the desired direction. Their report when they returned from session #2 corroborated the data. They were both excited, happier, and eager to receive their next assignment.

At this juncture two points should be emphasized. First, this "honeymoon effect" following the initial commitment to therapy is quite common; the phenomenon manifests itself in an initial "spike" in the SOC curve following the interpretive session. We think the nature of this session, with its emphasis on both verbal and written commitment and mutual responsibility, is largely responsible for this effect. Dennis and Pam responded in a fairly typical manner, and the initial change provides the therapist with an opportunity for capitalizing on the renewed collaborative spirit. Second, as we indicated in Chapter 5, it is important that the therapists not be excessively consumed by the honeymoon atmosphere that often accompanies these initial changes. The changes are often transient and cannot be expected to sustain themselves indefinitely. Not only must the therapist be prepared for backslides, but the couple must also be forewarned.

During session #2, Dennis and Pam were shown how to use the data from their home observations to produce increases in the rate of exchanged reinforcement. The basic strategy involved each of them scrutinizing the other's data, and in particular noting the behaviors that occur more or less frequently on days that were given relatively high satisfaction ratings. The next step was to form working hypotheses regarding which behaviors on their part serve as the best predictors of the other's daily satisfaction ratings. Finally, the hypotheses were to be tested by increasing the frequency of behaviors directly related to satisfaction, and decreasing the behaviors which appeared to correlate negatively with satisfaction. Then, if the partner's satisfaction ratings increase, the hypotheses have been confirmed. For example, in examining Pam's data, it appeared that she was happiest on days when there were high ratings

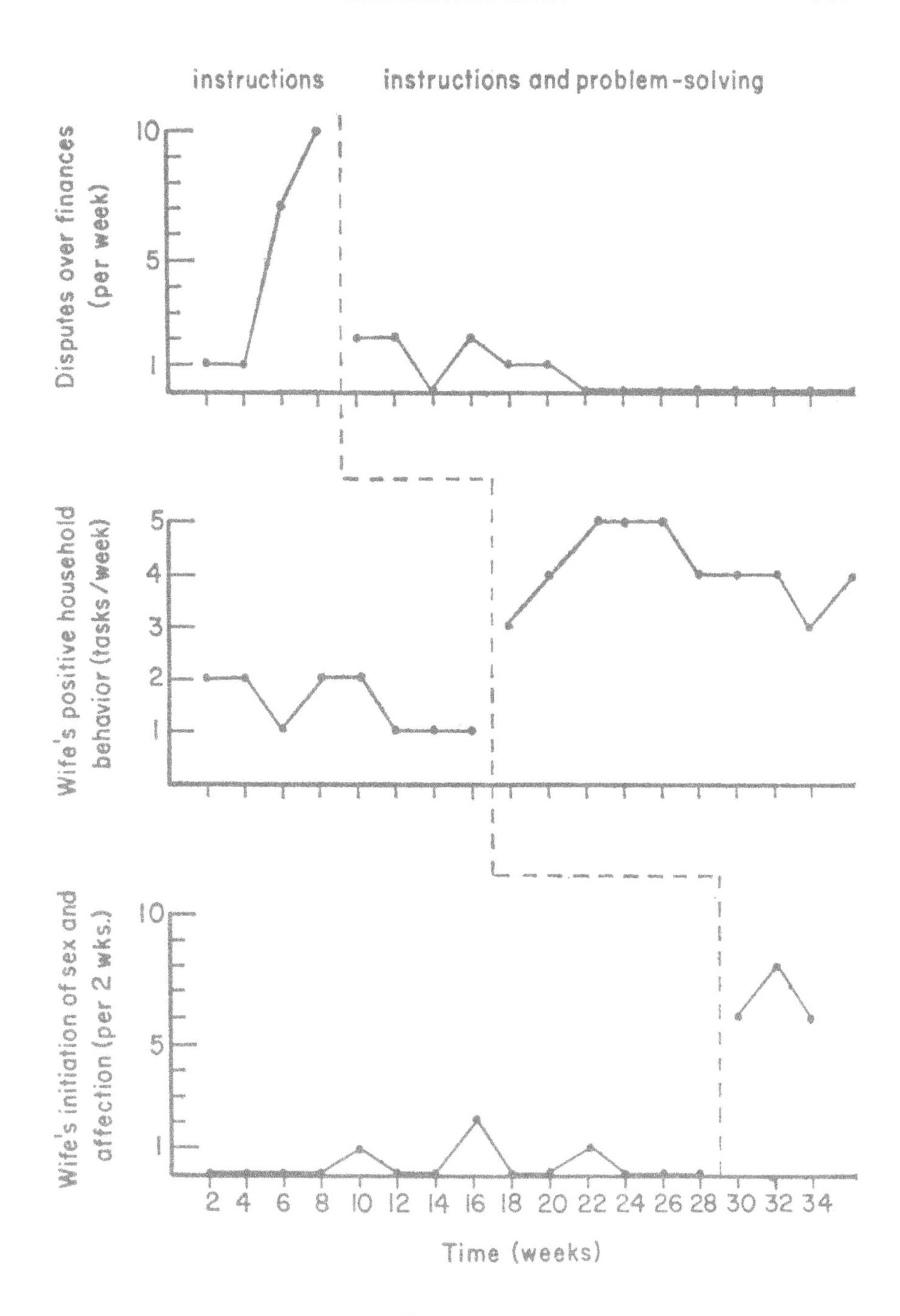
instructions
instructions and problem-solving
Disputes over finances (per week)
10
5
1
Wife's positive household behavior (tasks/week)
5
4
3
2
1
Wife's initiation of sex and affection (per 2 wks.)
10
5
1
2 4 6 8 10 12 14 16 18 20 22 24 26 28 30 32 34
Time (weeks)

FIGURE 2

TABLE 3

Frequency of Problem-Solving Behavior (PS), Marital Adjustment Scores (MAS), and Areas of Change (AC) Questionnaire Scores for Dennis and Pam at Pretest, Posttest, 6-month, and 1-year Follow-ups

		MEASURE			
		MAS	AC	Positive PS	Negative PS
Dennis					
	Pre	75	21	2.11	4.19
	Post	100	6	6.52	1.04
	6	117	8	—	—
	12	117	2	—	—
Pam					
	Pre	54			
	Post	109.5			
	6	93			
	12	129			

NOTE—All AC and PS scores base their unit of analysis on the couple, rather than on individual spouses; thus there is only one score for the couple as a whole on those measures. PS measures are expressed in terms of rate/minute.

of sexual, affectionate, and communication behaviors coming from Dennis. Thus, he focused on increasing the occurrence of those behaviors. Dennis, on the other hand, seemed to be happiest on days when Pam was engaged at home in instrumental tasks involving household management and child-rearing, and least happy on those days such activities were precluded by her involvement in community activities.

They both began to work independently on changing those behaviors which would presumably lead to an increase in the other's daily satisfaction rating. One fortunate characteristic of these behaviors was that they seemed to be functionally related to one another. Pam preferred to spend her time at home, but only when Dennis reinforced her with both verbal and physical attention. Similarly, Dennis tended to provide the benefits desired by Pam when she evidenced involvement in domestic tasks. In recent months, they were withholding these benefits from one another, awaiting the other's demonstration of love and good faith. Therapy induced them to simultaneously reverse this pattern, and for a month, the relationship steadily improved. However, as the paragraphs below indicate, there were aspects of their relationship difficulties which were not so easily reversed, and a crisis spurred on by one of these problem areas threatened to destroy the progress they had made during the two months since therapy had begun.

Sessions #4-8

Pam and Dennis had been deeply in debt for quite some time. In addition to the difficulties inherent in subsisting on one rather paltry income, they had been living beyond their means. They bought a house which they could not afford, and they also spent considerable money on weekends in order to socialize with their wealthier friends. Dennis had been aware of the extent of their indebtedness, but Pam had remained blissfully unaware of the problem, assuming that Dennis was keeping the books in order. During the two-week interval between sessions #4-5, a major creditor sent a letter to them which enumerated the debts and threatened to foreclose. Pam was shocked, becoming very depressed and angry, blaming Dennis both for his inadequacies as a financial manager and for his surreptitiousness. The crisis necessitated their borrowing $2,000 from a close friend and fundamentally altering their standard of living.

The immediate task in therapy was to prevent this crisis from undercutting the therapeutic progress to an excessive degree and to help negotiate a plan to remediate the financial crisis. The first task was dealt with by attempting to modify Pam's attributions regarding the meaning and implications of Dennis' behavior. The transcript below illustrates this process:

Pam: What bothers me most of all is the way you (*to Dennis*) kept this from me. All the while we were on Cloud 9 in here, you were sitting on a powder keg. He's (*to therapist*) been bullshitting me since we started this.

(Dennis was being quiet and unresponsive, staring down at his feet.)

Therapist: OK, I think I understand what's going on. Let me try and put this thing in perspective. First of all, let's all acknowledge the gravity of the situation. You two are in big trouble and you don't have the luxury of casting blame and pinning it on one another. Dennis, do you agree with Pam that your keeping this from her suggests that your effort in therapy was bullshit?
Dennis: No!
Pam: Then how do you explain yourself?
Dennis: (*after a long pause*) I was afraid to tell you.
Pam: Why?
Dennis: I was afraid you'd be acting just like you're acting.
Therapist: Now, I want you both to listen to me very carefully. There is no question about how this is a serious problem, and you (*to Pam*) are clearly justified in being upset with Dennis. But, and the "but" here is where you in particular need to listen, I don't share your interpretation of Dennis' behavior. It is his love for

> you and his fear of your anger and disapproval that made it so difficult to tell you about these financial hassles. I don't mean to justify the behavior. But his very concern for the relationship produced what you call deception. The better things get, the harder I'm sure it was to even conceive of telling you. You still should have told her, as I'm sure you know; but I wonder how many husbands in your shoes would have done the same thing you did. The issue is not whose fault this problem is, but how can you resolve this so that you're back on your feet, and how can you resume the considerable progress you were making before this happened?

About 45 minutes were spent in this vein, and the remainder of this session focused on resolving the financial crisis. In this session the couple was introduced to *problem-solving training*. In a step-by-step manner, over a period of four therapy sessions, the couple negotiated solutions to the financial crisis. In the process of accomplishing this, through feedback and coaching from the therapist, they began to adopt new, more effective problem-solving tactics. Problem-solving was highly appropriate for this couple. For one thing, prior to training they lacked a "solution-focus" when they discussed conflicts, opting instead for a backward-looking recapitulation of the past. In addition, Pam had placed Dennis in a no-win situation in their communication. She criticized him for not talking, and then when he did talk, she used her more sophisticated verbal skills to repudiate his remarks. The problem-solving guidelines increased her sensitivity to this problem. Finally, the structure of problem-solving was extremely useful to Dennis, providing him with an enhanced capacity for contributions to such discussions. In particular, paraphrasing and brainstorming served him well. The former facilitated his informing Pam that he was listening to and interested in what she was saying. Brainstorming undercut his tendency to censor himself before speaking.

The financial crisis was tackled by dividing it into a series of components. One involved the establishment of an austerity budget. Another focused on ways to supplement their income. A third dealt with the feasibility of Dennis returning to school. Gradually, as the change agreements brought order to a chaotic and anxiety-inducing life situation, the tension was alleviated and the relationship began to improve again.

Here is an example of one of their change agreements:

> Problem: We need extra funds to support the budget and we decided that Dennis would get a job for those extra funds.
>
> Solution: 1) Dennis would go to unemployment office (December 21) to see what is available and would return once a week until employment was found.

2) Dennis will go twice a week after work and file application even where employment was not available. There will be no follow-up unless advised by the employer.
3) Pam will look in the paper each day for leads for Dennis and free-lance work for herself.
4) Dennis will keep Pam posted about leads and applications and his feelings. Dennis will also provide feedback about leads he doesn't choose to pursue and why.

Although Dennis did not find a part-time job, he did decide to return to school on evenings. This soon led to additional income. More importantly, they both began to attack the problem with skill and foresight, and they communicated effectively in regard to a conflict area for the first time since their marriage began. As Figure 2 indicates, disputes over finances decreased and were gradually eliminated over a two-month period.

Sessions #9-12

The two primary problem areas focused on during the next two months of therapy involved Pam's household responsibilities (or what Dennis viewed as her inadequate execution of them), and disagreements regarding child-rearing issues. Dennis' concerns regarding household responsibilities had been assuaged to some degree; however he remained concerned that involvement in outside activities not infringe on the family's already greatly restricted time together. Little formal problem solving was necessary in regard to this issue, since it seemed to take care of itself as other aspects of the relationship gradually fell into place. However, several weeks were spent with Dennis and Pam applying their gradually emerging problem-solving skills to their interaction with the two children. Most of their concerns in this area centered around Pam's tendency to be erratic in her disciplinary tactics and Dennis' tendency to snap at and occasionally spank them. Their problem-solving discussions focused on arriving at a consistent set of contingencies which were agreeable to both, and standardizing their discrepant, and at times capricious, methods of discipline. An example of one of the change agreements formed during this phrase of therapy indicates another concern that they shared, an insufficient amount of quality time spent with the kids:

Problem: We don't spend enough quality time with the kids.
Solution: 1) After supper while the kids are getting ready for bed (during baths, etc.) we'll clear table, etc.
2) Then, till the kids go to bed (7:30-8:00) we'll play or

work as a group with no interruptions from TV or phone.
3) On Sunday, we'll seek some kind of church and then spend Sunday as a family day.

Later Phases of Therapy

After 12 therapy sessions, spanning about six months in time, the marriage had greatly improved, and the changes had begun to stabilize. The last five therapy sessions were devoted to three areas: 1) insuring that they shared quality time together despite their numerous obligations and hectic schedules; 2) improving their communication on matters related to sex; and most importantly, 3) *programming into their daily routine strategies which would ensure generalization.*

Their work on maximizing their mutual participation in reinforcing activities together focused on both the evenings during the week when they were home and on planning weekend activities that were inexpensive but enjoyable. The discussion of sex focused on ways to cope with Pam's more frequent desire for sex, which led to her desire to initiate it more often. Yet, her tendency to initiate sex was inhibited by Dennis' often rejecting responses. Their discussions about this problem produced an understanding that she could initiate sex, but that if Dennis was not interested he would respond in kind without "being totally rejecting." For example, in the past he had avoided an affectionate response to her sexual advances because he was afraid that such communication would be misinterpreted as sexual responsiveness. After discussing the problem, using their new problem-solving skills, the distinction between an affectionate, nonsexual response and a sexual response was clarified, and they were able to create an atmosphere which, as Figure 2 indicates, increased Pam's frequency of sexual initiation.

By now Dennis and Pam were handling their negotiations without much assistance from the therapist. They had been problem-solving at home as well as during therapy sessions. The only remaining question concerned how to facilitate a maintenance of treatment-derived gains. The primary strategy utilized was to gradually fade them from the therapy sessions, while substituting their own weekly meetings for biweekly therapist contacts. They set aside 90 minutes each Friday evening and evaluated the state of their marriage. During this time they enumerated the positive behaviors that had occurred during the week, evaluated the adequacy of their behavior change agreements, renegotiated agreements when necessary, and problem-solved any new conflict areas that had emerged since their last home therapy session. The idea was to allow them to become their own therapists, now that they had acquired the skills necessary to exert a therapeutic impact.

By the time they terminated, self-report, behavioral, and home observations all suggested substantial and sweeping improvements in the marriage. The target behaviors plotted in Figure 2 unmistakably suggest that behavior change was occurring, and the multiple baseline allows one to attribute these changes to problem-solving training. Their post-test self-report questionnaires were all within normal limits. Behavioral observations by trained observers, based on videotapes of laboratory problem-solving sessions, showed substantial increases in desirable problem-solving behaviors (solution focus, social reinforcement, compromise, etc.), and decreases in negative behaviors (criticism, complaint, etc.).

Follow-up reports at six months and one year following therapy termination suggested that treatment gains were maintained. Perhaps the enduring nature of the changes are best described by the wife in a letter to the therapist approximately one year following termination: "It is Christmas time, and we have money for presents and enough love and happiness to light up the state. With the exception of an occasional back-sliding, our marriage is great! The kids are growing big and emotionally sound and we're all looking forward to the best Christmas ever."

SUMMARY

A major contribution of behavioral, compared to other marital therapies, is that it offers couples long-range strategies to handle their relationships more effectively. In addition to dealing with immediate crises, a complete course of behavioral marital therapy includes the programming of skills that a couple can apply when their relationship falters. As exemplified by the first couple, premature termination in behavior therapy, as with all other therapies, carries the potential hazard of post-treatment deterioration. The fact that a spouse arrives at an important realization or engages in a new behavior by the end of therapy loses its significance unless it translates into more lasting change. Marital therapists of all persuasions bear equal responsibility in demonstrating that couples maintain their treatment gains over time.

CHAPTER 12

Conclusion: Marital Therapist as Scientist-Practitioner

THIS BOOK has been about treating couples in distress. Books such as this one are needed because couples seem to be making one another miserable at increasingly high rates. It is incumbent upon clinicians to do something with the couples who seek assistance from them, despite the lack of definitive experimental evidence in support of any marital therapy strategy at present. Books for clinicians will continue to be written as long as there is work for them to do. The careful, plodding pace of scientific research cannot possibly accommodate the immediate needs of the practitioner.

However, as we have interjected throughout the book, it is equally incumbent upon all of us to keep our commitment to any particular approach tentative until the results of controlled experiments confirm or repudiate our clinical intuition. As responsible representatives of the mental health professions, we are ethically bound to obey the directives of objective investigation in clinical practice. To offer our clients a treatment which has proven to be ineffective, or to practice a treatment in the absence of any supporting evidence when a treatment whose efficacy has been demonstrated is available, is a questionable ethical practice.

Although the task of empirical documentation is primarily for researchers, to a lesser extent practitioners can contribute significantly to the process. It is possible for a marital therapist to analyze and study his/her cases in a rigorous manner without any clinical liability, indeed, to the benefit of his/her clinical practice. Conducting one's clinical practice as a scientist not only may contribute to the advancement of marital therapy, but also will allow for a more objective, less biased evaluation of one's own clinical effectiveness. Moreover, an experimental analysis of individual cases will allow a practitioner to isolate the active ingredients of his/her treatment procedures, and separate them from whatever placebo effects or demand characteristics may be contributing to treatment efficacy.

Although the inclusion of scientific methodology in one's clinical practice will be somewhat costly, it is the only way that a clinician can receive accurate feedback about his/her effectiveness. Practitioners typically rely on their own inferences based on clients' self-report to assess the success of a particular case. As we mentioned in Chapter 10, even expert therapists overestimate their effectiveness, compared to the evaluation of clients and observers. Behavior therapists were not immune to this practice; in fact, they were even more grandiose in their overestimation than psychoanalytically oriented therapists. It is not particularly surprising that therapists tend to overestimate their positive impact on clients. Clients want to believe that they have benefited from therapy. They also want to please their therapists. The therapist does not need to be malevolent or Machiavellian to distort his/her degree of success; the perception of one's own skill and competence is of obvious importance to a therapist, and the judgment is usually subjective enough to allow such distortions to intrude. Follow-ups, which are rarely conducted by psychiatric facilities or by clinicians engaged in private practice, would provide an additional opportunity to appraise the effects of therapy. Maintenance of treatment gains is certainly expected in a successful therapy case, even though it is seldom assessed. Thus, therapists rarely receive any kind of feedback on this fundamentally important question.

Let us outline some of the tactics that therapists can use to more objectively appraise their work:

First, in their initial assessment of marital problems, they can make use of self-report measures of demonstrated reliability and validity. The "Locke-Wallace Marital Adjustment Test" (Locke & Wallace, 1959), the "Dyadic Adjustment Scale" (Spanier, 1976), the "Areas-of-Change Questionnaire" (Patterson, 1976), and the "Marital Status Inventory" (Weiss & Cerreto, 1975) are examples of useful self-report questionnaires which contain norms and have demonstrated their utility. These tests not only facilitate the task of assessment, but provide a basis for evaluating outcome, since they can be readministered at the conclusion of therapy.

Second, include in the initial assessment a baseline of the couple's complaints as they occur in the natural environment. Although couples are not truly objective observers of either their own or their partner's behavior, the collecting of data on the frequency, duration, or intensity of target behaviors as they occur outside of the therapy office provides the therapist with a very important and otherwise inaccessible perspective. This baseline not only aids in the selection of treatment goals, but also can serve as an ongoing method of evaluating progress. Couples can continue their recording throughout therapy, and as a result they receive constant feedback on their progress as does the therapist. The "Spouse Observation Checklist" (see Chapter 4) is a very useful device for such recording. The therapist's ingenuity comes into play both in operationalizing couples' complaints in terms that can be recorded and in prompting their compliance with the recording assignments (see Chapter 5).

Third, a truly ambitious scientist-practitioner would apply a multiple baseline analysis to the ongoing data collection (see Chapter 4), since only by the use of a single-subject experimental design can one truly isolate the impact of treatment on the couple's relationship. In practice, conducting such analyses is difficult, since the experimental demands of a multiple baseline design tend to conflict with clinical considerations. For example, a stable baseline is highly desirable prior to intervention, in order that the therapist can unambiguously assess the changes that occur upon the implementation of a treatment. However, clinical considerations seldom allow for the extensive period of baseline recording which is often necessary in order to arrive at stability. Another detriment to the conducting of a multiple baseline analysis in the clinical setting is the difficulty of identifying behaviors that are truly independent. To the extent that the behaviors being recorded are interrelated, it will be impossible to demonstrate the specific effects of one's treatment on a particular behavior. A final deterrent to single-subject experimental designs in outpatient clinical settings is the excessive variability of the situational variables which the behaviors under scrutiny are subjected to. On a day-to-day basis the couple is interacting in a variety of contexts, and conditions which influence the frequency of various relationship behaviors are not always constant from week to week. Since, in contrast to the highly controlled conditions found in inpatient settings, the therapist has less control over the behaviors that he/she is trying to influence, the behavior will fluctuate regardless of the impact of treatment. This will often render the data difficult to interpret by visual inspection.

Despite these various detriments to conducting a multiple baseline analysis of marital problems treated in an outpatient setting, such experimental rigor can be approximated, as our research has shown (Jacobson, 1977a, 1977b); and to the extent that it is possible, it is in the interest of the clinician to do so. Whenever possible, it is highly desirable to know which variables are accounting for positive changes occurring in therapy, both because such knowledge will lead to more efficient treatment strategies in future cases and because the active ingredients can be subsequently stressed in the later stages of therapy for the case which is currently being treated.

In approximating a multiple baseline design in a clinical setting, specific treatment techniques can be presented one at a time so that their impact on couples' behavior can be observed independently of other components of the treatment package. Although this may not always be the quickest way to provide benefit to the clients, in the long run they should benefit more, since the therapist will have a better idea of why change is occurring, and will be able to alter the treatment plan accordingly, by emphasizing effective elements and eliminating those which add little to the treatment's power. Similarly, if enough behaviors are being tracked simultaneously, it may be possible to assess effects similar to those gleaned from a multiple baseline analysis. For example, in the case of a particular couple, it may be that an intervention designed to improve communication may also affect the couple's sex life but will have minimal impact on their instrumental behavior, such as financial or household-related transactions. If a subsequent intervention designed to improve instrumental domains is successful, one can more confidently attribute both sets of changes to specific treatment effects.

Fourth, whenever possible, evaluate progress in therapy by means other than client self-report or inferences derived from couples' self-report. The ideal alternative to self-reports would be an unbiased, nonreactive, representative sample of a couple's relationship behavior in the natural environment. Since this is largely unfeasible even for researchers, it is hardly realistic to expect such an assessment from a practitioner. Nor is it realistic to expect a clinician to videotape couples in standardized problem-solving sessions before and after therapy, and to have these tapes rated by trained observers. However, it is reasonable and highly desirable, both in the assessment and in the evaluation of the effects of therapy, to observe the couple interacting with one another. It is critical that the therapist not be present during these interactions; the use of audiotape recording of the discussions makes this possible. It is also important that the therapist have some criteria for evaluating positive and negative communication, criteria decided upon prior to observing the behavior. We would recommend observing couples discussing problems in their relationships.

Fifth, set specific treatment goals against which both the therapist and the couple can evaluate the effectiveness of therapy. It is all too easy to find evidence for improvement at the conclusion of therapy, despite the failure of the treatment program to achieve the goals initially outlined. This post-hoc type of rationalization is not acceptable in research, it should not be acceptable to the practitioner, and it will not be acceptable to most clients.

Sixth, the success of therapy should be assessed from as great a variety of vantage points as possible. Self-reports questionnaires, behavior recorded by couples in the home, and observations of their interaction should all be included in an assessment of therapy progress. The more measures that converge in their assessment of improvement, the more confident a therapist can be that his/her work has been successful.

Seventh, conduct follow-ups up to at least a year following therapy termination. This need not involve anything more costly than mailing a self-report questionnaire to couples. Little elaboration is needed for this recommendation. The importance of follow-up information is paramount.

All seven of the above points, if adopted, would not only enhance the rigor of one's clinical practice, but also be consistent with what we believe is a therapist's responsibility to his/her clients. The first four guidelines, which collectively address the objectification of progress and would enhance the ability of both therapist and client to evaluate the success of therapy, are consistent with the ethical principle that the client has a right to an unbiased assessment of therapy outcome, to the extent that such an assessment is possible. Data collection is not simply a research strategy or an idiosyncracy of behavior therapy but a way of meeting the requirement of accountability to the consumers of our services. We recommend that pre- and posttest data be shared with clients.

The fifth suggestion, that goals be specified in advance of treatment, serves an additional function. With clear goals identified by the couple, the therapist is less likely to impose, inadvertently or otherwise, his views of the ideal relationship on the couple. The tendency of therapists to tacitly encourage the maintenance of relationships or advise couples on the basis of their own values rather than professional expertise has been discussed in previous Chapters (5 and 9). A clear therapeutic direction, with a constant monitoring of progress *as determined by the agreed upon direction,* is the best safeguard against such therapist impositions.

Finally, at some point in therapy it may become necessary for a therapist to acknowledge his/her inability to help a particular couple. To subject a couple to an interminable number of therapy sessions despite no signs of change is unfair to them. We have found that if no progress toward attainment of the treatment goals has occurred after 12 therapy sessions, there is little that we can do for the couple. If no change has occurred by that time, we will terminate under normal circumstances. Our point is that every therapist must admit defeat at times, and we all need to have some concrete criteria for deciding when to direct our healing skills elsewhere.

Thus, we think it is well within the realm of possibility for a marital therapist to be a scientist as well as a practitioner. In our creation of this book, we have tried to integrate these roles, and by doing so model our belief in their compatibility. The clinician and the applied researcher have much in common, and both deserve the insights which the other can provide. The assumption of both roles allows one to reap the rewards from both worlds, to the benefit of the scientific community, the community of practicing clinicians, and the unhappy community of distressed couples.

Bibliography

Ables, B. S. & Brandsma, J. M. *Therapy for Couples.* San Francisco: Jossey-Bass, 1977.

Alberti, R. E. & Emmons, M. L. *Your Perfect Right.* San Francisco: Impact, 1970.

Alkire, A. A. & Brunse, A. J. Impact and possible causality from videotape feedback in marital therapy. *Journal of Consulting and Clinical Psychology,* 1974, 42, 203-210.

Azrin, N. H., Naster, B. J., & Jones, R. Reciprocity counseling: A rapid learning-based procedure for marital counseling. *Behavior Research and Therapy,* 1973, 11, 365-382.

Bandura, A. Self-efficacy: Toward a unifying theory of behavioral change. *Psychological Review,* 1977, 84, 191-215.

Baum, W. M. The correlation-based law of effect. *Journal of the Experimental Analysis of Behavior,* 1973, 20, 137-153.

Beck, A. T. *Depression: Clinical, Experimental, and Theoretical Aspects.* New York: Harper & Row, 1967.

Beck, A. T. *Cognitive Therapy and the Emotional Disorders.* New York: International Universities Press, 1976.

Bergin, A. E. & Strupp, H. H. *Changing Frontiers in the Science of Psychotherapy.* Chicago: Aldine, 1972.

Berkowitz, L. Experimental investigations of hostility catharsis. *Journal of Consulting and Clinical Psychology,* 1970, 35, 1-7.

Bernal, M. E., Gibson, D. M., Williams, D. E., & Pesses, D. I. A device for recording automatic audio tape recording. *Journal of Applied Behavior Analysis,* 1971, 4, 151-156.

Birchler, G. R. Differential patterns of instrumental affiliative behavior as a function of degree of marital distress and level of intimacy. (Doctoral Dissertation, University of Oregon, 1972.) *Dissertation Abstracts International,* 1973, 33, 14499B-4500B. (University Microfilms No. 73-7865, 102).

Birchler, G. R., Weiss, R. L., & Vincent, J. P. A multimethod analysis of social reinforcement exchange between maritally distressed and nondistressed spouse and stranger dyads. *Journal of Personality and Social Psychology,* 1975, 31, 349-360.

Birchler, G. R. & Webb, L. J. Discriminating interaction in behaviors in happy and unhappy marriages. *Journal of Consulting and Clinical Psychology,* 1977, 45, 494-495.

Bowen, M. Family therapy and family group therapy. In: D. H. L. Olson (Ed.), *Treat-*

ing Relationships. Lake Mills, IA: Graphic Press, 1976.

CAMMERER, L. Family feedback in depressive illnesses. *Psychosomatics*, 1971, 12, 127-132.

CAMPBELL, D. T. & STANLEY, J. C. *Experimental and Quasi-Experimental Designs for Research*. Chicago: Rand McNally, 1963.

CARTER, R. D. & THOMAS, E. J. Modification of problematic marital communication using corrective feedback and instruction. *Behavior Therapy*, 1973, 4, 100-109.

CHRISTENSEN, A. Naturalistic observation of families: A system for random audio recordings in the home. *Behavior Therapy*, in press.

CIMINERO, A. R., NELSON, R. O., & LIPINSKI, D. P. Self-monitoring procedures in behavioral assessment. In: A. R. Ciminero, K. S. Calhoun, and H. E. Adams (Eds.), *Handbook of Behavioral Assessment*. New York: Wiley, 1977.

COLEMAN, R. E. & MILLER, A. G. The relationship between depression and marital maladjustment in a clinic population: A multitrait-multimethod study. *Journal of Consulting and Clinical Psychology*, 1975, 43, 647-651.

COTTON, M. C. *A Systems Approach to Marital Training Evaluation*. Unpublished doctoral dissertation, Texas Tech University, 1976.

DANAHER, B. G. Theoretical foundations and clinical applications of the Premack principle: Review and critique. *Behavior Therapy*, 1974, 5, 307-324.

EDMONDS, V. M., WITHERS, G., & DIBATISTA, B. Adjustment, conservatism, and marital conventionalization. *Journal of Marriage and the Family*, 1972, 34, 96-103.

EIDELSON, R. An affiliation-independence model of relationship formation. Unpublished manuscript, University of North Carolina, 1976.

EISLER, R. M. & HERSEN, M. Behavioral techniques in family-oriented crisis intervention. *Archives of General Psychiatry*, 1973, 28, 111-115.

EISLER, R. M., HERSEN, M., & AGRAS, W. S. Effects of videotape and instructional feedback on nonverbal marital interaction: An analog study. *Behavior Therapy*, 1973, 4, 551-558.

ELLIS, A. *Reason and Emotion in Psychotherapy*. New York: Lyle-Stuart, 1962.

ELLIS, A. Techniques of handling anger in marriage. *Journal of Marriage and Family Counseling*, 1976, 2, 305-315.

FELDMAN, L. B. Depression and marital interaction. *Family Process*, 1976, 15, 389-395.

FISHER, R. E. *The Effect of Two Group Counseling Methods on Perceptual Congruence in Married Pairs*. Unpublished doctoral dissertation, University of Hawaii, 1973.

FLOWERS, J. V. A simulation game to facilitate communication in marital therapy. Paper presented at the Western Psychological Association, Sacramento, 1975.

FOLLINGSTAD, D. R., HAYNES, S. N., & SULLIVAN, J. *Assessment of the Components of a Behavioral Marital Intervention Program*. Unpublished manuscript, University of South Carolina, 1976.

FOLLINGSTAD, D. R., SULLIVAN, J., IERACE, C., FERRARA, J., & HAYNES, S. N. Behavioral assessment of marital interaction. Paper presented at the Tenth Annual Convention of the Association for the Advancement of Behavior Therapy, New York, December, 1976.

FRAMO, J. L. Personal reflections of a family therapist. *Journal of Marriage and Family Counseling*, 1975, 1, 15-28.

FRANK, J. D. *Persuasion and Healing*. Baltimore: Johns Hopkins Press, 1961.

FRANKL, V. E. Paradoxical intentions: A logotherapeutic technique. *American Journal of Psychotherapy*, 1960, 14, 520-535.

FRANKL, V. E. Paradoxical intention and dereflection. *Psychotherapy: Theory, Research, and Practice*, 1975, 12, 226-237.

GELLES, R. J. *The Violent Home: A Study of Physical Aggression Between Husbands and Wives*. Beverly Hills, CA: Sage, 1972.

GINOTT, H. *Between Parent and Child*. New York: Macmillan, 1965.

GOLDFRIED, M. R. Behavioral assessment in perspective. In: J. D. Cone & R. P. Hawkins (Eds.), *Behavioral Assessment: New Directions in Clinical Psychology*. New York: Brunner/Mazel, 1977.

GOLDFRIED, M. R. & DAVISON, G. C. *Clinical Behavior Therapy*. New York: Holt, Rinehart, & Winston, 1976.

GOLDFRIED, M. R. & SPRAFKIN, J. N. *Behavioral Personality Assessment*. Morristown, NJ: General Learning Press, 1974.

GOLDSTEIN, M. K. Behavior rate change in marriages: Training wives to modify husbands' behavior. (Doctoral dissertation, Cornell University, 1971). *Dissertation Abstracts International*, 1971, 32, 548B. (University Microfilms No., 71-17, 094)

GORDON, T. *Parent Effectiveness Training*. New York: Wyden, 1970.

GOTTMAN, J., MARKMAN, H., & NOTARIUS, C. The topography of marital conflict: A sequential analysis of verbal and nonverbal behavior. *Journal of Marriage and the Family*, 1977, 39, 461-477.

GOTTMAN, J., NOTARIUS, C., GONSO, J., & MARKMAN, H. *A Couple's Guide to Communication*. Champaign: Research Press, 1976.

GOTTMAN, J., NOTARIUS, C., MARKMAN, H., BANK, S., YOPPI, B., & RUBIN, M. E. Behavior exchange theory and marital decision making. *Journal of Personality and Social Psychology*, 1976, 34, 14-23.

GREER, S. E. & D'ZURILLA, T. Behavioral approaches to marital discord and conflict. *Journal of Marriage and Family Counseling*, 1975, 1, 299-315.

GUERNEY, B. G. *Relationship Enhancement*. San Francisco: Jossey-Bass, 1977.

GURMAN, A. S. Contemporary marital therapies: A critique and comparative analysis of psychoanalytic, behavioral and systems theory approaches. In: T. J. Paolino, Jr. and B. S. McCrady (Eds.), *Marriage and Marital Therapy: Psychoanalytic, Behavioral and Systems Theory Perspectives*. New York: Brunner/Mazel, 1978.

GURMAN, A. S. & KNISKERN, D. P. Research on marital and family therapy: Progress, perspective, and prospect. In: S. L. Garfield and A. E. Bergin (Eds.), *Handbook of Psychotherapy and Behavior Change: An Empirical Analysis* (Second Edition). New York: Wiley, 1978.

GURMAN, A. S. & KNUDSON, R. M. Behavioral marriage therapy: I. A psychodynamic-systems analysis and critique. *Family Process*, 1978, 17, 121-138.

HALEY, J. Marriage therapy. *Archives of General Psychiatry*, 1963, 8, 213-234.

HALEY, J. *Uncommon Therapy: The Psychiatric Techniques of Milton H. Erickson, M.D.* New York: Norton, 1973.

HALEY, J. *Problem Solving Therapy*. San Francisco: Jossey-Bass, 1976.

HALLECK, S. L. *The Politics of Therapy*. New York: Science House, 1971.

HARRELL, J. & GUERNEY, B. Training married couples in conflict negotiation skills. In: D. H. L. Olson (Ed.), *Treating Relationships*. Lake Mills, IA: Graphic Press, 1976.

HEATH, S., KERNS, R., MYSKOWSKI, M., & HAYNES, S. N. The assessment of marital interaction in structured observation situations: Criterion-related validity and internal consistency. Paper presented at the Eleventh Annual Convention of the Association for the Advancement of Behavior Therapy, Atlanta, December, 1977.

HEINRICH, A. G. Personal communication. March, 1978.

HERRNSTEIN, R. J. On the law of effect. *Journal of the Experimental Analysis of Behavior*, 1970, 13, 243-266.

HERSEN, M. BARLOW, D. H. *Single Case Experimental Designs*. London: Pergamon, 1976.

HICKS, M. W. & PLATT, M. Marital happiness and stability: A review of the research in the sixties. *Journal of Marriage and the Family*, 1970, 32, 553-574.

HIGGINS, J. G. Social services for abused wives. *Social Casework*, 1978, 59, 266-271.

HOMANS, G. C. *Social Behavior: Its Elementary Forms*. New York: Harcourt Brace, 1961.

HOPS, H., WILLS, T. A., PATTERSON, G. R., & WEISS, R. L. *Marital Interaction Coding*

System. Unpublished manuscript, University of Oregon and Oregon Research Institute, 1972.

JACKSON, D. D. The study of the family. *Family Process,* 1965, 4, 1-20.

JACOBSON, N. S. Problem solving and contingency contracting in the treatment of marital discord. *Journal of Consulting and Clinical Psychology,* 1977, 45, 92-100. (a)

JACOBSON, N. S. The role of problem solving in behavioral marital therapy. Paper presented at the Annual Meeting of the Association for the Advancement of Behavior Therapy, Atlanta, December, 1977. (b)

JACOBSON, N. S. Training couples to solve their marital problems: A behavioral approach to relationship discord. Part I: Problem-solving skills. *International Journal of Family Counseling,* 1977, 5 (1), 22-31. (c)

JACOBSON, N. S. Training couples to solve their marital problems: A behavioral approach to relationship discord. Part II: Intervention strategies. *International Journal of Family Counseling,* 1977, 5 (2), 20-28. (d)

JACOBSON, N. S. Specific and nonspecific factors in the effectiveness of a behavioral approach to the treatment of marital discord. *Journal of Consulting and Clinical Psychology,* 1978, 46, 442-452. (a)

JACOBSON, N. S. A review of the research on the effectiveness of marital therapy. In: T. J. Paolino & B. S. McCrady (Eds.), *Marriage and Marital Therapy: Psychoanalytic, Behavioral and Systems Theory Perspectives.* New York: Brunner/Mazel, 1978. (b)

JACOBSON, N. S. A stimulus control model of change in behavioral marriage therapy: Implications for contingency contracting. *Journal of Marriage and Family Counseling,* 1978, 3, 29-35. (c)

JACOBSON, N. S. Contingency contracting with couples: Redundancy and caution. *Behavior Therapy,* 1978, 9, 679. (d)

JACOBSON, N. S. Behavioral treatments for marital discord: A critical appraisal. In: M. Hersen, R. Eisler, and P. Miller (Eds.), *Progress in Behavior Modification.* New York: Academic Press, in press. (a)

JACOBSON, N. S. Increasing positive behavior in severely distressed adult relationships: The effectiveness of problem-solving training. *Behavior Therapy,* in press. (b)

JACOBSON, N. S. & ANDERSON, E. A. The effects of behavioral rehearsal and feedback on the acquisition of problem-solving skills in distressed and nondistressed couples. Unpublished manuscript, University of Iowa, 1978.

JACOBSON, N. S. & BAUCOM, D. H. Design and assessment of nonspecific control groups in behavior modification research. *Behavior Therapy,* 1977, 8, 709-719.

JACOBSON, N. S. & MARTIN, B. Behavioral marriage therapy: Current status. *Psychological Bulletin,* 1976, 83, 540-556.

JACOBSON, N. S. & WALDRON, H. Toward a behavioral profile of marital distress. Unpublished manuscript, University of Iowa, 1979.

JACOBSON, N. S. & WEISS, R. L. Behavioral marriage therapy: "The contents of Gurman et al. may be hazardous to our health." *Family Process,* 1978, 17, 149-164.

JOHNSON, S. M. *First Person Singular: Living the Good Life Alone.* New York: Lippincott, 1977.

JOHNSON, S. M., CHRISTENSEN, A., & BELLAMY, G. T. Evaluation of family intervention through unobtrusive audio recordings: Experiences in "bugging" children. *Journal of Applied Behavior Analysis,* 1976, 9, 213-219.

JOHNSON, S. M. & LOBITZ, G. K. The personal and marital adjustment of parents as related to observed child deviance and parenting behaviors. *Journal of Abnormal Child Psychology,* 1974, 2, 193-207.

JONES, E. E., KANOUSE, D. E., KELLEY, H. H., NISBETT, R. E., VALINS, S., & WEINER, B. *Attribution: Perceiving the Causes of Behavior.* Morristown, NJ: General Learning Press, 1972.

KANFER, F. & GOLDSTEIN, A. P. (Eds.). *Helping People Change*. London: Pergamon, 1975.

KANFER, F. H. & GRIMM, L. G. Behavioral analysis: Selecting target behaviors in the interview. *Behavior Modification*, 1977, 1, 7-28.

KANFER, F. H. & SASLOW, G. Behavioral diagnosis. In: C. M. Franks (Ed.), *Behavior Therapy: Appraisal and Status*. New York: McGraw-Hill, 1969.

KAPLAN, H. S. *The New Sex Therapy*. New York: Brunner/Mazel, 1974.

KAZDIN, A. E. Reactive self-monitoring: The effects of response desirability, goal setting, and feedback. *Journal of Consulting and Clinical Psychology*, 1974, 42, 704-716.

KAZDIN, A. E. & WILSON, G. T. *Evaluation of Behavior Therapy: Issues, Evidence, and Research Strategies*. Cambridge: Ballinger, 1978.

KELLEY, H. H. & THIBAUT, J. W. *Interpersonal Relations: A Theory of Interdependence*. New York: Wiley, 1978.

KIMMEL, D. & VAN DER VEEN, F. Factors of marital adjustment in Locke's marital adjustment test. *Journal of Marriage and the Family*, 1974, 36, 57-63.

KIRWIN, P. Personal communication, 1974.

KLIER, J. L. & ROTHBERG, M. Characteristics of conflict resolution in couples. Paper presented at the Eleventh Annual Convention of the Association for the Advancement of Behavior Therapy, Atlanta, December, 1977.

KNOX, D. *Marriage Happiness: A Behavioral Approach to Counseling*. Champaign: Research Press, 1971.

LANG, P. J., MELAMED, B. G., & HART, J. A psychophysiological analysis of fear modifications using an automated desensitization procedure. *Journal of Abnormal Psychology*, 1970, 76, 220-234.

LAZARUS, A. A. *Behavior Therapy and Beyond*. New York: McGraw-Hill, 1971.

LEDERER, W. J. & JACKSON, D. D. *Mirages of Marriage*. New York: Norton, 1968.

LEVINE, P. M. & FASNACHT, G. Token rewards may lead to token learning. *American Psychologist*, 1974, 29, 816-820.

LEWINSOHN, P. M. A behavioral approach to depression. In: R. J. Friedman and M. M. Katz (Eds.), *The Psychology of Depression: Contemporary Theory and Research*. New York: Wiley, 1974.

LIBERMAN, R. P. Behavioral approaches to family and couple therapy. *American Journal of Orthopsychiatry*, 1970, 40, 106-118.

LIBERMAN, R. P., LEVINE, J., WHEELER, E., SANDERS, N., & WALLACE, C. Experimental evaluation of marital group therapy: Behavioral vs. interaction-insight formats. *Acta Psychiatrica Scandinavica*, 1976, *Supplement*.

LINEHAN, M. M. Issues in behavioral interviewing: In J. D. Cone and R. P. Hawkins (Eds.), *Behavioral Assessment: New Directions in Clinical Psychology*. New York: Brunner/Mazel, 1977.

LIPINSKI, D. P. & NELSON, R. O. The reactivity and unreliability of self-recording. *Journal of Consulting and Clinical Psychology*, 1974, 42, 118-123.

LOBITZ, W. C. & LOPICCOLO, J. New methods in the behavioral treatment of sexual dysfunction. *Journal of Behavior Therapy and Experimental Psychiatry*, 1972, 3, 265-271.

LOCKE, H. J. & WALLACE, K. M. Short marital adjustment and prediction tests: Their reliability and validity. *Marriage and Family Living*, 1959, 21, 251-255.

LOVE, L. R. & KASWAN, J. W. *Troubled Children: Their Families, Schools, and Their Treatments*. New York: Wiley, 1974.

MACE, D. R. Marital intimacy and the deadly love-anger cycle. *Journal of Marriage and Family Counseling*, 1976, 2, 131-137.

MAHONEY, M. J. *Cognition and Behavior Modification*. Cambridge: Ballinger, 1974.

MAHONEY, M. J. & THORESON, C. E. *Self-Control: Power to the Person*. Monterey, CA: Brooks-Cole, 1974.

MARGOLIN, G. A sequential analysis of dyadic communication. Paper presented at the

Annual Meeting of the Association for the Advancement of Behavior Therapy, Atlanta, December, 1977.

MARGOLIN, G. A multilevel approach to the assessment of communication positiveness in distressed marital couples. *International Journal of Family Counseling*, 1978, 6, 81-89. (a)

MARGOLIN, G. The relationship among marital assessment procedures: A correlational study. *Journal of Consulting and Clinical Psychology*, 1978, 46, 1556-1558. (b)

MARGOLIN, G. Conjoint marital therapy to enhance anger management and reduce spouse abuse. *American Journal of Family Therapy*, in press.

MARGOLIN, G., CHRISTENSEN, A., & WEISS, R. L. Contracts, cognition, and change: A behavioral approach to marriage therapy. *The Counseling Psychologist*, 1975, 5, 15-26.

MARGOLIN, G., OLKIN, R., & BAUM, M. *The Anger Checklist.* Unpublished inventory, University of California, Santa Barbara, 1977.

MARGOLIN, G. & WEISS, R. L. Communication training and assessment: A case of behavioral marital enrichment. *Behavior Therapy*, 1978, 9, 508-520. (a)

MARGOLIN, G. & WEISS, R. L. Comparative evaluation of therapeutic components associated with behavioral marital treatment. *Journal of Consulting and Clinical Psychology*, 1978, 46, 1476-1486. (b)

MARTIN, D. *Battered Wives*. San Francisco: Glide, 1976.

MASTERS, W. H. & JOHNSON, V. E. Counseling with sexually incompatible marriage partners. In: R. Brecher and E. Brecher (Eds.), *An Analysis of Human Sexual Response*. New York: Signet, 1966.

MASTERS, W. H. & JOHNSON, V. E. *Human Sexual Inadequacy*. Boston: Little, Brown, 1970.

MCLEAN, P. D. Therapeutic decision-making in the behavioral treatment of depression. In P. O. Davidson (Ed.), *The Behavioral Management of Anxiety, Depression, and Pain*. New York: Brunner/Mazel, 1976.

MEICHENBAUM, D. A cognitive-behavior modification approach to assessment. In: M. Hersen and A. S. Bellack (Eds.), *Behavioral Assessment: A Practical Handbook*. New York: Pergamon, 1976.

MEICHENBAUM, D. H. *Cognitive Behavior Modification*. New York: Plenum, 1977.

MEISSNER, W. J. The conceptualization of marriage and marital disorders from a psychoanalytic perspective. In: T. J. Paolino, Jr. and B. S. McCrady (Eds.), *Marriage and Marital Therapy: Psychoanalytic, Behavioral and Systems Theory Perspectives*. New York: Brunner/Mazel, 1978.

MILLER, S., NUNNALLY, E. W., & WACKMAN, D. B. Minnesota Couples Communication Program (MCCP) Premarital and marital groups. In: D. H. L. Olson (Ed.), *Treating Relationships*. Lake Mills, IA: Graphic, 1976.

MINUCHIN, S. *Families and Family Therapy*. Cambridge, MA: Harvard University Press, 1974.

MISCHEL, W. *Personality and Assessment*. New York: McGraw-Hill, 1968.

MORSE, W. H. & KELLEHER, R. T. Schedules as fundamental determinants of behavior. In: W. N. Schoenfeld (Ed.), *The Theory of Reinforcement Schedules*. New York: Appleton-Century-Crofts, 1970.

MURSTEIN, B. I. & BECK, G. D. Person perception, marriage adjustment and social desirability. *Journal of Consulting and Clinical Psychology*, 1972, 39, 396-403.

NADELSON, C. Marital Therapy from a psychoanalytic perspective. In: T. J. Paolino, Jr. and B. S. McCrady (Eds.), *Marriage and Marital Therapy: Psychoanalytic, Behavioral and Systems Theory Perspectives*. New York: Brunner/Mazel, 1978.

NAPIER, A. Y. The rejection intrusion pattern: A central family dynamic. *Journal of Marriage and Family Counseling*, 1978, 4, 5-12.

NOTZ, W. W. Work motivation and the negative eff:ects of extrinsic rewards: A review with implications for theory and practice. *American Psychologist,* 1975, 30, 884-891.

NOVACO, R. W. Treatment of chronic anger through cognitive and relaxation controls. *Journal of Consulting and Clinical Psychology,* 1976, 44, 681.

O'LEARY, K. D. & TURKEWITZ, H. Marital therapy from a behavioral perspective. In: T. J. Paolino and B. S. McCrady (Eds.), *Marriage and Marital Therapy: Psychoanalytic, Behavioral, and Systems Theory Perspectives.* New York: Brunner/Mazel, 1978.

OLSON, D. H. Marital and family therapy: Integrative review and critique. *Journal of Marriage and the Family,* 1970, 32, 501-538.

OLTMANNS, T. F., BRODERICK, J. E., & O'LEARY, K. D. Marital adjustment and the efficacy of behavior therapy with children. *Journal of Consulting and Clinical Psychology,* 1977, 45, 724-729.

ORDEN, S. R. & BRADBURN, N. A. Dimensions of marriage happiness. *American Journal of Sociology,* 1968, 73, 715-731.

OVERALL, J. E., HENRY, B. W., & WOODWARD, A. Dependence of marital problems on parental family history. *Journal of Abnormal Psychology,* 1974, 83, 446-450.

PATTERSON, G. R. *Families: Applications of Social Learning to Family Life.* Champaign: Research Press, 1971.

PATTERSON, G. R. Some procedures for assessing changes in marital interaction patterns. *Oregon Research Institute Research Bulletin,* 1976, 16, No. 7.

PATTERSON, G. R., COBB, J. A., & RAY, R. S. A social engineering technology for retraining the families of aggressive boys. In: H. E. Adams and I. P. Unikel (Eds.), *Issues and Trends in Behavior Therapy.* Springfield, IL: C. C. Thomas, 1973.

PATTERSON, G. R. & HOPS, H. Coercion, a game for two: Intervention techniques for marital conflict. In: R. E. Ulrich and P. Mountjoy (Eds.), *The Experimental Analysis of Social Behavior.* New York: Appleton-Century-Crofts, 1972.

PATTERSON, G. R., HOPS, H., & WEISS, R. L. A social learning approach to reducing rates of marital conflict. In: R. Stuart, R. Liberman, and S. Wilder (Eds.), *Advances in Behavior Therapy.* New York: Academic, 1974.

PATTERSON, G. R., RAY, R. S., SHAW, D. A., & COBB, J. A. *Manual for Coding of Family Interactions.* Oregon Research Institute, 1969.

PATTERSON, G. R. & REID, J .B. Reciprocity and coercion: Two facets of social systems. In: C. Neuringer and J. L. Michael (Eds.), *Behavior Modification in Clinical Psychology.* New York: Appleton-Century-Crofts, 1970.

PATTERSON, G. R., WEISS, R. L., & HOPS, H. Training of marital skills: Some problems and concepts. In: H. Leitenberg (Ed.), *Handbook of Behavior Modification.* New York: Appleton-Century-Crofts, 1976.

PAUL, G. L. Behavior modification research: Design and tactics. In: C. M. Franks (Ed.), *Behavior Therapy: Appraisal and Status.* New York: McGraw-Hill, 1969.

PETERSON, D. R. *The Clinical Study of Social Behavior.* New York: Appleton-Century-Crofts, 1968.

PREMACK, D. Reinforcement theory. In: D. Levine (Ed.), *Nebraska Symposium on Motivation: 1965.* Lincoln: University of Nebraska Press, 1965.

RAPPAPORT, A. F. Conjugal relationship enhancement program. In: D. H. L. Olson (Ed.), *Treating Relationships.* Lake Mills, IA: Graphic, 1976.

RAPPAPORT, A. F. & HARRELL, J. A behavioral exchange model for marital counseling. *The Family Coordinator,* 1972, 22, 203-212.

RESICK, P. A., SWEET, J. J., KIEFFER, D. M., BARR, P. K., & RUBY, N. L. Perceived and actual discriminations of conflict and accord in marital communication. Paper presented at the Eleventh Annual Convention of the Association for the Advancement of Behavior Therapy, Atlanta, December, 1977.

RIMM, D. C. & MASTERS, J. C. *Behavior Therapy: Techniques and Empirical Findings.* New York: Academic Press, 1974.

ROBINSON, E. A. & PRICE, M. G. Behavioral and self-report correlates of marital satisfaction. Paper presented at the Annual Meeting of the Association for the Advancement of Behavior Therapy, New York, December, 1976.

RUBINSTEIN, D. & TIMMINS, J. F. Depressive dyadic and triadic relationships. *Journal of Marriage and Family Counseling*, 1978, 4, 13-24.

SAGER, C. *Marriage Contracts and Couple Therapy: Hidden Forces in Intimate Relationships.* New York: Brunner/Mazel, 1976.

SATIR, V. *Conjoint Family Therapy.* Palo Alto: Science & Behavior Books, 1967.

SCHACHTER, S. & SINGER, J. E. Cognitive, social, and physiological determinants of emotional state. *Psychological Review*, 1962, 69, 379-399.

SELIGMAN, M. E. P. *Helplessness: On Depression, Development, and Death.* San Francisco: W. H. Freeman & Co., 1975.

SIDMAN, M. *Tactics of Scientific Research: Evaluating Experimental Data in Psychology.* New York: Basic Books, 1960.

SKINNER, B. F. *Science and Human Behavior.* New York: MacMillan, 1953.

SKINNER, B. F. *Beyond Freedom and Dignity.* New York: Knopf, 1971.

SLOANE, R. B., STAPLES, F. R., CRISTOL, A. H., YORKSTON, N. J., & WHIPPLE, K. *Psychotherapy Versus Behavior Therapy.* Cambridge: Harvard University Press, 1975.

SLUZKI, C. Marital therapy from a systems theory perspective. In: T. J. Paolino, Jr. and B. S. McCrady (Eds.), *Marriage and Marital Therapy: Psychoanalytic, Behavioral, and Systems Theory Perspectives.* New York: Brunner/Mazel, 1978.

SPANIER, G. B. Measuring dyadic adjustment: New scales for assessing the quality of marriage and similar dyads. *Journal of Marriage and the Family*, 1976, 38, 15-28.

STEINGLASS, P. The conceptualization of marriage from a systems theory perspective. In: T. J. Paolino, Jr. and B. S. McCrady (Eds.), *Marriage and Marital Therapy: Psychoanalytic, Behavioral and Systems Theory Perspectives.* New York: Brunner/Mazel, 1978.

STRAUS, M. A. Leveling, civility, and violence in the family. *Journal of Marriage and the Family*, 1974, 36, 13-29.

STUART, R. B. Operant interpersonal treatment for marital discord. *Journal of Consulting and Clinical Psychology*, 1969, 33, 675-682.

STUART, R. B. An operant interpersonal program for couples. In: D. H. L. Olson (Ed.), *Treating Relationships.* Lake Mills, IA: Graphic, 1976.

STUART, R. B. & STUART, F. *Marital Pre-Counseling Inventory.* Champaign: Research Press, 1973.

TAVORMINA, J. B. Basic models of parent counseling: A critical review. *Psychological Bulletin*, 1974, 81, 827-835.

THARP, R. G. Psychological patterning in marriage. *Psychological Bulletin*, 1963, 60, 97-117.

THIBAUT, J. W. & KELLEY, H. H. *The Social Psychology of Groups.* New York: Wiley, 1959.

THOMAS, E. J. *Marital Communication and Decision-Making.* New York: Free Press, 1977.

THOMAS, E. J., CARTER, R. D., GAMBRILL, E. D., & BUTTERFIELD, W. H. A signal system for the assessment and modification of behavior (SAM). *Behavior Therapy*, 1970, 1, 225-259.

THOMAS, E. J., WALTER, C. L., & O'FLAHERTY, K. A verbal problem checklist for use in assessing family verbal behavior. *Behavior Therapy*, 1974, 5, 235-246.

TODD, F. J. Coverant control of self-evaluation responses in treatment of depression: A new use of an old principle. *Behavior Therapy*, 1972, 3, 91-94.

TSOI-HOSHMAND, L. Marital therapy: An integrative behavioral-learning model. *Journal of Marriage and Family Counseling*, 1976, 2, 179-191.

TURKEWITZ, H. & O'LEARY, D. K. A comparison of communication and behavioral marital therapy. Paper presented at the Eleventh Annual Convention of the

Association for the Advancement of Behavior Therapy, Atlanta, December, 1977.
VINCENT, J. P., WEISS, R. L., & BIRCHLER, G. R. A behavioral analysis of problem solving in distressed and nondistressed married and stranger dyads. *Behavior Therapy*, 1975, 6, 475-487.
WEISS, R. L. *Marital Interaction Coding System-Revised.* Unpublished manuscript, University of Oregon, 1975.
WEISS, R. L. The conceptualization of marriage from a behavioral perspective. In: T. J. Paolino, Jr. and B. S. McCrady (Eds.), *Marriage and Marital Therapy: Psychoanalytic, Behavioral and Systems Theory Perspectives.* New York: Brunner/Mazel, 1978.
WEISS, R. L. & AVED, B. M. Marital satisfaction and depression as predicators of physical health status. *Journal of Consulting and Clinical Psychology*, 1978, 46, 1379-1384.
WEISS, R. L. & BIRCHLER, G. R.: *Areas of Change.* Unpublished manuscript. University of Oregon, 1975.
WEISS, R. L. & BIRCHLER, G. R. Adults with marital dysfunction. In: M. Hersen and A. S. Bellack (Eds.), *Behavior Therapy in the Psychiatric Setting.* Baltimore: Williams & Williams, 1978.
WEISS, R. L., BIRCHLER, G. R., & VINCENT, J. P. Contractual models for negotiation training in marital dyads. *Journal of Marriage and the Family*, 1974, 36, 321-331.
WEISS, R. L. & CERRETO, M. *Marital Status Inventory.* Unpublished manuscript, University of Oregon, 1975.
WEISS, R. L., HOPS, H., & PATTERSON, G. R. A framework for conceptualizing marital conflict, a technology for altering it, some data for evaluating it. In: L. A. Hamerlynck, L. C. Handy, and E. J. Mash (Eds.), *Behavior Change: Methodology, Concepts, and Practice.* Champaign, IL: Research Press, 1973.
WEISS, R. L. & MARGOLIN, G. Marital conflict and accord. In: A. R. Ciminero, K. S. Calhoun, & H. E. Adams (Eds.), *Handbook for Behavioral Assessment.* New York: Wiley, 1977.
WEIMAN, R. J. *Conjugal Relationship Modification and Reciprocal Reinforcement: A Comparison of Treatments for Marital Discord.* Unpublished doctoral dissertation, Pennsylvania State University, 1973.
WILLS, T. A. WEISS, R. L., & PATTERSON, G. R. A behavioral analysis of the determinants of marital satisfaction. *Journal of Consulting and Clinical Psychology*, 1974, 42, 802-811.
WILSON, G. T. & EVANS, I. M. Adult behavior therapy and the client-therapist relationship. In: C. M. Franks and G. T. Wilson (Eds.), *Annual Review of Behavior Therapy: Theory & Practice*, Vol. IV. New York: Brunner/Mazel, 1978.
WOLPE, J. & LAZARUS, A. A. *Behavior Therapy Techniques.* New York: Pergamon, 1966.
WOLPE, J. & RACHMAN, S. Psychoanalytic "evidence," a critique based on Freud's case of Little Hans. *Journal of Nervous and Mental Disease*, 1960, 131, 135-147.
YATES, A. J. *Behavior Therapy.* New York: Wiley, 1970.

Index

For Product Safety Concerns and Information please contact our EU
representative GPSR@taylorandfrancis.com
Taylor & Francis Verlag GmbH, Kaufingerstraße 24, 80331 München, Germany

mcontent.com/pod-product-compliance
nt Group UK Ltd.
Keynes, MK11 3LW, UK
525
1B/185